Models of Practice in Occupational Therapy

Models of Practice in Occupational Therapy

Kathlyn L. Reed, Ph.D., OTR
Professor and Chairperson
Department of Occupational Therapy
College of Allied Health
University of Oklahoma
Health Sciences Center
Oklahoma City, Oklahoma

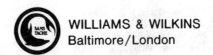

WILLIAMS & WILKINS
Baltimore/London

Editor: George Stamathis
Copy Editor: Andrea Clemente
Design: James R. Mulligan
Illustration Planning: Reginald Stanley
Production: Carol L. Eckhart

Copyright ©, 1984
Williams & Wilkins
428 E. Preston Street
Baltimore, Md. 21202, U.S.A.

Made in the United States of America

Library of Congress Cataloging in Publication Data

Reed, Kathlyn L.
   Models of practice in occupational therapy.

   Includes index.
   1. Occupational therapy. I. Title.
RC487.R43 1983   615.8'515   83-6905
ISBN 0-683-07206-4

Composed and printed at the
Waverly Press, Inc.
Mt. Royal and Guilford Aves.
Baltimore, Md. 21202, U.S.A.

Preface

The purposes of this book are to (a) provide a common framework for reviewing theoretical and practice models, (b) review the existing models of practice in occupational therapy according to the framework, (c) summarize a "state of the art" in occupational therapy practice model development and (d) suggest some directions for future development of and research on theoretical and practice models in occupational therapy. The book is intended to be useful to the advanced student, practitioner and researcher as a text or reference to a wide area of occupational therapy literature, both historical and current. The student will learn how practice models are built and what composes a number of old and new practice models in occuaptional therapy. The practitioner can compare and contrast existing models to determine which are most consistent with the practice setting in which the practitioner works. If none are useful the model building chapter may provide a framework for development. For the research therapist the models provide a ready source of literature review on many of the major models which have been or are used currently in occupational therapy practice.

The book is organized into chapters which address the role of models in theory development and review existing practice models in occupational therapy. Each chapter on specific models of practice outlines the assumptions, concepts, assessment instruments, and intervention strategies which appear in the literature. Additional information from non-occupational therapy sources is included in some sections to clarify some assumptions and concepts. In each case the author has attempted to organize, analyze and synthesize both the historical and current literature relative to the model. The author hopes that the identification and discussion of known models of practice will facilitate further research and development of knowledge as to what occupational therapy practice is and can become. In particular there is a need to further develop and refine the models and theories of occupational therapy practice to provide a more substantial case and rationale for research into the unique role of occupational therapy as a useful service to people who want or need to maintain, improve, or regain health and independent functioning through the use of occupation.

Contents

CHAPTER 1

Terminology: Definitions and Descriptions

In any field of study, understanding the language and terminology is basic to the comprehension of the subject matter. Although the scientific community prides itself on striving toward precision of study, the language which must communicate the facts and discoveries is frequently less than clear. One area in which the language is unclear concerns the use and definition of terms. The lack of common usage of such words as model, theory, paradigm and frame of reference makes understanding more difficult and communication uncertain. Although there is no way to unscramble the multiple usages of the same term and multiple terms for the same thought, it is possible to become more cognizant of the problem. The purpose of this chapter is to discuss and describe some of the common terms used in building, describing and analyzing models.

MODELS

A model is a device for generating ideas, for guiding conceptualization and therefore, for generating explanation (1). In other words, a model is a physical or symbolic representation of an object or idea. Models can be grouped into three general types. These are iconic, analogue and symbolic (1). Iconic models, such as a photograph or map, visually or pictorially represent certain aspects of a system. Analogue models employ one set of properties to represent another set of properties which the system being studied possesses. For example, the flow of water through pipes may be considered an analogue of the "flow" of electricity through wires. Symbolic models use symbols to represent or designate properties of the system under study, such as the use of mathematic equations.

Models also can be classified according to their level of abstraction (2). At the lowest level are isomorphic models. True isomorphic models are replicas to scale and function of a real phenomena such as a miniature electric train or scaled version of a steam driven engine. Many models at this level are not true isomorphic models but do attempt to reproduce the most relevant and important features for the purpose of permitting a more careful examination of the phenomena. Examples include models of the heart and a kidney machine. In the middle are the descriptive models which present the structure of the relationship and reality as opposed to the features. An organization chart of a hospital or diagram of the four chambers of the heart are examples. At the highest level are the abstract models. These models represent reality symbolically. Examples include mathematical, statistical and schematic models.

A third way to classify models is based on the metaphor used (3). The most general or meta models are machine and organism. The machine model views humans as performing tasks assigned without question or reason as a mechanical device would do. Organism models view humans as open, self maintaining and self regulating biological systems. Other metaphors have been used as meta models. Examples are contextualistic models which are based on the historical event, and formistic which is based on perception and discrimination (4). Under the general or meta models which are based on philosophy are the more explicit or super models and finally, the specific practice models.

Apostel (5) lists nine specific functions of models in the empirical sciences. These functions can be summarized as follows: A model can achieve the following.

1. Explain a domain of facts for which no theory has been developed (theory formation)
2. Simplify the assumptions of a theory in which the formulation is too difficult to use in basic hypothesis (simplification)
3. Provide an interpretation of two existing theories so their similarities can be understood (reduction)
4. Fill in a missing part of a incomplete theory (extension)
5. Compare a newer more specific theory to an older more general theory (adequation)
6. Yield explanations about facts within an existing theory (explanation)
7. Act as a practical size to provide information relative to a theory concerning a very large or very small object (concretization)
8. Function as a representation of visualization of the theory (globalization) and
9. Bridge the gap between theoretical concepts and observational levels by illustrating the relationship between the two (action or experimentation).

All of these functions will be addressed to one degree or another in the chapters that follow. In particular, the function of theory formation will be emphasized. Because of this emphasis it is necessary to further define some subtypes of models. A conceptual model is a graphic or schematic representation of a concept (6). Thus, a conceptual model diagrams or describes a single concept. A theoretical model uses a symbolic approach to analyzing the relationship between concepts or illustrates an hypothesis based on the concepts (7).

The use of any model is itself based on certain assumptions or givens. Griffiths (8) has suggested that the use of a model is based on the following assumptions:

1. The world is knowable in general.
2. Order can be imposed on the phenomena under study.
3. Models are culture bound.
4. All models are constructs of systems.

In other words, models are not independent entities. They must relate to the situation or phenomena under consideration. However, the latitude of conformity in a model is generally greater than that allowed in a theory. Conditions for using a theoretical model according to Black (9) are:

1. We have an original field of investigation in which *some* facts and regulations have been established in any form, ranging from disconnected items and crude generalizations to precise laws.
2. A need is felt for further scientific mastery of the original domain.
3. We describe some entities (objects, materials, mechanism, systems, structures) belonging to a relatively unproblematic, more familiar or better organized secondary domain.
4. Explicit or implicit rules of correlation are available for translating statements about the secondary field into corresponding statements about the original field.
5. Inferences from the assumptions made in the secondary field are translated by means of the rules of correlation and show independently checked against known or predicted data in the primary domain.

Theoretical or conceptual models may be illustrated in several ways. The more common illustration methods are described by Lippitt (10) as:

1. A graphic model—usually a two- or three-dimensional diagram such as that used to portray a stock market trend, or the relationship between temperature and humidity or the number of crimes in a particular city over a time period.
2. A pictorial model—attempts to transmit an idea by means of illustrating a real life situation, such as a cartoon that demonstrates pictorially what might result from unsafe practices.
3. A schematic model—for example, an organization chart that depicts the authority relationship within an organization, a flow chart showing the movement of information or a PERT chart demonstrating time phasing.
4. A mathematic model—mathematical symbols are used to depict factors in the real world to facilitate the study of interrelationships of a situation where quantification is possible.
5. A simulation model—approximates the real life situation, frequently in three-dimensional space, and usually is less abstract, such as a trainer system for learning to drive an automobile or fly an airplane.
6. A scale model—duplicates the features of real world object or situation in as many ways as practical or possible, such as a replica of a steam driven locomotive or miniature version of the White House.

Scale, pictorial, and simulation models are examples of the iconic model group. Graphic and schematic models are examples of an analogue model group, while the mathematic model is a type symbolic model group.

Models provide certain advantages, according to Lippitt (10). These are:

1. Models allow experimentation without risk.
2. Models are good predictors of system behavior and performance.
3. Models promote deeper understanding of a system.
4. Models permit the relative significance of various factors to be determined.
5. Models predicate the type and amount of data which should be collected and analyzed.
6. Models permit consolidation of the change problem as a whole.

On the other hand, there are some disadvantages. Disadvantages of using models based on Lippitt (10) are:

1. A model may induce one to overgeneralize or oversimplify a theory or concept.
2. There may be a tendency to make the theory or concept fit the model rather than trying to fit the model to the theory.
3. The relationship between the variables of model, or the nature of the constraints, may be incorrect or misleading, which could lead to unproductive research or conclusions.
4. A model may not be properly validated or understood and thus could result in work or effort being expended on an invalid model or misinterpretations of the model.
5. A model may have no intrinsic means of evaluating its worth or usefulness in relationship to a theory or concept.
6. A model may be overcomplicated by excessive details that convey no meaning or distort the meaning.
7. A model may be used or applied where it is not applicable because the assumptions on which the model is based are not transferable.
8. A model may be incomplete or fail to include pertinent factors of the theory or concept it represents.
9. Model building may divert useful energy into nonproductive activity.

In summary, a model is a device used to represent or stand for an object or idea through the use of a physical or symbolic form. Models are useful in suggesting ideas or methodologies, providing alternatives, and analyzing situations and conditions. Conceptual or theoretical models are subtypes of models which relate to theory building and explanation. Models may be illustrated in several ways. The method depends on the model builders choice. Although models are useful, there are certain disadvantages or drawbacks including overgeneralization, logic fallacy, incorrect linkage, inaccurate representation and invalid construction.

THEORY

The word theory also has several definitions (11). Four of these definitions can be described briefly while the fifth requires more elaboration. The more popular definition of the word theory in everyday language is that of a mere hypothesis, conjecture or guess. A statement is made which consists of relating a few variables which pertain to an event or situation. For example, the statement might be, "My theory is that he did not come to the meeting because he never received the announcement." The "theory" is of limited value even if true because it pertains to a specific set of circumstances.

A second use of the word theory is a mental plan of how to do something. Generally the plan is vague in terms of concepts and descriptions of the events or things which will be effected by the plan. For example, the "theory" is to reduce the number of automobile accidents by half by getting rid of all the drunk drivers. On the surface this "theory" may sound like a good idea but in reality it will not work as stated. Specifically, what is meant by the phrase "getting rid of" and how will it be done? Better formulation of this "theory" could upgrade its acceptability.

A third use of the term "theory" is to describe the art or science of knowing the principles and methods as opposed to "practicing" which consists of applying the skills. For example, many educational courses are divided into theory and practice courses. Theory courses are taught through the methods of lecture or discussion primarily, whereas practice courses are taught through demonstration and performance.

Fourth, the term "theory" may be used to describe a summary statement of the principles or laws which make up a given explanation of a phenomena. The statement may be verbal or mathematical. For example, the equation $E = MC^2$ is a summary equation of the theory of relativity. The summary may be an adequate description of the "theory" if one is familiar with the physical assumptions, concepts and interrelated principles involved. Otherwise the summary is an inadequate explanation and fails to communicate the full theory of relativity. In other words, the summary of a theory is acceptable to those "in the know" but unacceptable to those not familiar with the subject matter.

Finally, the word theory can be used to define "a set of interrelated constructs (concepts), definitions and propositions (assumptions) that present a systematic view of phenomena by specifying relations among variables, with the purpose of explaining and predicting the phenomena" (12). In other words, the theory describes the "formulation of apparent relationships or underlying principles of certain observed phenomena which has been verified to some degree" (13). In this text the word theory will be used to refer to the interrelation of assumptions, concepts and definitions in some form or another.

Types of Theories

Reynolds (11) suggests that there are three types of theories which interrelate assumptions, concepts and definitions. The three types vary as to how the set of statements are organized. The types are called set of laws, axiomatic and causal process.

SET OF LAWS

The criteria for a set of laws theory are:

1. Only those statements that can be considered laws are acceptable.
2. All laws must be supported by empirical research.

3. Concepts used in laws must have operational definitions that allow their identification in concrete situations.
4. Only relational statements should be included as laws.

A fifth criterion could be added but is subject to controversy. Some scientists suggest that the relationship must be causal, while others accept a relationship which indicates an association. Most theories of occupational therapy do not seem to be formulated as a set of laws.

AXIOMATIC FORM

The criteria for an axiomatic theory are:

1. A set of definitions including theoretical concepts, both primitive and dervied (nominal), and operational definitions.
2. A set of existence statements that describe the situations in which the theory can be applied, sometimes referred to as the *scope conditions*, since they describe the scope of conditions to which the theory is considered applicable.
3. A set of relational statements, divided into two groups:
   a. Axioms—a set of statements from which all other statements in the theory may be derived.
   b. Propositions—all other statements in the theory, all derived from combinations of axioms, axioms and propositions, or other propositions.
4. A logical system used to
   a. relate all concepts within statements and
   b. derive propositions from axioms, combinations of axioms and propositions, or other propositions.

The differences between axiomatic and set of laws theories are that in axiomatic theories:

1. It is not necessary for all concepts to be measurable, since some can be derived from others.
2. The number of statements can be smaller because it is not necessary to describe a relationship between every pair of concepts.
3. Research may be more efficient because the empirical support for any one statement tends to provide support for the entire theory.
4. The form permits examination of all of the consequences of the assumptions or axioms, not just those that can be stated as laws.

In general, however, the axiomatic form is difficult for practice fields to follow because of the difficulty in deciding what statements are axioms and which are propositions.

CAUSAL PROCESS

Most theories in occupational therapy would fit into this type of theory construction. The characteristics are:

1. A set of definitions, including those of theoretical concepts, using both primitive and derived (nominal) terms and operational definitions.

2. A set of existence statements that describe those situations in which one or more of the causal processes are expected to occur, or will be "activated."
3. A set of causal statements with either deterministic or probabilistic relations that describe one or more causal processes or causal mechanisms that identify the effect of one or more independent variables on one or more dependent variables.

Differences between causal process and axiomatic theories are:

1. All statements in the causal process theory are considered to be of equal weight, not as axioms and propositions.
2. All statements are presented as a causal process, not an existence situation.

DiRenzo (1) stresses that theories are not models. Models may describe, generate ideas, suggest explanations, interpretations or methodologies but do not meet the criteria of a theory. The function of a theory then is to provide an explanation and assert that a truth actually exists. Thus, a model does not fit the requirements of a theory. Rather a theory makes use of a model as a basis for explanation to bridge one theory to another or to describe a component within a theory.

PARADIGMS

In the scientific community a paradigm is a new idea, conceptualization or orientation. Reynolds (11) suggests there are three types of paradigms which are classified according to their degree of newness.

Kuhn Paradigms

A Kuhn paradigm is named for T. S. Kuhn who originally suggested the definition and criteria for such a paradigm which he called a scientific revolution. He defines a paradigm as accepted examples of scientific practice which include law, theory, appreciation and instrumentation (14). The criteria for a paradigm are:

1. It represents a radically new conceptualization of the phenomena.
2. It suggests a new research strategy or methodological procedure for gathering empirical evidence to support the paradigm.
3. It tends to suggest new problems for solutions.
4. Application of the new paradigm frequently explains phenomena that previous paradigms were unable to explain.

Examples include Darwin's theory of evolution and Freud's theory of personality. Both fit the criteria because they present a "unique and unprecedented orientation toward the phenomena, a dramatic break with past and existing orientations" and involve a major shift in research strategy including new research techniques. It is doubtful that any theory of occupational therapy would qualify as a Kuhn paradigm.

Paradigms

The basic difference between a Kuhn paradigm and a paradigm is a matter of degree. The major characteristics of a paradigm are:

1. The conceptualization represents a unique description of the phenomena, but a *dramatic* new orientation or "world view" is absent.
2. Although new research strategies may be suggested, dramatic new procedures or methodologies are absent.
3. The new conceptualization may suggest new research questions.

Some theories of occupational therapy may qualify as paradigms, such as Reilly's occupational behavior model which is discussed in Chapter 9.

Paradigm Variations

Once a paradigm has been presented, other theorists may attempt to redefine, rework or expand on the original idea. Such refinements are called paradigm variations. Paradigm variations may change the emphasis but not the basic conceptualization of a phenomena described in a theory. Most theories in occupational therapy are examples of pattern variations. Examples include Azima's object relations model which expands on Freud's theory and Fidler's communication model which expands Sullivan's theory of interpersonal relationships.

Paradigm Acceptance

Describing the types of paradigms does not specify how a paradigm comes to be accepted. Reynolds (11) suggests the acceptance of a paradigm is influenced by two factors. One factor is the terminology used to define or describe the concepts. If the concepts are not part of the existing knowledge of the community to which the theory is addressed, practitioners will be slow to accept the paradigm. People seem to relate to what they know and tend to resist or have difficulty learning new concepts. The second factor relates to degree of newness of the paradigm, especially its degree of departure from existing knowledge. A new or radical departure may be met with hostility or skepticism for some years before acceptance begins to occur. However, novelty is not a guarantee of acceptance. Many new ideas are presented, but only a few turn out to have the makeup of a new paradigm which will actually advance the world of knowledge about a particular phenomena.

A paradigm is not generally the same as a model. Usually a model has a limited purpose to represent or explain selected ideas or concepts. As a rule, therefore, a model is not as comprehensive as a paradigm which includes one or more types of theories, research methodologies and instrumentation.

Likewise, a paradigm is not the same as a theory. As with a model a theory may be contained within a paradigm. Often several theories may be contained within a paradigm because the theories are based on ideas and themes which are incorporated into the paradigm. The paradigm, however, contains aspects that are not contained in a theory, such as research strategies or instrumentation.

FRAME OF REFERENCE

A frame of reference can be described as an individual, a sociological or methodological term (15). Allport (16) uses the individual approach when he says a frame of reference "has to do with any context whatever that exerts a demonstrable influence upon the individual's perception, judgment, feeling or actions." Ackerman and Lohnes (17) use the sociological approach by stating that a frame of reference "implies a manner of thinking and speaking that is common to a particular discipline or background." Holzner (18) states that in terms of methodology such as model building, a frame of reference is "a set of basic assumptions necessary to determine the subject matter to be studied and the orientation toward such study." Consistent in all three definitions is the idea that a frame of reference involves a background mechanism which is based on perceptual, cognitive, psychological and social factors and which leads to the development and use of a standard, schema or set of facts to judge, control or direct some action or expression. In model building a frame of reference tends to determine which aspects of philosophy and reality the modeler will use as the basis for the model. The sources of such a frame of reference may be an existing philosophy, theory, practice, knowledge or research findings. These sources may be accepted in toto, in part or refuted. However, as a selected collection, they form the base and parameters on which the specific assumptions and concepts of the model itself are founded.

Thus, a frame of reference is not the total model but does form a part of the model building process. A frame of reference likewise is not a theory because it is only a mechanism which can be used to explain the relationship of the theory to the action. A frame of reference consists primarily of previously existing assumptions which are drawn together but does not include concepts and definitions as well so that the relationships between variables can be explained or predicted with some precision or degree of probability.

Furthermore, a frame of reference is not a paradigm because a frame of reference by definition relates to existing attitudes, feelings or thoughts which are already known to exist, while a paradigm is designed to explain the previously unexplained phenomena and to provide a unique description of a phenomenon.

SUMMARY

For the purposes of this book, the term model was selected because some of the material collected and discussed is at the beginning stages of theory development. Also, some material has been drawn from a variety of sources and combined because the author thought the material could be fitted together to make a more adequate theory base. However, some missing links are evident and the presentation is not systematic and interrelated at this time. Thus, the term model is used to review materials at a pre-theory or early paradigm level. In some cases theories or paradigms ultimately may be derived, while in other cases the materials may not be developed beyond the existing level because time and events have overtaken the ideas initially presented. The use of such old ideas is for historical reference primarily.

The term model also permits the materials to be presented in a uniform style and to note where further information or better organization is needed in a format that is less formal than might be used in a theory orientation format. In some cases figures and drawings have been included which the author felt might promote understanding of the interrelations of stated concepts.

In summary, models, theories, paradigms and frames of reference all have a place in model and theory analysis. Models serve the widest variety of roles. They can be organized into at least three hierarchies and become a number of formats or illustrations as outlined in Table 1.1. This text, however, is most concerned with meta, theoretical and conceptual models.

The term "theory" also has a number of definitions and a hierarchy of use as summarized in Table 1.2. Ideally, many of the models presented in this text may someday become fully integrated theories with an interrelated formulation of ideas and beliefs. At present, however, most are missing aspects of formulation necessary to satisfy the requirements of a documented theory.

Table 1.3 summarizes the use of the terms "paradigm" and "frame of reference." Paradigms can be analyzed in terms of a hierarchy. However, frames of reference are not hierarchical because they are used in different situations. Of most concern to this text is the methodological use of a frame of reference.

The four terms can be further summarized by examining them in relation to each other. Figure 1.1 illustrates the use of the terms in relation to the text. The final objective or goal is to develop a number of theories for occupational therapy. However, the first step must be the collection and analysis of a variety of models which this text addresses. At the same time, existing frames of reference which underlie models, theories and paradigms can be discussed. Paradigm identification and analysis is explored only briefly.

Table 1.1
Summary Analysis of the Word "Model"

A. Hierarchy of types of representation	B. Hierarchy of level of abstraction
1. Iconic	1. Isomorphic
2. Analogue	2. Descriptive
3. Symbolic	3. Abstract
C. Hierarchy of use of metaphor	D. Format/illustrations not
1. Conceptual	hierarchical
2. Theoretical	1. Graphic
3. Meta or metaphysical	2. Pictorial
	3. Schematic
	4. Mathematical
	5. Simulation
	6. Scale

Table 1.2
Summary Analysis of the Word "Theory"

A. Uses in language
  1. Hypothesis, guess
  2. Plan
  3. Knowledge
  4. Summary statement
  5. Interrelated formulation

B. Types of organization
  1. Causal process
  2. Axiomatic form
  3. Set of laws

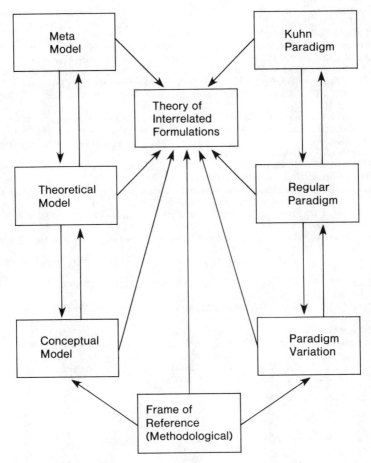

Figure 1.1.   The interrelation of words and terms.

Table 1.3
Summary Analysis of Paradigm and Frames of Reference

Paradigms	Frame of Reference
Hierarchy of types of use 1. Paradigm variations 2. Paradigm—regular 3. Kuhn paradigm	Types of perspectives 1. Individual 2. Sociological 3. Methodological

References

1. Di Renzo GJ: Toward explanation in the behavioral sciences. In Di Renzo GJ: *Concepts, Theory and Explanation in the Behavioral Sciences.* New York, Random House, 1966, pp 248–249.
2. Brodbeck M: Models, meaning and theories. In Gross L: *Symposium on Sociological Theory.* Evanston, Ill, Row, Peterson, 1959.
3. Reese HW, Overton WF: Models of development and theories of development. In Goulet LR, Baltes PB: *Life Span Developmental Psychology.* New York, Academic Press, 1970.
4. Pepper SP: *World Hypotheses.* Berkeley, Calif, University of California Press, 1942.
5. Apostel L: Towards the formal study of models in the non-formal science. In Kazemir BH, Vuysje D: *The Concept and the Role of the Model in Mathematics and Natural and Social Sciences.* Dordrecht, Holland, Reidel Publication, 1962, pp 1–3.
6. Wolman BP: *Dictionary of Behavioral Science.* New York, Van Nostrand Reinhold, 1973, p 241.
7. Miller N: Comments on theoretical models. *J Pers* 20:82, 1951–1952.
8. Griffiths DE: Some assumptions underlying the use of models in research. In Culberton JA, Hencley SP: *Educational Research: New Perspectives.* Danville, Ill, Interstate Printers & Publishers, 1963, pp 125–26.
9. Black M: Models and Metaphors: *Studies in Language and Philosophy.* Ithaca, New York, Cornell University Press, 1962.
10. Lippitt GL: *Visualizing Changes: Model Building and the Change Process.* La Jolla, Calif, University Associates, 1973, pp 33, 78–81, 82.
11. Reynolds PD: *Primer in Theory Construction.* Indianapolis, Bobbs, Merrill, 1971, pp 10–11.
12. Kerlinger N: *Foundations of Behavioral Research* , 2nd ed. New York, Holt Rinehart & Winston, 1973, p 11.
13. *Webster's New Twentieth Century Dictionary*, 2nd ed. New York, Simon & Schuster, 1979.
14. Kuhn TS: *The Structure of Scientific Revolutions*, 2nd ed. Chicago, University Press, Chicago, 1970, p 10.
15. Gould J, Kolb WL: *A Dictionary of the Social Sciences.* New York, Free Press, 1964, p 120.
16. Allport G: The psychologist's frame of reference. *Psychol Bull* 37:24, 1940.
17. Ackerman WB, Lohnes PR: *Research Methods for Nurses.* New York, McGraw Hill, 1981, p 12.
18. Holzner B: Frame of reference. In Gould J, Kolb WL: *A Dictionary of the Social Sciences.* New York, Free Press, 1964, p 120.

CHAPTER 2

Model Building in a Practice Profession

BUILDING A BASIC MODEL

One way to approach the analysis of models is to explore how a model is developed in the first place. Although the exact process any given model builder uses may vary, some identifiable phases must be completed. There appear to be five phases which can be identified by examining the products or outcomes which are produced (Fig. 2.1). These five phases are frame of reference, statement organization, descriptor organization, logical deductions and conclusions or outcomes specified in the model.

In phase one the frame of reference is identified from the knowledge or beliefs which the model builder decides are relevant to the model. Such beliefs may be drawn from many sources, but those that seem most relevant to occupational therapy include beliefs about human potential, health status, occupational roles, therapy process, effects of disease, etc. Statements based on these beliefs become the assumptions of a model and form the second phase. An assumption is a statement that something is true (believed) for the purpose of theoretical or model development (1).

Assumptions are identified in many forms. The model builder may call the assumptions axioms, premises, propositions, postulates, suppositions, tenets, or theses. Various authors choose to describe the forementioned terms in different words or phases, but they serve the same function of organizing the beliefs into a concise form and priority of concern. If a model builder does not fulfill the first two phases the model will suffer from a loss of continuity with the third phase.

The third phase is the descriptor organization which defines the concepts of the model and states the interrelations of the parts. A concept is an idea, thought or notion (2). This phase is accomplished first through the identification and definition of concepts and then through organizing the concepts into a system or structure. Concepts are the principal building material of a model. They must be consistent, however, with the assumptions or the model will not be well integrated. Concepts often appear as vocabulary words.

There are three major types according to Marx (3). One, concepts can refer to things (objects, organisms) and properties of things. Examples include splints, adapted eating utensils, built-up handle, rocker knife and swivel spoon. Things and properties of things are thus nouns or adjectives. Two, concepts may refer to events (things in action) and properties of events. Examples include actions such as roll over, play, talk, eat, reach, or descriptions such as sadly, friendly, slowly. Most behavioral concepts must be described by some verb, adverb or both. The third type

13

MODELS OF PRACTICE

Figure 2.1. Terms and phases in model theory building. (Adapted from R. M. Thomas: *Comparing Theories of Child Development.* Belmont, Calif, Wadsworth, 1979.)

	Phase 1: Frame of Reference	Phase 2: Statement Organization	Phase 3: Descriptor Organization	Phase 4: Logical Deductions	Phase 5: Conclusions/ Outcomes
Products of the phase (output)	Assemble philosophical background	Organize the assumptions which are central to the model	Organize the concepts which describe the model	Develop hypotheses which state questions or suggest answers	Organize principles (maxims and laws)
The model builder's behavior (input)	Identify a certain philosophy from existing knowledge	Accept certain beliefs as being true (self-evident)	Defines the parts of the model	Suggest relationships or outcomes which might be expected if the model is accurate (represents real world)	Draws generalization from evidence collected to test accuracy of the model
Method	State the frame of reference	State the assumptions in a concise form and order of priority	State the interrelations of the parts as a system or structure	Perform research studies	Summarize the principles

Figure 2.2. Relationships between concepts. (Reproduced with permission from M. E. Hardy (5).)

Nature of Relation[a]	Meaning
Symmetrical	If A, then B; if B, then A
Asymmetrical	If A, then B; but if no A, no conclusion about B
Causal	If A, always B
Probabilistic	If A, probably B
Time order	If A, later B
Concurrent	If A, also B
Sufficient	If A, then B, regardless of anything else
Conditional	If A, then B, but only if C
Necessary	If A and only if A, then B

[a] The relations are not all mutually exclusive.

of concept describes the relationships among things, events and their various properties. The term construct may be used to refer to this abstract level of concept. Examples include habit, personality, anxiety, socialization, and competence. Such concepts are broad and often are difficult to describe in the precise terms needed for research designs. Concepts may be specific to the profession or may be borrowed from other disciplines. A model builder may use any combination of discipline-specific or borrowed concepts to build a model.

The fourth phase is called the logical deduction phase. The purpose of this phase is to suggest relationships or outcomes which might be expected if the model is an accurate representation of the real world. The outcome of the phase is one or more hypotheses which state questions or suggest answers. Actually, model builders rarely state a formal hypothesis which is defined as a conjectural statement of the relation between two or more variables (4). Rather, persons interested in doing research on the concepts of the model are more likely to develop a formal hypothesis. The model builder, however, may provide some suggestions within the description of the model.

Hardy (5) has outlined nine possible relationships between concepts. The nine are labeled symmetrical, asymmetrical, causal, probabilistic, time order, concurrent, sufficient, conditional and necessary (Fig. 2.2). Clarification of the relationships appear in Roy and Roberts (6).

In a symmetrical relationship the concepts are reciprocal so that either may lead to the other. For example, it may be possible to state that an increased number of skills leads to an increased level of performance or that an increased level of performance leads to an increased number of skills. If both statements can be shown to occur, then the relationship between the concepts of skill and performance are symmetrical. If, however, only one statement can be shown to occur, then the relationship is asymmetrical. For example, if an increase in the number of skills leads to an increased level of performance but an increase in the level of performance does NOT lead to an increased number of skills, then the relationship is asymmetrical. It can be assumed further that an increase in the number of skills is the result of other factors or concepts, such as practice, experience or opportunity.

A causal relationship shows an invariant and consistent link between two concepts. For example, if the statement could be shown to always occur that an increased number of skills would lead to an increased level of performance, then the relationship would be causal. Obviously such a consistent relationship is difficult to find in the study of human behavior. Usually a number of factors may result in a similar outcome. Levels of performance may be influenced by motivation, physiological factors or environmental situations. Thus, causal relationships are rare in models or theories of human behavior phenomena. On the other hand, probabilistic relationships are much more common. For example, if the number of skills is increased it is probable the level of performance also will be increased.

Both time order and concurrent types of relationship refer to the sequence of an occurrence. In a time order relationship the statement could be made that if the number of skills is increased, later there would be an increased level of performance. Obviously the critical variable is the amount of time delay between the two concepts. In contrast, a concurrent relationship would state that as the number of skills increased, the level of performance would increase at the same time. Thus, the time factor must be simultaneous. Sufficient, conditional and necessary are relationships that demand, or are influenced by, other factors. A sufficient relationship means that the relationship occurs or exists regardless of any other factors. For example, an increase in the number of skills could be said to influence the level of performance regardless of anything else. If the connection between skill and performance can be established no matter what other circumstances may exist, then the relationship is sufficient.

A conditional relationship, however, demands a third factor. For example, if the increased numbers of skills leads to an increased level of performance only when the desire to perform (motivation) reaches a certain point, then a conditional relationship exists. Skill and performance are dependent on motivation to determine the outcome of skill and performance.

Finally, a necessary relationship is said to occur when the first factor must be present for the second to occur. For example, if an increased number of skills must occur for the performance level to increase, then the number of skills is necessary in the level of performance. A necessary relationship occurs only when the first condition must occur in order to obtain the second.

To repeat, there are nine possible relationships of a concept to another. The relationships are important in analyzing assumptions and in selecting hypotheses to be tested. However, one should be aware that the nine relationships may occur in combination and are not, therefore, mutually exclusive. For example, it is possible to have an asymmetrical relationship which is probabilistic. To illustrate, skill probably will influence performance. However, the asymmetrical and probabilistic relationship may not occur unless a conditional factor such as feedback occurs. Thus, performance probably will influence skill if feedback is given as to type of skills needed.

Finally, the fifth phase involves reaching conclusions and specifying outcomes. This phase includes the drawing of generalizations from evidence collected to test or estimate the accuracy of the model. The conclusions can be stated as principles. A principle is a working hypothesis or guideline of scientific investigation (7). Usually a principle is based on research and testing, but model builders may become impatient and state hypotheses as principles because the model builder is convinced of their truth even if others may want to reserve judgment until more evidence is available. Generally, principles can be defended with better evidence than a well meaning intention.

In summary, model building is composed of five phases which form a sequence of interlocking systems. Although a model builder may not complete all of phase one before proceeding to the next, a good model ultimately will have identifiable products or outputs at each stage. The frame of reference, assumptions and concepts are crucial to exploring, organizing and developing the model, while hypothesis and principles are important to test the value of the model in describing the phenomena or aspect which the model is supposed to elucidate. Development of a model can be considered stage one in model building while testing can be called stage two. Stage three is the final stage in which the model is organized and may be used as a theory. Figure 2.3 illustrates this building process.

BUILDING A PRACTICE MODEL

In a practice profession, however, a good model at this stage is not sufficient to guide an intervention program. The model must undergo further expansion and elaboration. The model in Figure 2.4 shows the additional phases which must be delineated in order to use a model in the practice arena. Figure 2.5 shows the outline of those phases in comparison to Figure 2.3. The additions form another layer of model development which includes expected results of intervention, assessment techniques, implementation strategies plus the same items of logical deductions and conclusions or outcome.

Expected results of intervention are stated as general objectives and goals. All practice models must have as one goal: the changing or modifying of human structure, function or behavior. Otherwise, a practice model is unnecessary. Actually general objectives and goals are similar to assumptions. They state what the model builder believes or assumes will happen if certain conditions exist and certain strategies are used to change or modify the existing conditions. For example, if the basic model states that stresses and forces are involved in bone growth and development, one could assume that too much stress or force could break a bone. The practice model then states that a broken bone can be mended, and the result will be a bone that functions as it did before the fracture.

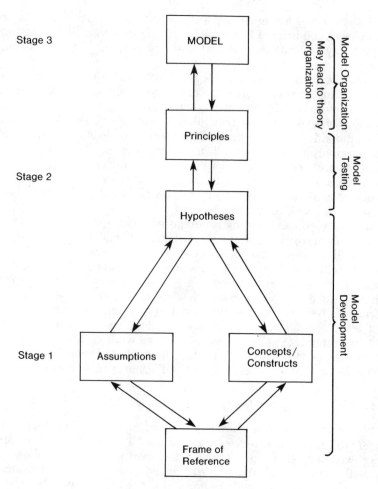

Figure 2.3. Building a model.

The second phase of practice model building identifies the assessment or evaluation techniques which will record changes related to the objectives or goals of intervention. Thus, in applying a practice model the first step is to decide whether intervention is needed by determining if change has occurred. To use a particular model the change should be within the arena which the model purports to provide intervention strategies. Thus, the assessment tools and techniques must detect changes which the intervention model addresses. In the case of a fracture an x-ray, palpation or perhaps observation will assess the fracture and provide the information on which to initiate an intervention strategy. For occupational therapy the assessment tools have included standardized and nonstandardized tests, observation reports and interview forms. What type of instrument is used depends often on the type of information sought. For

Figure 2.4. Terms and phases in practice model building.

	Phase 1: Expected Results of Intervention	Phase 2: Assessment Instruments	Phase 3: Intervention Strategies	Phase 4: Logical Deductions	Phase 5: Conclusions Outcome
Product	Stated as objectives or goals	Tests Standardized Nonstandardized Observation reports Interview forms	Media, or modalities Methods or techniques Equipment and supplies Basic or prerequisite skills	Hypotheses Stated questions Stated answers	Intervention principles
Model builders behavior	Believes that behavior can be changed in certain ways or directions by using certain means	Record behavior and analyze that which seems to be important or related to the objectives and goals	Uses selected approaches to attempt to change behavior in the direction of the objectives and goals	Suggests relationships or outcomes which might be expected if the model is effective in bringing about change in the direction of the objectives or goals	Draws generalizations from the evidence collected to test or estimate the accuracy of the model

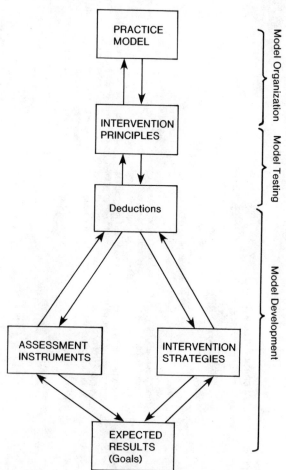

Figure 2.5. Putting a practice model together.

example, current behavior can be assessed by observing and measuring the behavior directly. However, past events require either a reporting or interviewing format. The choice of assessment technique therefore is crucial to the acquisition of useful assessment information. The type of assessment also is important. Children may have more difficulty accepting a fixed presentation sequence at a desk or table for 1½ hours. An adult, on the other hand, may have some difficulty in performing a task with many gross motor items, such as rolling or creeping on the floor. Thus, finding the right kind of an assessment instrument can be the key to compiling a useful data base on which to plan an intervention program.

After the assessment instruments are developed the implementation strategies can be selected and identified which the model builder believes will facilitate the changes specified in the objectives and goals. The strategies may include modalities, media, methods, techniques, equipment and basic skills. All, however, must have some identifiable relationship to the objectives and goals.

Modalities and media provide the means or agent through which change is expected to occur. In other words modalities and media are what we use in an intervention program. They include activities of daily living tasks, manual arts, creative crafts, education materials, prevocational tools, and avocational activities. Methods and techniques provide the specific approaches to the use of the modality or medium, in other words, how we use the modality or medium. Learning one-handed dressing skills, practicing prehension patterns, or planning a woodworking project are all examples of specific methods or techniques. Equipment specifies the things or objects that are needed to perform method or technique used within the modality or medium. Usually equipment is considered to be nonhuman objects and external to the body. Examples include tools, toys, wheelchairs, splints, and games. Some items, however, may be considered as nearly human and may be internal or in the body, such as a hip replacement. The unit is nonhuman because it is made of metal and plastic. However, once it is in place the unit becomes very much a part of the human body. Thus, some equipment may be easier to identify than others.

Basic skills are those which are considered to be prerequisite to the performance of more complex activities. Sometimes model builders specify the basic skills when describing a particular method or technique. In such cases no further delineation is needed. However, other model builders do not mention that some skills are needed before a particular method or technique can be used. In these cases the practicing therapist must be alert to the need to supply the missing specifications. Otherwise a very good intervention approach may be misapplied or fail. A simple example of a basic skill is hand to mouth range of motion and coordination. Without this basic skill, independent self-feeding and teeth brushing cannot be achieved. Therefore, a good model builder will specify which basic skills if any, are needed to facilitate the performance of a particular intervention approach.

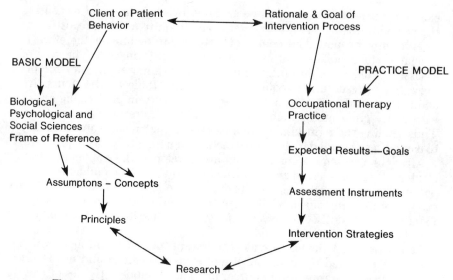

Figure 2.6.   Interrelation of client behavior and intervention process.

In phase four the model builder repeats the phases outlined in the basic model. Once again logical deductions must be derived, hypotheses formed, research performed, results analyzed and finally, phase five occurs in which conclusions and outcomes are determined upon which principles can be stated relative to the accuracy of the intervention process in producing the change stated in the expected results.

It should be noted that the process of model building and research analysis does not occur always in the sequence outlined in this chapter. The sequence provides an ideal process but perhaps more importantly, it provides a framework for determining the progress of a model in reaching the final goal of becoming a valid and reliable theory. A model with missing or incomplete phases is an incomplete model and would become an inadequate theory. Either the original model builder needs to provide more information, or other persons will have to complete the missing phases. Another alternative is to abandon the model altogether as not workable or unsuitable.

INTEGRATING BASIC AND PRACTICE MODELS

Ultimately, basic and practice models should be integrated into a single model or theory. This final step is important for consistency and to provide a cross-check through testing and research for accuracy. Figure 2.6 illustrates the interaction points between the basic model and the practice model. These interaction points occur between the client's behavior and rationale for intervening, and between the behavioral principles and selected intervention strategies. If the client's behavior fits the rationale for intervention and principles of behavior can be changed through the intervention strategies in the direction of the

  I. Frame of Reference—Includes historical review of beliefs and values which the model builder proposed or borrowed to build the model.
 II. Assumptions—Includes the statements of beliefs or values about man, health, occupation, and therapy which the model builder proposed as rationale for the model.
III. Concepts—Includes the ideas and definitions which form the core of the model.
 IV. Expected Results—States the objectives, goals and outcomes proposed in the model.
  V. Assessment Instruments—Lists and briefly discusses the methods of assessment developed or suggested by the model builder to collect data and information for determining whether problems exist and what intervention strategies to use.
 VI. Intervention Strategies—Lists the media or modalities, methods, techniques or approaches, equipment and prerequisite skills.
VII. Summary—Summarizes the key aspects of the models.
VIII. Critique—Assesses the strengths and weaknesses of model.

Figure 2.7.   Outline for the review of models.

intervention goal, then the integrated model is consistent and accurate in purpose and goal.

Throughout the review of models a consistent outline will be followed. This outline includes the frame of reference, assumptions and concepts followed by expected results, assessment instruments, intervention strategies and finally, a summary and critique. The outline is shown in Figure 2.7.

References

1. Chaplin JP: *Dictionary of Psychology*, revised ed. New York, Dell, 1975, p 42.
2. Gould J, Kolb WL: *A Dictionary of the Social Sciences*, New York, Free Press, 1964, p 120.
3. Marx MH: The general nature of theory construction. In Marx MH: *Theories in Contemporary Psychology*. New York, Macmillan, 1963, pp 9–10.
4. Kerlinger N: *Foundations of Behavioral Research*, 2nd ed. New York, Holt Rinehart & Winston, 1973, p 14.
5. Hardy ME: The nature of theories. In Hardy ME: *Theoretical Foundations for Nursing*. New York, MSS Information Corporation, 1973, pp 10–22.
6. Roy C, Roberts SL: *Theory Construction in Nursing: An Adaptation Model*. Englewood Cliffs, NJ, Prentice-Hall, 1981, pp 2–4.
7. Wolman BB: *Dictionary of Behavioral Science*. New York, Van Nostrand Reinhold, 1973, p 288.

CHAPTER 3

The Use of Models in a Practice Profession

In the opinion of the author models in a practice profession such as occupational therapy should attempt to accomplish the following:

1. Identify the frame of reference that underpins the practice of the profession.
2. Provide a means of organizing and arranging the assumptions, concepts and definitions which appear to support the practice of the profession.
3. Identify that which is unique to the practice of the profession and therefore distinguishes occupational therapy from other professions in medicine and health fields.
4. Be a guide for the advancement of occupational therapy research.
5. Provide a logical rationale for specialization practice while not losing the essence of occupational therapy.
6. Permit change elaboration and refinement as time and knowledge advance.
7. Help explain occupational therapy to other professions and consumers.
8. Indicate the areas of commonality with other helping professions which enable occupational therapy to work with other professionals in the practice area.
9. Be an aide to the development and refinement of theories of practice in occupational therapy.

FRAME OF REFERENCE

As discussed in Chapter 1, a frame of reference is the belief or value system upon which the model is built. A frame of reference should be broad enough to encompass the philosophical statements which underpin the concepts but not so broad that many other models for other professions can be built upon the same framework. Of course there can be some overlapping. Indeed some overlapping, especially in the area of assumptions, seems necessary so that the practice area of the professions can understand and relate to each other.

ASSUMPTIONS, CONCEPTS AND DEFINITIONS

As stated in Chapter 2, assumptions are broad, general statements that are considered to be true for the purpose of model or theory development. The statements usually are drawn in part from the frame of reference.

The assumptions are used in a model and they need to be comprehensive enough to address all areas of concern to the model. As with the frame of reference, the assumptions should relate both to the areas which are unique to the professions as well as to those which interrelate the profession with others. When assumptions and concepts are interrelated, they form the basis for an explanation of a model and eventually a practice model.

As stated in Chapter 2, concepts are the organizing ideas of a model and of a theory mediated by a word, symbol or sign which may combine several elements from different sources into a single motion. "Concepts are formed by a process of abstraction which is then followed by a process of generalization" (1). The abstraction sorts out the relevant clues which make up the concept, and the generalization permits the application of the clues to new objects or situations. For example, the concept of self maintenance involves those activities which are performed on a regular or routine schedule for the purpose of keeping the body in good health and in condition to perform other activities. Thus, eating fits the idea of self maintenance as does mobility because both result in keeping the body in good health and in condition to perform.

Definitions give the formal or significant meaning to a work or phrase. When a definition is stated clearly in a model or theory it becomes a concept.

UNIQUENESS

It is important to describe and delineate what is unique about occupational therapy so that the profession can be separated from other disciplines as well as integrated into the whole field of disciplines concerned with medicine and health. In general there is some agreement that occupational therapy is concerned with the role of occupation in human endeavors and is a health-related field which specializes in dealing with humans who may lose, have lost, or not acquired, certain skills which are assumed to contribute to living as "normal" persons and functioning to a certain level of capacity in the environment. The exact role of occupation in terms of its relationship to health, range of specialization, types of skills which can be gained or regained and contribution toward reaching normalcy or obtaining functional capacity in an environment remain unresolved. Lack of specificity as to exactly what constitutes occupational therapy hinders acceptance of the profession as an applied discipline which can influence positively the state of a person's health and function. A model can be useful in illustrating a description and delineation of the unique character of occupational therapy.

RESEARCH

Good research depends in part on articulated assumptions and concepts which can be operationally defined or measured. A model provides a method for organizing portions of practice and application into identifiable problems which then can be stated and hypotheses can be developed. Through research the objectives and goals can be validated and the efficacy of occupational therapy can be advanced. Thus, the development of a model or models provides a useful first step in the quest toward achieving a scientific rationale for the practice of occupational therapy.

SPECIALIZATION

A model also can provide an understanding of how different areas of occupational therapy practice all fit together so that the essence of the field is maintained regardless of how diversified or specialized the practice arena becomes.

Specialization can serve a useful purpose of expanding knowledge and skill in certain select areas of practice. However, specialists must be careful not to lose the core of occupational therapy lest the practice infringe upon other professional territory and go out of the realm of occupational therapy. A good model can help practitioners identify both the scope and the limitations of occupational therapy in both theory and practice.

CHANGE

No profession can afford to stand still in face of advances. Changing technology, society and culture demand that the profession be responsive to and be able to change without losing its major identifying characteristics. A model can assist in the change process by indicating where expansion can occur and the directions in which such expansion can occur. Again the change must be accomplished without loss of the essence or core concepts. Thus, those characteristics which are most central to the model should appear in the center of the model and be identified clearly.

COMMUNICATING TO OTHERS

Communication about the theory and practice of occupational therapy continues to be a major problem. Both consumers and other professionals have a difficult time grasping the essence of occupational therapy. The profession must become more descriptive, and occupational therapists must become more articulate in describing the field. The essence of occupational therapy appears to be that of understanding how humans use occupations to aid their adaptation to the environment and in how to adapt the environment to meet human needs through the use of these occupations. The central focus of occupational therapy becomes the application of the knowledge of occupations to meet the needs of humans who may lose, have lost or never learned how to use for themselves the occupations as tools in the adaptation process. A better model of how occupational therapy "works" is one way to bridge the communication gap so that other professionals and consumers will understand more of the purpose and significance of occupational therapy.

COMMONALITIES

As indicated under frame of reference a profession must have some commonalities with other professions in order to work in harmony with them. The commonalities which serve as bridges to the professions are found most frequently in the frame of reference and assumptions, but some may occur in the concepts as well. There may be, for example, similarities in the belief and value systems. Thoughts about the worth of human and of humans as energy systems are specific examples of such overlapping areas. A model can facilitate the identification of such commonalities by permitting a means of comparison which can be visually inspected as well as verbally discussed.

DEVELOPING THEORIES FOR PRACTICE

Finally a model should serve as an aid to the development and refinement of practice models. There are several levels of theories which a model can support. Dickoff and James (2) suggest four general levels. These levels include (a) factor isolating, (b) factor relating, (c) situation relating and (d) situation producing. Factor isolating or naming theories attempt to depict, describe and classify the ideas and concepts which characterize an area of interest, such as the practice of hand rehabilitation. Examples of ideas or concepts might include such terms as arches of the hand, patterns of grasp, web space and dynamic splints.

Factor relating or descriptive theories suggest how the concepts may be interrelated or correlated. In the example of hand rehabilitation, a factor-relating theory would describe the relationship of the web space to the opposition of the thumb and fingers and suggest that there may be a correlation between the maintenance of web space to the functional skill of opposition.

The third level of theory is called situation producing or predictive theory. This level specifies the nature of the relationship such as causal, associational, inhibitory, or catalytic. In the previous example a situation-producing theory would state that there is a direct and positive correlation between the amount of flexible web space and the ability to oppose the thumb against the finger pads of all four fingers.

A situation-producing theory is the fourth level. This level is also called prescriptive, normative or goal-directed theory. Such a theory evaluates action itself in contrast to the previous level which evaluates the products of action. Thus, situation-producing theories are most useful to the practitioner. In the example of hand rehabilitation, a situation-producing theory might state that the goal of the hand therapist is to achieve or maintain the normal amount of web space in order to provide functional opposition of the thumb and fingers. The theory would specify also the procedures for accomplishing the goal.

In summary, models can serve the profession of occupational therapy in several ways. A frame of reference model would identify the beliefs and values which underpin the field of occupational therapy. Models of assumptions and concepts can illustrate the proposed relations of ideas on which occupational therapy is based. A model can represent the unique characteristics of occupational therapy and be used to identify and select research strategies. A model may visually diagram an area of specialization within the parameters of occupational therapy or show

how change has occurred within the field. Models can be used to point out commonalities with other disciplines to facilitate communication. Finally, models can illustrate the development of practice models.

In critiquing the models presented in this book, the following questions based on the nine usage statements will be discussed.

1. Is the model based on a frame of reference consistent with the values and beliefs of occupational therapy?
2. Are the assumptions, concepts and definitions identified and defined clearly and are they relevant to occupational therapy?
3. Does the model identify an unique aspect of occupational therapy or identify occupational therapy as a unique profession?
4. Can or has the model been used as a guide for research in occupational therapy?
5. Does the model permit specialization without losing the core of occupational therapy?
6. Can the model be elaborated and refined?
7. Is the model useful in explaining occupational therapy to others?
8. Does the model provide a common thread to other practice disciplines?
9. Can the model assist in the development and refinement of practice models in occupational therapy?

References

1. Chaplin JP: *Dictionary of Psychology*, revised ed. New York, Dell, 1975, p 105.
2. Dickoff J, James P: A theory of theories: A position paper. *Nurs Res* 17:198–203, 1968.

CHAPTER 4

Characteristics and Sources of a Good Model

In Chapter 3, models were examined in terms of their usefulness to occupational therapy. In this chapter models are reviewed in terms of their general characteristics which are important in any area of model building for theory development.

The following characteristics are based on Thomas (1) and Overton and Reese (2).

1. *A model should accurately reflect the facts of human performance in the real everyday world.* Models are subject to three errors in this standard. First is that the model is based on circumstances and generalizations which go beyond the data available regarding the facts of performance studies. For example, Gesell (3) states the children in one study were above average in intelligence and had parents who were highly cooperative yet he generalized that all children were like those in the study. Might children with lower intelligence and less cooperative parents give somewhat different performances? Second, a model may be developed in part on data which were studied but the conclusions were then extended to other areas of interest to the modeler. For example, data may be based on studies of fine motor development, but the conclusions speak to the development of social interaction skills. A third source of error is to mix previous experience with current observations. For example, in studying the development of play skills, the observer must be careful not to "color" the observations with memories of the observer's childhood play.

2. *A model should be understandable to a person who is reasonably competent, i.e., has a command of language, logic and analysis.* In particular the reader should be able to understand (a) the basic philosophy and assumptions on which the model is built, (b) the definitions of terms and concepts used in the model, (c) what events or facets of the real world are referred to in the model, and (d) how the explanations and predictions about human performance and occupation are derived logically from the assumptions and concepts. Although the standard may appear straightforward and simple, it is frequently difficult to achieve. Model builders may think their presentation is clear but in fact the model is obscure and confusing. A model is more believable if it is also comprehensible. On the other hand, the reader has a responsibility to understand the basics of model building, use of mathematical symbols and logic analysis. Building and comprehending models is a two way street.

3. *A model should explain why past events occurred, predict future events and, if possible, predict specific individual performance rather than general group performance.* It is usually easier to explain the past because

the data are available for analysis. Predicting general future events is not too difficult since the law of averages will prove some events correct unless the predictions are outlandish. What is difficult is to predict with some degree of accuracy what will happen to individual performance. Yet in practice this is the information needed to develop and implement an effective treatment plan for each event.

4. *A model should offer practical guidance in solving everyday problems in human performance which can be used by therapists, clients, parents, spouses and friends.* A model is more useful if it can be applied to the daily problems of living, such as reaching for and grasping a fork, and not just a "trick" motion such as extending the arm overhead to open the hand (Souque's phenomenon). Also, a model is more useful if it can, in part, be understood and applied by nonprofessionals. A model which works for therapists but is incomprehensible and unusable by anyone else is of little use. Human performance which can be obtained only in the therapy environment is probably of limited value except as part of an evaluation procedure.

5. *A model should be internally consistent.* Models can be presented in words, symbols or diagrams. One model may be used to complement or reinforce the other. However, the reader should not have to jump back and forth or totally ignore aspects of the model in order to understand it.

6. *A model should be economical,* that is, it should use as few concepts and assumptions as possible and use simple mechanisms to explain the phenomena of human performance. This standard is often referred to as the law of parsimony. The purpose of the standard is to encourage the selection of explanations needed to define and describe events, but not to exceed the evidence with elaborate, complex and confusing explanations. In other words, if two explanations of a phenomenon fit the facts equally well, the better choice is the simpler explanation because more people will understand and will be less confused.

7. *A model should stimulate the discovery of knowledge, including the creation of new research techniques.* If the model is to be of value to the discipline it should lead to the discovery of new knowledge. Such efforts may include the development of new techniques to study the phenomena described in the model. As the phenomena are explored further, understanding of the field should occur. Thus, a model can be evaluated in terms of the techniques, efforts, and knowledge which are produced as a result of the model.

8. *A model should explain human performance and occupation in a way that makes good sense and is self-satisfying.* This standard includes in part many of the previous standards but also includes the intuitive emotional aspects which are not readily identifiable. Practitioners are more likely to accept a model that "rings true" or "feels right" than one that "just does not fit." A good model is pleasing and sells itself as well as being subjectable to research and analysis. In the final analysis a

model must depend on self conviction for its ultimate acceptance or rejection.

9. *A model should provide an explanation of the phenomena being studied in regard to four causal determinants: material, efficient, formal and final.* Material cause is the internal substance which causes the organism or object to change. Examples include physiologic, neurologic, or genetic processes which result in behavior change. Efficient cause is the external agent, antecedent condition or independent variable which changes the organism or object. Examples include physical or social environment, age or economic factors. Formal cause is the pattern, structure, organization or form of the organism or object. Examples in the psychological structure are id, ego and superego, the cognitive sequence of sensory motor, concrete and abstract or the organization of body from cephal to caudal. Final cause is the end toward which the organism or object develops or moves. Examples include maturity, differentiation, hierarchical integration or self actualization. It will be observed in Chapter 5 on Meta Models that organismic models use all four causes. Especially important are formal and final because they specify the purpose or teleology of existence. In contrast, mechanistic models state only the material and efficient causes. An illustration of how the four causes could be incorporated into a theory relevant to occupational therapy might be as follows: the neuromuscular system (material) interacting with the physical and social environments (efficient) organizes sensory information into effective motor acts (formal) for the purpose of achieving adaptive responses in the organism (final). Another example might be the individual (material), interacting with physical, social and cultural environments (efficient), develops and organizes occupational performance (formal) to achieve adaptive behavior (final). It should be clear that material and efficient causes are causes of *being* (givens, prerequisites), while efficient and final causes are causes of *becoming* (direction, order and goal of change).

These nine characteristics will not be reviewed in detail for each model analyzed. Instead only the relevant concerns will be discussed if there seems to be a major missing characteristic which seriously reduces the model's effectiveness. The reader, however, may want to examine a model with the following questions in mind which are based on the nine characteristics.

1. Does the model reflect the real world of human performance?
2. Is the model clearly understandable?
3. Does the model explain the past and predict the future in practical terms?
4. Is the model practical for application?
5. Is the model internally consistent?
6. Is the model economical (parsimonious)?
7. Is the model useful in stimulating further study, research and understanding?

8. Is the model intuitively self-satisfying?

9. Does the model explain the causes of the phenomena being studied?

SOURCES OF MODELS

At this point it should be evident that models can be derived from many sources. These sources include practical experience, new knowledge, reexamination of old models, interest in exploring new areas, attempts to consolidate several existing models or attempts to explain future trends or events. Many model builders are simply trying to explain what they observe in their everyday practice as therapists. Such attempts are often overlooked or not recognized initially until others also report similar finds.

New knowledge is a frequent source of new models. The neurophysiologic model of facilitation and inhibition of the central nervous system is an example of a model built on new knowledge gained from the fields of neurology, physiology and anatomy (see Chapter 12). Reexamining old models can be a fruitful source of ideas for better models. An example is the reexamination of the Meyer-Slagle model of habit-training. Although some of the application techniques in a mental institution are now used more by nursing than occupational therapy, the concepts of time organization and habits of activity can be redeveloped into a new model, temporal adaptation, which may use the profession well (see Chapter 11). Interest in exploring new areas is also an obvious source for new models. For example, models for practice in education need to be developed. Models used in medical and rehabilitation facilities are not applicable for schools because the basic assumptions and purpose are different. Schools are designed primarily to educate. Therapy may be a secondary concern. On the other hand, hospitals and rehabilitation facilities are designed primarily to improve health and function with education as a secondary concern. Models need to fit the circumstances to which they are applied.

Consolidation of existing models is a useful approach to model building, especially if the consolidated model makes use of the best aspects of the several models from which it is drawn. One area that could use a consolidated model is the neurophysiologic techniques. Presently, practitioners have to draw upon several sources to develop a complete treatment or management program. There is a danger that the indexing of techniques without the guidance that an integrated model can provide will result in less effective or countereffective treatment. A comprehensive model could consolidate the assumptions, concepts and techniques so as to aid the practitioner in preparing an effective program for each client. The consolidated model could provide an additional benefit by making the theory and techniques more understandable.

Finally, models can be useful in explaining future trends or events. Prevention as a practice area is an example of a trend that can be helped by model building. When an unfamiliar trend or event is introduced, one of the principal problems is to cite examples of what should or could be clear in the practice arena. Models can be useful in suggesting what practice might look like and in outlining the steps needed to actually decide what approaches to try in setting up a program.

In summary, models come from many sources and serve many purposes. Models can look backwards at what practice was, models can reflect what practice is now, and models can look forward to what practice can or may become. The major information can be gathered, sorted and analyzed in an organized manner which permits analysis and comparison with other models.

References

1. Thomas RM: *Comparing Theories of Child Development.* Belmont, Calif, Wadsworth, 1979.
2. Overton WF, Reese HW: Models of development; methodological implications. In Nesselroade JR, Reese HW: *Life Span Developmental Psychology—Methodological Issues.* New York, Academic Press, 1973.
3. Gesell A, Ilg FL: *Child Development: An Introduction to the Study of Human Growth.* New York, Harper, 1949.

CHAPTER 5

Meta Models

As stated in Chapter 1, models can be classified based on different metaphors. Table 5.1 outlines the types of metaphors and levels of models used in this book to illustrate the impact of models on occupational therapy practice. In this chapter, the meta models will be discussed, while the following chapters examine the super models, health and rehabilitation models, and occupational therapy models.

Models have varied traditionally according to two major themes, the organismic and the mechanistic models. As was noted in Chapter 1, these two meta models are considered to be antithetical to each other. In other words, any model or theory based on one cannot use any concept from the other without violating the division between the two. The best a model or theory can do is to reach the halfway point between the two opposites. Figure 5.1 and Table 5.2 outline the various philosophical and conceptual differences between the two meta models. It should be kept in mind, however, that no model builder encompasses all of the issues listed into one model. The list is provided for discussion and examination relative to the total profession of occupational therapy and not to any one or group of models or theories.

INTERNAL VS. EXTERNAL LOCUS OF CONTROL (1, 2)

This issue concerns whether behavior is based on changes within the person or changes external to the person. Models based on internal locus of control are consistent with the organismic model, while those which assume that the locus of control is external to the individual follow the mechanistic model. Generally developmental approaches such as those of Gesell and Piaget* are considered organismic because the processes of maturation, assimilation and accommodation depend on the person's internal sources of stimulation (growth and cognition) as the primary source of change.

In contrast, behavioristic approaches such as those of Skinner are considered examples of the mechanistic model because the constructs of social learning and behavior modification are controlled by stimuli external to the individual. The issue of internal or external locus of control probably is the key or central point in models built to examine human performance.

QUALITATIVE VS. QUANTITATIVE CHANGE (1–3)

Qualitative changes based on the organismic model are characterized as stages or levels of development which are defined or delineated unique behaviors occurring at each stage or level. Qualitative changes based on

---

* For general references, see Bibliography.

Table 5.1
Overview of Model Levels

Title	Type		Information Provided
Meta models	Organismic	Mechanistic	Primarily concerned with philosophical issues
Super models	Humanism Development Systems Holism	Reductionism Behaviorism Psychoanalysis	Provide general guidelines for observing human performance as it occurs
Health models (samples)	Wholistic health Developmental Biopsychosocial	Biomedical Rehabilitation Behavior modification	Provide general guidelines for intervention
OT theoretical models (samples)	Occupational behavior Occupational model Human development through occupations	Orthopaedic Kinesiology Object relations Learning theory	Provide guidelines for observing human performance through the use of occupations
OT practice	Stated in review of each model	Stated in review of each model	Provide specific guidelines for the assessment and the management through occupational therapy intervention

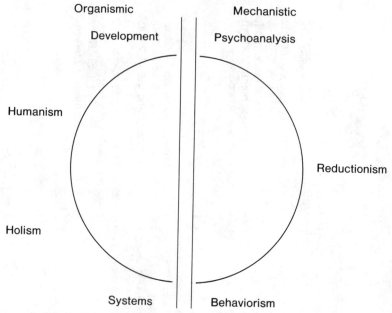

Figure 5.1. Model of meta and super model relationships.

the mechanistic model examine the cumulative effects of specific behaviors within periods of the life-span. In other words the changes are in the operational efficiency. An example of qualitative changes can be found in Piaget's stages of cognitive adaptation. The sensorimotor, concrete operation and formal operation periods are all characterized by specific subperiods of behavior which are unique to that period. An example of a qualitative process is the process of learning as proposed by behaviorists. Basically, learning is the same process throughout life, but the accumulated experience enables the learner to become more efficient in interacting with the environment and thus learn more complex sequences of behavioral responses.

END POINT VS. NO END POINT (1, 2)

In the organismic model there is an end point to the progression of change. This end point provides a goal, purpose and direction to the change which can be identified. The most common end point is some type of maturity. For example, in Piagetian theory the formal operations stage is the end point. In Erickson's theory, the eighth and final stage of ego integrity vs. despair is the end point.

On the other hand, the mechanistic model has no end point. Behavior is considered to be a function of the situation and thus the goal, purpose and direction may change, depending on the environmental conditions

Table 5.2
Metamodels: Contrasting Views between Major Philosophies

Organismic	Mechanistic
1. *Internal locus of control* (1, 2) Activity generated from within; individual is active and dynamic	*External locus of control* Activity result of outside forces; individual is reactive, passive and a robot.
2. *Qualitative* (1–3) Stages, levels, milestones, phases, ages, periods	*Quantitative* Cumulative effect
3. *End point* (1, 2) Fixed process	*No end point* Additative line or product
4. *Discontinuous change* (1–3) Patterns of behavior irreversible	*Continuous change* Patterns of behavior are reversible
5. *Emergence or constructivism* (1, 2) Behavioral or functional change is a transformation and is irreducible	*Reductionistic* Any change in the organism can be reduced to more elementary form
6. *Holistic* (1–3) Whole is different or greater than sum of parts	*Elementaristic* Whole is equal to the sum of parts
7. *Structure-function* (1–3) Function determines structure	*Antecedent-consequent* All behavior caused by environmental forces
8. *Structural change* (1–3) Change is determined by the form of the organization	*Behavioral change* Change is determined by efficient cause
9. *Open system* (4, p. 39) Interacts with the environment	*Closed system* Does not interact with the environment
10. *Age restriction* (1, 2) Chronological age is used as boundaries for stages or levels	*No age restriction* Chronological age is an increasing continuum of time
11. *Free will* (5, p. 931; 6, p. 15) Man is able to choose and exercise volitional control	*Determinism* All events follow natural laws which man does not control
12. *Universality* (1, 2) Behavior characteristics of all organisms	*Relativity* Behavior characteristic of individual only
13. *Heredity* (7) Inherent, genetic, nature and primarily responsible for man's behavior	*Environment* Nurture is primarily responsible for man's behavior
14. *Rationalism* (6, pp. 30, 186) Reason is source of knowledge	*Expiricism* Experience is source of knowledge
15. *Man is responsible* (6, p. 14) Responsible for individual action	*Man is irresponsible* Is not responsible for self
16. *Steady state* (4) Achieves balance in spite of input and output, a dynamic process	*Equilibrium* Achieves balance through a static process

Table 5.2—*Continued*

Organismic	Mechanistic
17. *Equifinality* (4, p. 132) Alternate route may have the same outcome	*Finality* The outcome is determined by initial conditions
18. *Negentropy* (4, p. 41) Individual can increase amount of free energy	*Entropy* Amount of free energy is limited
19. *Autonomous activity* (4, p. 209) Individual can initiate action	*Dependent activity* Individual is conditioned to do certain actions.
20. *Moral values* (5, p. 395; 6, p. 16; 8) Have knowledge of right and wrong	*Amoral* No need to know right and wrong
21. *Symbolic activity* (4, p. 215) Individual seeks symbolic activity	*Nonsymbolic activities* The environment controls the type of activity
22. *Critical periods* (7, p. 136) Certain times in development most favorable for learning	*Noncritical periods* Learning is possible at any age
23. *Emotionalism* (6, p. 38) Feelings, affect and mood are part of organism	*Unemotional* Feelings, affect and mood are not necessary
24. *Monism* (8, p. 81) Mind and body are one	*Dualism* Mind and body are separate
25. *Subjectivism* (8, p. 88) Concerned with inner processes of thought and feeling	*Objectivism* Concerned with external actions and responses
26. *Tension seeking* (9, p. 55) Man seeks situations which increase tension in the body-need induction	*Tension reducing* Man tries to reduce the tension which arises in the body-need reduction
27. *Fluid dimensions* (8, p. 122; 10, p. 89) of time and space	*Fixed dimensions* of time and space
28. *Pull motivation* (9, p. 300) Emphasis on purpose, value and needs, "carrot" theories	*Push motivation* Emphasis on drive, motive, and stimulus, "pitchfork" theories
29. *Unidirectional* (1, 2) Development of progression of complexity and expansion	*Alternating directional* Developmental progression and regression are equal possibilities
30. *Present, future-oriented* (1) Time perspective is looking ahead	*Past-oriented* Time perspective is looking backward

present at the time. Again, behaviorists' theories such as those of Skinner, Bijou and Watson are examples.

DISCONTINUOUS VS. CONTINUOUS CHANGE (1–3)

Theories based on discontinuity organize the changes observed in the individual into stages, levels, periods, milestones, phases or ages. Each stage represents a distinct organization of the total individual into something that was not present before. In contrast, theories based on continuous approach proposed that change is a steady, cumulative process which is based on identifiable units of previous development. Examples of stages can be found in Piaget's levels of cognitive adaptation or Erickson's eight stages of life. Continuous change is evident in the theory of behaviorism. Change occurs whenever the environmental conditions are such that events prior to, or rewards given after, a response alter the nature of that response. Thus change can be increased or decreased, brought about or extinguished.

EMERGENCE VS. REDUCTIONISM (1, 2)

Emergence or constructivism is the process of changing the structure and function into something that did not exist before. The organismic model is based on the concept that as stages or levels occur, the changes that occur reorganize the total individual into a different system.

In contrast, reductionism is the process of reducing any higher level or more complex behavior into a lower level or simpler behavior. The reductionistic approach is basic to the mechanistic assumption that all behavior can be changed from one form to another and back again. In physics and chemistry the basic level is atoms and molecules; in physiology, the cell is a basic unit and in behavior, a stimuli response sequence is the basic unit. Again, stage theories such as those of Piaget and Erickson are examples of emergence, while Freudian and Skinnerian theories are examples of reductionism as is the biomedical model of disease and pathology.

HOLISM VS. ELEMENTARISM (1–3)

Holism is the assumption that the organism as a whole is different from the sum of its parts. In other words an individual has characteristics as a total human being which are not present *per se* in any of the specific parts. On the other hand, elementarism is the assumption that the organism is the sum of its parts. That is when all the elements of a person are put together the total person can be observed; conversely any part of a person can be observed by examining the elements in that part. Thus any part of a person's behavior can be studied by examining the elements or units which make up the behavior.

STRUCTURE-FUNCTION VS. ANTECEDENT-CONSEQUENT ANALYSIS (1–3)

Structure-function is basically the assumption that a person has functions, objectives or general purpose which is carried out or contained within a structure. Thus, the functions are enumerated and structure identified which serve the functions. The results delineate the process by which functions can occur and achievement obtained.

Antecedent-consequent proponents assume that behavior is a function of altering the events which occur before a response or changing the events that occur after a response. Thus no specific structure is needed since the generating force leading to behavior is external to the individual.

STRUCTURAL CHANGE VS. BEHAVIOR CHANGE (1–3)

The organismic model assumes that change occurs in the form, structure or organization of the individual and that the changes are directed toward an end state or goal. Actual change may or may not be observable to others. In some cases, the person's word must be accepted.

In contrast, the mechanistic model assumes that change is evident through the behavioral response that is made and can be observed by others. Change has occurred when the individual responds differently to the situations or events which exist in the environment. Thus change is measured by the degree of difference in a response from previous behavior.

OPEN VS. CLOSED SYSTEM (4)

An open system maintains itself by exchanging matter with the environment and by continuously building up and breaking down components. Humans are considered to be open systems in the organismic model because each individual is capable of taking in nutrients and information, converting the inputs into useful products and putting out energy, responses or waste. Thus there is a constant interchange between the individual and the environment.

On the other hand, a closed system does not interact with the environment. Technically no materials enter or leave. A human functions as if there were no need to interact with the environment. Although no theory proposes that humans are totally closed systems, there is in the mechanistic model a view that supports interaction only for the purpose of tension reduction. In other words, a person only interacts with the environment when tissue or bodily needs arise.

AGE RESTRICTIONS VS. NO AGE RESTRICTION (1, 2)

Theories developed from the organismic model often make use of chronological age as a restriction, limit or boundary for stages and levels. The assumption is that chronological age is a guide to the determination of structural changes within the individual. In the mechanistic model age is not considered a change agent because age can be reduced to time and time simply provides more opportunity for the environment to change behavioral responses.

FREE WILL VS. DETERMINISM (5, 6)

The organismic model contains the assumption that humans are capable of choosing those activities and behavior which are needed or desired. In other words, each person is capable of guiding or directing the self through the use of volitional control. This capacity for self-direction is in contrast with the assumption of determinism. Determinism is based on the assumption that all facts and events are controlled by natural laws. By deduction it follows that human behavior and activity follow the same natural laws, and therefore an individual's behavior and activity are directed by situations over which a person has little control. Thus, the individual is much like a pawn who reacts rather than an originator who acts on the environment.

UNIVERSALITY VS. RELATIVITY (1, 2)

Universality is based on the assumption that some behavior or activity is common to all human beings or at least to all biologically intact human beings. Universality is supported by genetic inheritance which may be common or similar to all humans living or yet to be born. The inheritance includes a number of preprogrammed units which provide the basic sets of behavior or outline the parameters. On the other hand, relativity is based on the assumption that behavior is dependent on the environmental conditions. The rationale would be that similar environmental conditions exist to which similar responses are given. The same reasoning suggests that individual differences occur because different environmental conditions exist for each individual.

HEREDITY VS. ENVIRONMENT (7)

The organismic model is basically built on the assumption that heredity is the critical component in determining behavior. Heredity is controlled by genes and expressed through maturation. Environment is considered to facilitate the maturation of behavior by some theorists such as Piaget. However, the structural organization of behavior is present at birth. Environment provides the activity to interact with the existing organization. Followers of the mechanistic model in contrast believe that environment is the key to building behavior repertoires. Behavior is learned and acquired through socialization and education.

RATIONALISM VS. EMPIRICISM (5, 6)

Theories based on the organismic model assume that reason and intuition are the primary sources of knowledge. Rationalism permits the individual to know reality independent of experience. In other words, the intellect is the true source of reality rather than the senses. Through the use of reason and intuition a person has the authority and ability to determine one's own course of action.

In contrast, the mechanistic model is based on empiricism in which all knowledge is assumed to come from experience and observation. Thus, the senses are the source of knowledge and truth, and the brain is a blank tablet (tabula rasa), which must depend on external information for its knowledge.

RESPONSIBLE VS. IRRESPONSIBLE (6)

The organismic model is organized to assume that humans are rational and thus capable of reason and responsibility. That is, humans can think for themselves, determine the results of their actions, choose a course of action and accept the consequences for that choice. In contrast, the mechanistic model has a basic assumption that man is irresponsible and unable to direct self activities without assistance and control. Reason is considered impossible because a person does not initiate action but only reacts to activity as it exists.

STEADY STATE VS. EQUILIBRIUM (4)

A steady state is achieved by reaching a constant internal and external balance, while at the same time continuously exchanging and using component materials. Thus, the individual is able to maintain the self in spite of building up and breaking down and importing and exporting nutrients and information. In the organismic model the individual is viewed as able to maintain the integrity of the self while continuously seeking to interact with the environment.

Equilibrium is the process of maintaining a balance among bodily processes. When equilibrium mechanisms are working, changes in the internal or external environmental stimulate other processes to counter-act those changes through a feedback system that leads to the restoration of balance. The mechanistic model is based on the assumption that the individual will seek equilibrium and only interacts with the environment to achieve the elements needed to restore the balance.

EQUIFINALITY VS. FINALITY (4)

Equifinality is the capacity of the individual organism to reach the same goal from different starting points and in different ways. The organismic model is based on the assumption that the individual has the capacity to organize the self in a number of different ways which will all reach the same or similar end point.

In contrast, finality as an assumption in the mechanistic model states that end or final state is determined by the initial conditions. Thus, the individual has no real capacity to alter or change either the direction or end point which will be achieved.

NEGENTROPY VS. ENTROPY (4)

In the process of negentropy or negative entropy the system is able to take in more energy than is needed to convert the energy source into a usable energy form. Thus, the individual has a net gain in energy resources which can be used to build the system as well as maintain it. The organismic model has adopted the assumption that each individual is capable of achieving negentropy and thus is able to progress through maturation and learning to higher levels of organization and differentiation.

In contrast, the mechanistic model follows the assumption that the body has a relatively fixed quantity of energy available. As the energy is used, the amount of entropy, conversion of energy, increases which in turn increases the amount of disorder over time. Thus, the body continues to function until it breaks down, but it cannot expand or improve because of the original limitation of energy available.

AUTONOMOUS VS. DIRECTED ACTIVITY (4)

Basic to the organismic model is the assumption that humans are capable of performing autonomous behavior, that is, behavior which is initiated within the individual. This assumption of self-initiated action permits the individual to take charge of the self and be responsible for the actions taken.

On the other side, the mechanistic model is based on the assumption that all activity is caused by events external to the individual, thus the individual is responding rather than initiating. There is little need for initiating action because the environment provides the necessary stimulation to produce the behavior needed.

MORAL VALUES VS. AMORAL (5, 6, 8)

Within the organismic model moral values are considered essential and part of a person's responsibility. Moral values include a sense of ethics which describes right and wrong actions. These actions are theoretically both possible, but the ethical responsibility will enable the person to choose the right action.

In contrast, the mechanism model has no scope of values or ethics because none are needed. Humans are not considered to be making choices but responding according to learned behavior. If the behavior is rewarded it will be continued; if not, it will be extinguished. Teaching a person the "right thing to do" is simply a case of rewarding the behavior that is wanted so the person will continue to perform that behavior.

SYMBOLIC VS. NONSYMBOLIC ACTIVITY (4)

The organismic model includes the assumption that humans use symbols to convey their activity and that much of activity in which humans engage is at the symbolic level. After the basic physiological and psychological needs are met, the individual engages in symbolic behavior. This engagement may continue without any observable or known cause other than simply for the pleasure of involvement.

By comparison the mechanistic model does not recognize symbolic activity. What appears as symbolic activity can be understood at a lower level. What appears as "activity for its own sake" is simply behavior for which the cause is unclear or unidentified at this time. All behavior has a cause because all behavior follows the natural laws of cause and effect.

CRITICAL PERIODS VS. NONCRITICAL PERIODS (7)

Critical periods as an assumption of the organismic model states that there are certain times in the life of individuals which are optimal for learning specific adaptive behaviors. It follows then that if the critical period age is past, optimal learning will not occur and may never occur. Thus, it is important to provide opportunities for learning adaptive behaviors during the critical period for maximum results.

In contrast, the mechanistic model is based on the assumption that the individual is plastic and is therefore able to learn behaviors at any chronological age. The important factor is the amount of reinforcement provided. Sufficient reinforcement will produce the desired adaptive behavior no matter when the learning occurs during the natural history of the individual.

EMOTIONALISM VS. UNEMOTIONALISM (6)

Feelings, affect and mood are considered as impacting the thought and reasoning processes within the organismic model. Thus, emotion is an integral assumption in which the individual's behavior might be affected by the emotional content. In contrast, the assumption of the mechanistic model is that machines are affected by observable physical forces. An individual thus can be understood entirely from the outside without reference to inner states, such as feelings or emotions.

MONISM VS. DUALISM (8)

A basic assumption of the organismic model is that mind and body operate together and that there is no real distinction between the mind, body and spirit. Thought and reason are not considered as separate functions but as expressions of the whole of which thought and action are aspects.

In comparison, the mechanistic model is based on the assumption that the mind and body are separate. Body became the more important of the two because it could be studied objectively. Soma could be studied as a machine, while psyche could not and thus was ignorable. Furthermore, machines, and thus, individuals can be understood entirely without reference to internal energy sources.

SUBJECTISM VS. OBJECTISM (8)

The organismic model is based on the organism as the sphere of concern. Thinking and reasoning as action potentials are subjective or difficult to discern with the senses. Thus, much of the focus of the individual must be inferred from observation or obtained through interview. Generalizations from one person to the next are risky at best.

In contrast, the mechanistic model operates on the basis that external actions are the major sphere of concern. What can be verified through senses is important. Sensory based data can be observed, quantified, and measured. Generalities of behavior can be obtained by using the normal curve of distribution and standard deviations.

TENSION SEEKING VS. TENSION REDUCING (9)

Tension seeking involves the active exploration of the environment in an attempt to learn about and master the unknown. In tension-seeking behavior, the person deliberates by and consciously risks some degree of potential harm or displeasure in order to gain greater satisfaction. In contrast, tension reduction is directed toward decreasing the scope of interaction with the environment so as to reduce a designated drive, such as hunger, safety, or belonging. Activity is focused on the target, and when the objective is obtained behavior ceases and does not generally reappear until the drive reappears. On the other hand, tension-seeking behavior such as learning a new skill may lead to a further expansion of behavior to learn yet another skill or perfect the first one. Tension-seeking behavior thus expands the behavior repertoire, whereas tension-reducing behavior tends to become sterotyped and limited.

FLUID DIMENSION VS. FIXED DIMENSION OF TIME AND SPACE (8, 10)

The organismic view recognizes that time and space have psychological and sociocultural dimensions as well as physical dimensions. Such dimension may change, depending on the situation and interpretation by the individual. Time may appear to go by slowly if little activity is occurring or rapidly if the person is busily involved. For younger people, the present is all important, whereas for the older persons the past may be more easily remembered.

In contrast, the mechanistic view states that time and space are absolute quantities and values. Failure to adhere to the values is evidence of loss of reality or failure to understand reality. The person is expected to conform to the values of time and space as stated by the physical sciences. Such a view persists in mechanistic philosophy, even though experiments have illustrated the fallacy in such logic.

PULL MOTIVATION VS. PUSH MOTIVATION (1)

The organismic philosophy includes ideas related to purpose, value or need as the motivational forces which direct human action. Kelly, a psychologist, calls these "carrot" theories because they depend on the person's willingness to seek out action and "go for" the carrot on the stick.

On the other hand, there are motivational concepts which are described as drives, motives or stimuli. These concepts are associated with the mechanismic view that a person must incur a motivational force from the internal or external environment in order to become activated. Kelly describes such theories as "pitchfork" theories because the source of energy seems to push a person from the rear to get moving.

UNIDIRECTIONAL DEVELOPMENT VS. ALTERNATING DIRECTIONAL DEVELOPMENT (1, 2)

The organismic view assets that development change is cumulative and irreversible. The organism through the process of development expands and increases in complexity. As the change occurs, the organism progresses in only one direction, forward and onward. Behavior that appears to be from a younger period is described as due to temporary instability, especially in times of stress where older patterns of behavior are more sure.

In contrast, the mechanistic philosophy states that behavior change can be forwards or backwards. Behavior may regress to a more primitive or immature form that the person supposedly had "outgrown." Such behavior is most likely to appear in situations of anxiety or crisis. In psychoanalytic literature such regression is a mechanism available to the ego whenever it is unable to cope with the present situation.

PRESENT, FUTURE-ORIENTED VS. PAST-ORIENTED (2)

Models based in the organismic framework tend to view the present and future time frame as most important when viewing an individual's situation. The focus is on what the person can do and has potential for doing. Thus, the past may or may not be indicative of the person's total being. Therefore, use of past history should be interpreted with caution because it may be irrelevant or misleading. Instead, much more useful information may be obtained by discovering how a person views the current situation and what plans or interests the person has for the future.

The opposite position is that the past is all important because infancy and early experience shape the total potentials or significantly influence all later action. Like the machine a person is able to do only what the person was built to do. The building blocks were set in early life. The objective of later life is to understand and use what was built in the early childhood.

THE INFLUENCE OF THE META MODELS ON OCCUPATIONAL THERAPY

Occupational therapists began working within the organismic model based on the humanistic philosophy as illustrated in the moral treatment approach and the theory of psychobiology developed by Adolph Meyer. Practice was concerned with organizing the individual's daily activities, treating the individual with respect, and promoting socially acceptable behavior. As the influences of Gesell began to affect practice in the 1930s and 1940s, the organismic model remained, although the focus of intervention changed to the following stages of development.

In the 1940s and 1950s the pressure of medical specialization in rehabilitation and psychoanalytic theory began to push the organismic orientation into a second rate position. Behavior was assessed in discrete units, such as range of motion in degrees, muscle strength in pounds and analysis of specific past events. The concentration on observable details and regressive behavior sometimes ignored the whole person with feelings and thoughts. Practice was to be oriented to research methods designed to find the statistical laws of human behavior. Health was the absence of disease or trauma. The shift from organismic to mechanistic models became evident. During the 1960s and 1970s, occupational therapy in psychiatry began to resist the move to the mechanistic model. Developmental ideas began to reappear. At the same time, occupational therapy in physical dysfunction tried to embrace the mechanistic model. Thus, the neurobehavioral approaches, such as progressive resistive exercise, active and passive range of motion became popular. Some sensorimotor concepts followed the reductionistic philosophy also.

Beginning in the 1960s, however, there were a few examples of a resurgence of the organismic model. The occupational behavior model (Reilly) is most notable. In the seventies, there were more models based on adaptation such as the recapitulation of ontogenesis (Mosey) and the lecture on adaptation by King. The concepts of humanism, holism, competence and occupation became, once again, more visible as spheres of influence in occupational therapy. Occupational therapy has begun to reassert its rightful heritage.

References

1. Looft WR: Socialization and personality throughout the life span; an examination of contemporary psychological approaches. In Baltes PB, Schaie KW: *Life Span Developmental Psychology.* New York, Academic Press, 1973, pp 25–82
2. Friedrich D: *A Primer For Developmental Methodology.* Minneapolis, Burgess Publishing, 1972, pp 3–8.
3. Reese HW, Overton WF: Models of development and theories of development. In Goulet LR, Battes PB: *Life Span Development Psychology.* New York, Academic Press, 1970, pp 115–145.
4. Bentalanffy LV: *General Systems Theory.* New York, Braziller, 1968.
5. Solomon RC: *Introducing Philosophy : Problems and Perspectives,* 2nd ed. New York, Harcourt, Brace, Jovanovich, 1981.
6. Blackham HJ: *Humanism,* 2nd ed. New York, International Publications Service, 1976.
7. Thomas RM: *Comparing Theories of Child Development.* Belmont, Calif, Wadsworth Publishing, 1979, p 29.
8. Lamont C: *The Philosphy of Humanism,* 6th ed. New York, Frederick Ungar Publishing, 1982, pp 12–14.
9. Hergenhahn BR: *An Introduction to Theories of Personalities.* Englewood Cliffs, NJ, Prentice-Hall, 1980.
10. Capra F: *The Turning Point: Science, Society and the Rising Culture.* New York, Simon and Schuster, 1982.
11. Kelly G: *The Psychology of Personal Constructs,* Vol 1. New York, Norton, 1955, pp 36–38.
12. Arndt WB: *Theories of Personality.* New York, Macmillan, 1974, p 53–64.

CHAPTER 6

Super Models

Over the years many models have been used as frames of reference for the development of practice models and theories in occupational therapy; however, six major "super" models appear most frequently. These are the humanistic, reductionist, developmental, psychoanalytic, behavioristic and system models. A seventh, the holistic model, seems to be emerging. Each of these "super" models has provided a framework through which to examine the role of occupational therapy as a practice discipline (Table 6.1). An analysis of the models themselves illustrates both the similarities and differences. To facilitate the comparison, the same questions have been posed and answered (1). The first is concerned with how the model explains its view of an individual as a being in the world, in terms of what impacts upon the individual, what the individual impacts upon and how the individual is put together as a biological unit. The second question asks how the model accounts for stability and change under the conditions defined as normal in the context of the model. The third question is concerned with the source "of change and causes that create 'normal' change." A fourth question asks what the model assumes about goals in terms of the direction of "normal" change and who establishes the goals. Fifth, what are the symptoms that something is wrong or abnormal and what are goals and strategies of intervening. Finally, what is the place and role of the change agent.

HUMANISTIC MODEL

This appears to be the earliest model on which occupational therapy practice was based. Its roots go back to the era of "moral treatment" in the 1800s. The model was based more on common sense than on scientific fact and is consistent with the assumptions of the organismic meta model. Humanism was based on the equality of men and their ability for rational thought. Humans were believed to be subject to the natural universal laws which governed their activity. If the environment in which they lived was basically good, then the individual would grow and become a righteous individual.

The key to *stability* was a well organized routine of wholesome activities. Positive *change* occurred as the child learned new activities and incorporated these into the routine. The *source of change* was stress caused by social pressures to change behabior. The *goal* was to organize the habits and activities required by the social and physical environment. *Intervention* was needed when the external pressures became so great that the organized routine became disorganized. Thus, the *goal of intervention* was to restore or maintain the habits into a functional routine again. The *strategy of intervention* was to treat the individual as a functioning person, to organize the surroundings so that the person was

Table 6.1
Overview of Philosophy and Models Related to Occupational Therapy

Meta Models	Organismic				Mechanistic		
Super models	Humanism	Development	Systems	Holism	Reductionism	Behaviorism	Psychoanalysis
Health models	Milieu	Health development	a. Biopsychosocial b. Health education	a. Wholistic health b. High level wellness	a. Biomedical b. Bio rehabilitation c. Public health	a. Behavior modification b. Impaired health c. Social rehabilitation	Psychoanalytic process
OT theoretical models (samples)	a. Moral treatment b. Pseudopharmacology	a. Occupational behavior b. Adaptation c. Sensory integration d. Activity therapy			a. Orthopaedic b. Kinesiology	"Learning theory"	a. Object relations b. Communications
Assessment instruments (samples)	Activity analysis	Case study/history Interest checklist Activity configuration			(Prevoc eval) (ADL checklist) (Reflex test)	(Behavior analysis)	Activity batteries
Expected outcome	Balance of occupational performance				Restoration of specific performance areas		

comfortable, and to organize the person's time into purposeful activity (2). Ideally, the *change agent* was a part of the situation whose role was to organize and facilitate the activities in which the person engaged.

This model is the basis for the theory of occupation presented by Adolph Meyer and the habit training approach of Eleanor Clarke Slagle. Susan Tracy and William R. Dunton, Jr. also followed the general concepts of the humanistic model (see Chapters 11 and 13).

REDUCTIONISTIC MODEL

In contrast to the humanistic model, the reductionistic model is based on the mechanistic model. It is also intertwined in the scientific method. Basically, reductionism attempts to explain a complex whole in terms of its simpler elements (3). Thus, the reduction model would see a person as a collection of cells which are composed of biochemical properties. *Stability* is achieved through homeostasis or the balance between dynamic forces. *Changes* occur through the chemical processes which maintain, enlarge or reduce the body structures. The *source of change* is cell division or enlargement through the action of mitosis or catabolism. The *goal* of change is to achieve equilibrium by altering the internal processes. *Intervention* occurs when disease or trauma alters the cellular structure. The *goal of intervention* is to destroy or get rid of pathogens or correct structures through the use of drugs or surgery. If neither is successful, custodial care is employed. The *change agent* works outside the treatment setting as one who determines an external diagnoser and actor. The reductionist model has been used as the framework for the orthopedic and kinesthetic models (see Chapter 12). These models helped occupational therapy achieve some recognition in the medical community because they were more "scientific" than humanism.

DEVELOPMENTAL MODEL

The developmental model is based on the view of the individual as undergoing a progressive and continuous change from birth to death (4). *Stability* is discussed in terms of phases, stages, levels or periods which an individual attains or should attain. *Change* is therefore a constant factor, and although there are similarities among individuals, the developmental model recognizes individual differences and uniquenesses. The *source of change* is within the basic nature of the organism and is caused by maturation or learning. The direction is ontological, because the individual tends to follow the developmental pattern of the species. The *goals* are determined by both inherited and environmental influences. Here, variations of the developmental model have a wide range of explanations as to how many goals are achieved as a result of heredity vs. environment. *Intervention* is needed when there is a defined discrepancy between the actual development and the supposed potential for development based on some reference point such as chronological age. The *goal of intervention* is to remove the blockage so that development can continue. In some cases the blockage may be circumvented. The *strategies* are aimed at promoting the attainment of higher responses. The *change agent* remains outside the situation as an external diagnoser but does act as a facilitator when environmental changes are being used in the intervention process.

Developmental models have been very popular in the practice of occupational therapy. Therapists have borrowed from the theories of Gesell, Piaget and others. They also have provided their own such as these of Ayres, Mosey and Llorens (see Chapters 11, 12, and 13). Thus, the impact of the developmental model on occupational therapy practice has been significant since the 1940s.

PSYCHOANALYTIC MODEL

The psychoanalytic model is based on the mechanistic meta model and the general assumption that behavior is controlled by childhood anxieties and defensive maneuvers which are unconscious (5). However, Freud could not explain change through the mechanistic model so he borrowed the concept of development from the organismic view. *Stability* is obtained through the personality structure of the id, ego, and superego. *Change* occurs as the individual progresses through the psychosexual stages of development which include the oral, anal, phallic, latency and genital periods. The *source of change* is attributed to life energy which has two causal forces. These are aggression and sex or also called death and life. The direction of the *goal* is instinctual and set by early experience with parents. *Intervention* is considered when symptoms of inadequate defense mechanisms occur. The *goal of intervention* is to help the person gain insight and understanding. *Strategies* include the use of techniques such as free association, repression, identification and transference. The *change agent* functions outside the intervention process and acts in the role of a listener or clarifier. Occupational therapy models based on the psychoanalytic model include those of Azima and Fidler and Fidler (see Chapter 13).

BEHAVIORISTIC MODEL

In the behavioristic model behavior is seen as lawful, orderly and controllable (6). *Stability* is obtained through behavioral control and is *changed* through reinforcement or reward. The *source of change* is learning caused by tension reduction which is determined by observed behavior. The direction of *goals* is determined by emergent or engineered situations set by environmental forces. *Intervention* is recommended when behavior is either excessive or deficient according to some standard. The *goal of intervention* is to establish or reestablish the correct amount of behavior. *Strategies* include shaping, chaining, generalization and extinction. The *change agent* may function outside or as part of the situation, depending on the role taken in the intervention process. The role may be as a facilitator to help the patient develop a self-controlled change program or as a controller who provides the reinforcements or rewards. The article by Smith and Tempone (7) and Mosey's action-consequence chapter (8) are based on the behavioristic model. These have not been reviewed in the text because occupational therapists have not added anything to the existing model.

THE SYSTEM MODEL

The system model grew as a reaction against the reductionist model. It is based on the view that the whole is not the same as the sum of its parts (9). Thus, an individual is not the sum of a series of biochemical cells but rather a significant whole. *Stability* is achieved through structural integration of the parts into a cohesive whole. *Change* is derived from the structure. The *source of change* is structural stress. The cause is tension which is external to the individual. The direction of *goals* is emergent and thus dependent on the situation or vested interest. Symptoms which may require *intervention* include stresses and strains which are internal and tensions which are external. The *goal of intervention* is to achieve adjustment or adaptation with the the physical, physiological and sociocultural environments. *Strategies* are aimed at altering the inputs into the systems in the hopes of changing the output. Feedback is a particularly important input. The *change agent* may be inside or outside the system and may assume the role of internal or external diagnoser and actor.

System models have become widely known to occupational therapy in the past several years. However, the primary occupational therapy models which are based on the systems model are Reilly's occupational behavior and Kielhofner's model of human occupation (see Chapter 9).

HOLISTIC MODEL

This model is emerging but has had an effect on the occupational therapy literature. Much of the thinking comes from the group relations literature, including small group, assertiveness training and consciousness raising. The major theme centers on the concept that a person can change behavior by, or through, their own actions, beliefs and values (10). *Stability* is obtained through the individual's satisfaction with the level of mastery or achievement obtained. *Change* is the result of self-induced and self-controlled action. The *source* of change is primarily the self, although the change agent may act as a partner. The causal force is rational, conscious choice. The direction or *goal* is determined by deliberate selection set by the individual or by a collaborative process. *Intervention* is begun when there is a perceived need on the part of the individual, although the change agent may act as a clarifier. The *goal of intervention* is self-improvement. *Strategies* usually involve some sort of "trying it out" situation. Thus, simulation, "dry runs" or supervised real events can be used. The *change agent*, when involved, is part of the situation and participates in the here and now settings with the individual.

One model which makes use of the general ideas of the holistic model is that of Watanabe. Such a model tends to stress cognitive skills and responsibility for self behavior.

In summary, there are seven models which have been or are being used to develop practice models in occupational therapy as outlined in Table 6.2. One additional note is important. Super models are not necessarily mutually exclusive. Thus, some practice models may make use of more than one super model. This multiple use seems to be popular with the developmental and systems models. It is not unusual to see the word adaptation included in a developmentally based model and stages appearing in a systems based model. Whether such crossing over into other frames of reference will cause problems in verifying practice models remains to be determined. At present the cross-reference seems to provide adequate explanations for model and theory-building purposes.

Table 6.2
Models Change[a]

Assumptions and Approaches to:	Humanistic Model	Reductionist Model	Developmental Model
1. View of the individual	Person's environment influences and alters function	Humans can be reduced to the least common denominator	Humans grow, develop and elaborate
2. Content			
Stability	Routine activity	Homeostasis	Phases, stages
Change	Integrate new habits	Chemical processing	Constant and unique
3. Causation			
Source of change	Stress	Cell division and enlargement	Nature or organism
Causal force	Social pressures	Mitosis	Maturation, learning
4. Goals			
Direction	Organized habits	Achieve equilibrium	Ontological
Set by	Social and physical environment	Internal process	Inherited and environmental influence
5. Intervention			
Confronting symptoms	Disorganized habits	Disease, trauma	Discrepancy between actuality and potential
Goals of intervening	Restore and maintain habits	Destroy pathogens; correct structure	Removal of blockages
Strategies	Activity in normal settings	Drugs, surgery, custodial care	Promote higher level response
6. Change agent			
Place	Part of situation	Outside	Outside
Role	Participate facilitator	External diagnoser and actor	External diagnoser, facilitator

Table 6.2—*Continued*

Assumptions and Approaches to	Psychoanalytic	Behavioristic
1. View of the individual	Behavior is controlled by unconscious anxieties and defenses	Behavior is lawful, orderly, and controllable
2. Content		
Stability	Personality structure	Behavior control
Change	Psychosexual stages	Reinforcement, reward
3. Causation		
Source of change	Life energy	Learning
Causal force	Aggression, sex, death, life	"Tension reduction"
4. Goals		
Direction	Instinctual	Emergent or engineered
Set by	Early experience with parents	Environmental forces
5. Intervention		
Confronting symptoms	Inadequate defense mechanism	Excessive or deficient behavior
Goal of intervening	Insight, understanding	Correct amount of behavior
Strategies	Free association, repression	Shaping, chaining, generalization, extinction
6. Change agent		
Place	Outside	Outside or part of situation
Role	Listener, clarifier	Controller or facilitator

Assumptions and Approaches to:	Systems Model	Holistic Model
1. View of the individual	Whole of a person is different from sum of parts	Person can change behavior by self initiated action, belief and values
2. Content		
Stability	Structural integration	Satisfaction, achievement "frozen parts"
Change	Derived from structure	Induced, controlled
3. Causation		
Source of change	Structural stress	Self and change agent
Causal force	Tension reduction	Rational choice
4. Goals		
Direction	Emergent	Deliberate selection
Set by	"Vested interest" situational	Individual or collaborative process

Table 6.2—*Continued*

Assumptions and Approaches to:	Systems Model	Holistic Model
5. Intervention		
Confronting symptoms	Stress, strains and tensions	Perceived need
Goals of intervening	Adjustment, adaptation	Improvement
Strategies	Alter inputs, *i.e.*, feedback	Try out
6. Change agent		
Place	Inside or outside the "target" system	Part of situation
Role	Internal or external diagnoser and actor	Participant in here and now

[a] Adapted from R. Chin (1).

References

1. Chin R: The utility of system models and developmental models for practitioners. In Bennes WG, Benne KD, Chin R: *Planning of Change*. New York, Holt, Rinehart & Winston, 1961, p 212
2. Bockhoven JS: *Moral Treatment in Community Mental Health*. New York, Springer, 1972, p 12.
3. Sloane EH: Reductionism. *Psychol Rev* 52:217, 1945.
4. Chaplin JP: *Dictionary of Psychology*, revised ed. New York, Dell, 1975.
5. Million T: *Theories of Psychopathology*. Philadelphia, Saunders, 1967, p 139.
6. Hall CS, Lindzey G: *Theories of Personality*, 2nd ed. New York, Wiley, 1970, pp 480–481.
7. Smith AR, Tempone VJ: Psychiatric occupational therapy within a learning theory context. *Am J Occup Ther* 22:415, 1968.
8. Mosey AC: *Three Frames of Reference for Mental Health*. Thorofare, NJ, CB Slack, 1970, pp 84–131.
9. Laszlo E: *The Systems View of the World*. New York, Braziller, 1972, p 28.
10. Tubesing NL: *Whole Person Health Care: Philosophical Assumptions*. Hinsdale, Il, Wholistic Health Center, 1977, pp 6–7.

CHAPTER 7

Health and Rehabilitation Models

Over the years philosophy and science have provided the rationale for the development of several general health and intervention models. Occupational therapy has been made a part of these models with varying degrees of success. The following chapter is a review of the existing health and intervention models designed to influence the state of a person's health and the impact of each model on the practice of occupational therapy.

As in Chapter 6, comparison of the models has been achieved by answering the same questions for each model. The questions used in analyzing health models were adapted from Siegler and Osmond (1). The questions include: what is the view of health and illness; what is the rationale for intervention; what is the expected result or outcome; and what are the roles of the healer, subject and society. Nine models are reviewed and are summarized in Tables 7.1 and 7.3 to 7.6. They include the biomedical, impaired, biopsychosocial, public health, moral, wholistic, health development, health education and prevention, and high level wellness models. These nine seemed to represent the primary health models which have served as frames of reference. A tenth model is offered as an example of how occupational therapy can relate to health for occupational therapy models. In addition, two rehabilitation models are presented to complete the health views influencing occupational therapy.

BIOMEDICAL MODEL (Table 7.1)

The biomedical or pathologic model of health is based on the mechanistic and reductionistic models. That is, health is the result of actions by external agents over which the individual has little control, such as bacteria, fungi, viruses and mechanical forces. The agents may invade, cut, tear or separate the body or its parts. Furthermore, health is analyzed by reducing all body function to the chemical and physical properties through the study of molecular biology. Thus, the view of health is based on the maintenance of the norm of measureable biological variables (2). It follows that nonhealth would be the result of disordered biological or somatic processes which are called diseases or traumatic states.

The rationale for intervention is based on the assumption that a disordered biological state can be corrected. Prognosis depends on how well the healer feels able to bring about the correction. Goals based on the model include treating the disease, restoring health and preventing death. The practitioner's role is based on the physician's right to confer on the subject (patient) the sick or well role based on the existence or lack of disease. To fulfill the duties of the role, the physician must diagnose and recommend treatment in the forms of advice, surgery or drugs. The subject's role in this model includes the right to exemption

56

Table 7.1
Health Models

	Biomedical or Pathology	Impaired Health or Chronic
View of health	Maintenance of the norm of measurable biological (somatic) variable and absence of disease	Permanently handicapped, disabled or insane but depends on performance
Cause of nonhealth status	Disordered biological (biochemical or neurophysiological) process-disease, trauma	Unimportant-relative health status will be confined by society and the individual
Rationale for intervention by healers	Disease can be treated by connecting the biochemical or neurophysiological process	Assure that person is impaired only and not sick; assist in gaining functional independence
Expected results A. Prognosis B. Goals	No promise but usually hope is offered that person will get well; treat disease, restore health or prevent death	No change in health status is expected, provide rehabilitation and protection at reduced functional level
Practitioner's role A. Rights B. Duties	Confine the sick and well roles Make a diagnosis, recommend treatment (surgery or drugs)	Confine the impaired role; prescribe rehabilitative services
Subject's role A. Rights B. Duties	Exemption from normal responsibilities; seek help, follow orders, get well	Expect protection from abuse exploitation and persecution; behave as much as possible like a normal person
Society's role A. Rights B. Duties	Protection from sick people Provide medical care	Protection from impaired persons who are dangerous; provide rehabilitation services

from normal responsibilities while sick. At the same time, however, the subject is expected to seek the physician's advice, follow the physician's orders and get well. Society's role is based on the right to protection from sick people who might spread the disease. To fulfill the right, society has a duty to provide and sanction medical care services.

Over the years occupational therapists have found the medical model offers some problems as a frame of reference for occupational therapy (3, 4). First, occupational therapy does not deal with any drugs or surgery. Treatment through occupational therapy is not directed at microorganisms or injurious agents. Rather, occupational therapy is concerned with what happens, or may happen, to the person after the disease or injury. The aftereffects and sequelae rather than the causes are the domain of occupational therapy. The occupational therapist looks at the functional level of the individual who has had a disease or injury and attempts to determine what activity will be needed to help the person learn or relearn the skills of functional performance. Thus, studying the disease or injury is not useful to the occupational therapist. What is useful is an analysis of the aftereffects and the development of techniques to reduce, eliminate or minimize the aftereffects.

The second problem with the biomedical model is the focus only on biological causative agents. The biomedical model is designed to focus attention on the individual organism as the site of the problem, that is, the disease or injury is perceived to be located in the biological environment. This focus directs treatment to the individual and away from the sociocultural environment. Occupational therapy does have some effect on the biological structure of the organism but a large part of the treatment is directed toward facilitating the person's interaction with the sociocultural environment. The focus is on assisting the person to adjust to the sociocultural environment *and* to adjust the sociocultural environment to the person whenever possible. The concern for helping the individual to function in the sociocultural environment makes working within the biomedical model difficult, since there may be no follow through on the part of the physician.

A third problem is that occupational therapists may work with people who have no identifiable disease or injury. Children with development delay of unknown origin, people who are bothered by the hassle of living but have no organic disorder and the elderly who have lost their direction for living after retirement do not conform to the biomedical model. There is no specific etiology. Thus the treatment tends to become diffuse and ultimately ineffective as seen by the large institutions and nursing homes which continue to care for the physical body but leave the person to struggle for self-fulfillment with limited success. Although occupational therapy can be of real assistance to such persons, the opportunity is denied or restricted because of limited funds and resources and because the outcome is not as well documented as is the outcome of treatment for some specific pathologies.

A fourth problem concerns the treatment itself. The biomedical model can in many cases state in advance that the treatment will be successful in eliminating the disease or injury. An inflamed appendix can be surgically removed. Antibiotics will kill bacteria. A broken bone can be realigned so it will heal. There is little such perfect prediction that an occupational therapist can make. Will the child with spastic cerebral palsy be able to print the letters of the alphabet? Will the adolescent who broke his neck be able to dress himself? Will the woman who suffered brain damage be able to fix a meal? The answer cannot be stated in advance. Many of the tasks which occupational therapists help people to learn or relearn must be accomplished in a series of steps. The steps may be accomplished quickly or slowly, in a continuous forward pattern or with a few backslides. The course itself may be fairly short or very long. Insurance companies and other payers find such unpredictability difficult to reconcile in setting rate structures.

A fifth problem concerns the tendency of the biomedical model to foster a dependency role for the person receiving treatment. Therefore, when the person comes to occupational therapy there is a preset expectation on the part of the individual that the occupational therapist will take charge. Although the occupational therapist may be quite capable of taking charge, such an authoritarian approach is of limited value in accomplishing the objectives and goals most often established in occupational therapy for functional independence. Rather the preferred approach is generally one in which the occupational therapist works with the person as a facilitator rather than as a boss. The person therefore is expected to participate in setting the objectives and goals and in determining the methods which will be used to try to achieve the objectives and goals. This approach of joint participation is true even with children, although the degree to which the children can participate may be different from that of an adult. In other words, occupational therapists as a rule are striving to facilitate independence and not further dependence.

In summary, the biomedical model places some restrictions on occupational therapy practice which can have negative effects in the application of occupational therapy principles. These include an orientation to acute disease conditions rather than sequelae, biological focus but not sociocultural environment focus, specific etiology rather than problems in living, predictable outcomes vs. uncertain attainment, and dependence vs. independence. These and other factors are summarized in Table 7.2.

IMPAIRED MODEL

The impaired or chronically disabled model appears to be based on the organismic and humanistic models, but the frame of references is not clearly identified since the model is new (5, 6). Thus, the focus of control is primarily within the person who can be expected to be responsible for personal behavior. In the impaired model, the view of health is based on a feeling state and a performance criterion which supercedes the acknowledged permanent impairment. If the person acts as if sick and incapacitated, health is poor. On the other hand, if the person acts as if well and functions as if normal, then health is good. Basically then health status is the result of social convention rather than diagnosis tests (7).

The purpose of intervention in the impaired model seems to be to encourage or assist the person to gain functional independence. At the same time, there is a need to check the person to be sure that no new or recurring illness has occurred. Thus the practitioner's role includes the right to confine the impaired role and the duty to prescribe rehabilitation services to promote functional independence. At the same time, the

Table 7.2
Some Differences between the Biomedical
and Occupational Therapy Models

Topic	Biomedical Model	Occupational Therapy Model (Unspecified)
Definition of health	Health is defined as an absence of disease	Health is defined as presence of competent adaptive occupational behavior
Description of health	Health is descriptive as a passive, dependent process	Health is described as an active process called occupational performance
View of mind and body	Dualism of mind and body	Monism or unity of mind and body
Assessment standards	Uses minimum standards as basis of evaluation	Uses optimum standards as basis of evaluation
Intervention approach	Intervention by drugs and surgery	Intervention through learning tasks
Outcome criteria	Cure and control of biological problems	Palliative and decontrolling of biopsychosocial problems
View of problem area	Disorder is disease and lack of homeostasis of biochemical processes	Disorder is occupational dysfunction and lack of integration in adaptive skills
Effective range	Useful in controlling infections with single cause, acute diseases	Useful in dealing with chronic and multifactor disorders
Predictability of outcome	General good	Highly variable

subject has a right to expect protection from abuse, exploitation and persecution and a duty to behave as much as possible like a normal person (1). Society's role consists of the right to protect itself from impaired persons who may be dangerous to others by doing activities for which the skills do not exist or have not been relearned. The duty is to provide rehabilitative services in which the person can learn to function.

The impaired or chronically disabled model seems to hold some possibilities as a frame of reference for occupational therapy. First, the social response patterns which Gordon (5) identified are consistent with objectives and goals commonly used in occupational therapy. Specifically, Gordon lists the following responses in his study. (a) Impaired persons were to be encouraged to do things for themselves in terms of seeking physical comfort. (b) They were to be encouraged to do some sort of useful work in terms of achieving social responsibility. (c) They were to be encouraged to talk about any changes in their condition but not to bother others with every ache and pain in terms of sharing information. These statements seem to reflect a common agreement between the impaired model and occupational therapy practice. Second, the interaction pattern between the healer (practitioner) and subject (client) is consistent with the philosophy of occupational therapy. Namely, the impaired or chronic model is based on the assumption that the patient or client "is an active participant in his medical care" (6). Occupational therapists have stressed that the patient or client should participate actively in the planning and implementing of the individualized occupational therapy program. Third, the impaired or chronic model includes recognition of social adjustment, including problems in role identification and self concept (6). Heard (8) has addressed these problems in her practice model for occupational therapy. Fourth, there is a recognition that treatment or intervention may need to go beyond the hospital to the home in order to consider the client's total living situation. Occupational therapists have been concerned with home management techniques and architectural barriers for many years.

Although several favorable comments have been cited there is one important negative concern. This concern centers on the fact that American society has not developed a social definition of impaired or chronic roles. In order for occupational therapy to work successfully within a model based on the impaired model the profession will need to assist other professions in conveying to society that the impaired role is a legitimate one and that it is different from the sick role assumed under the biomedical model.

BIOPSYCHOSOCIAL MODEL (Table 7.3)

The biopsychosocial model of health is based on the organismic and systems models. It recognizes that individuals control the expression of disease in different ways and that analysis through a systems approach permits the understanding that a change in any subsystem may affect the whole system. Health, therefore, is the result of the interaction of biological, psychological and sociocultural factors (2). Nonhealth or disease is a result of the same factors. The rationale for intervention is to use the knowledge of the interacting system to aid the person toward regaining health. Prognosis depends on the complexity of the factors and the skills of analysis. The goal is to restore or maintain health.

The practitioner's role usually is fulfilled by a physician and involves determining if a person is sick or has a problem in living or both. At the same time the duty is to determine why and in what ways the person is sick or has problems in living (2). Based on the information, a treatment program is planned. The subject's right is to get an accurate diagnosis by providing information. The duties include trusting the healer's judgment and following the treatment program. Society has a right to expect that healers and subjects will work to maintain health. Thus, the duty of society is to provide health and treatment services.

According to Mosey (4), the biopsychosocial model provides a number of advantages as a frame of reference for occupational therapy. One is that the model focuses on the body, mind and environment as sources of information about a client. Biologic aspects include the anatomy and physiology underlying occupational therapy practice. Psychologic aspects concern the growth and development issues within occupational therapy practice, while the sociologic aspects address the interaction of role relations and group process which are incorporated into occupational therapy practice. Another advantage is the focus on the teaching-learning process which addresses the problems of working together to solve problems in learning. The process permits attention to be directed toward adding to as well as deleting from an individual's repertoire of skills. In addition, the biopsychosocial model can be clearly separated from the biomedical model to facilitate the clarification of occupational therapy roles from medical roles. Finally, the model does not depend on a hospital base for explanation but can be applied to many community settings.

A major drawback mentioned by Mosey is the concentration on the teaching aspects. She feels some occupational therapists might object to the strong emphasis on the teaching role rather than the treating role. Another possible drawback is the concern that some occupational therapists may feel the model requires operant conditioning techniques. However, as pointed out in Chapter 6, operant conditioning or behavior modification is incompatible with this model, since it is based on the mechanistic metamodel. Nevertheless, ruling out a model as a frame of reference does not rule out use of some techniques. Reinforcement techniques could be compatible with the biopsychosocial model if the focus of control is retained by the client and not by the therapist. Thus, the client must set the type and schedule of reinforcement alone or with the assistance of a therapist.

PUBLIC HEALTH MODEL

The public health model is based on the mechanistic and reductionistic models as was the biomedical model. The major difference is that the goal of public health officials is to preserve the health of a group of people, whereas the clinician in the biomedical model is concerned with one person (1). Another difference is that the public health officer has the force of law to back up orders, whereas the clinician can give advice but cannot force a person to take advice. Health in the public health model is the result of controlling disease causing agents by elimination, neutralization or spatial segregation (quarantine). Nonhealth occurs when people encounter disease-causing agents. Most often the sources are air, water, food, sewage, insects or contaminants. Intervention is designed to inform people as to how diseases can be prevented and good health promoted. The prognosis depends on how well the orders are followed, but the goals remain to prevent disease and promote health.

The practitioner (public health official) expects that directives will be implemented. Duties include constant inspection of the environment for disease-causing agents or conditions which support the spread of disease-causing agents. However, the individual is rarely considered. Instead society as a group is the subject. Society expects that the official will

Table 7.3
Health Models

	Biopsychosocial	Public Health
View of health	Determined by interaction of biological, psychological and sociocultural factors	Degree to which disease-causing agents are controlled
Cause of nonhealth status	Same as above; health and nonhealth are a continuum	Disease-causing agents in the air, water, food, sewage, etc.
Rationale for intervention by healers	Knowledge can be used to assist people in restoring and maintaining health	Knowledge can be used to prevent the spread of disease and promote normal health
Expected results A. Prognosis B. Goals	Depends on complexity of factors; restore or maintain health	Depends on how well orders are followed; prevent disease, promote health
Practitioner's role A. Rights B. Duties	Determine whether a person is sick or has a problem in living or both; determine why and in what ways person is sick/has problems in living, develop treatment plan	Expect that health directives will be implemented; constantly inspect environment for disease-causing agents
Subject's role A. Rights B. Duties	Get an accurate diagnosis; provide information; trust healer's judgment and follow treatment program	Not part of the model; healer does not deal with individuals *per se*
Society's role A. Rights B. Duties	Maintenance of health; provide health and treatment services	Information and concern about health issues; preserve health, follow orders and advice

provide information about health issues and will act to preserve health. In turn, society's duty is to follow the orders and advice.

Occupational therapists must be careful to differentiate between the public health model and the health education and prevention model. The public health model has the same types of limitations for occupational therapy as the biomedical model. It is concerned primarily with acute contagious diseases, not with chronic, noncontagious conditions. The focus is on biological agents. Social factors are relevant only to the extent that they affect biological transmission. Thus people are quarantined, told to wash their hands after eliminating and instructed on how to dispose of garbage because these actions slow down the transmission of disease. There are, of course, social consequences of preventing disease, but the social good is secondary to the biological containment. There is no concern in the public health model for people with "problems in living." The model is designed to deal only with disease, primarily contagious, and with prevention of the same diseases. Occupational therapists must be careful not to broaden the prevention concept beyond that which is met. Screening clinics for tuberculosis is an example of a prevention program within the public health model, but a screening clinic for developmental delay is not. The latter is an example of a program in the health education model. Finally, the public health model provides no direct intervention services which are ongoing. Its intervention program is limited to giving immunizations and providing information upon request. There are no continuing programs for the individual management of disease conditions. A person would be referred to a physician for management of a diseased condition. Thus, the public health model offers little as a frame of reference for occupational therapy. It has been presented to clarify the difference between it and the health education and prevention model which is discussed later in this chapter.

MORAL MODEL (Table 7.4)

The moral or milieu model is based on the organismic and humanistic models. It is a very old model which has undergone several periods of popularity and decline. Thus, its form has changed over the years. Siegler and Osmond (1) suggest that there are actually five subtypes of the model. One is the rehabilitative moral model which focuses on techniques for helping a person to relearn socially acceptable behavior. The second subtype is the deterrent moral model which uses punishment as a means of stopping misbehavior. For example, a patient could be told that if he misbehaves once more he will be signed up for five electric shock treatments. The third subtype is the retributive moral mode in which the punishment is designed to fit the crime. For example, a patient may be told that every time he bites someone else, he will be confined to a quiet room for 6 hours. Subtypes two and three are different because the retributive model is based on a demonstration of guilt, whereas the deterrent model requires no such demonstration but only the performance of behavior displeasing to someone else. The fourth subtype is the preventative moral model which assumes that behavior learned as a youngster will be carried out as an adult. Thus masturbation done as a child was considered to cause insanity in an adult. Finally, the fifth moral model is the restitutive moral model in which the person repays society for some wrongdoing. An example might be volunteering for charity work to repay society for "putting up with" the bad behavior exhibited during a mental health crisis. Although the focus of this section will be on the rehabilitative moral model, the other four subtypes are important to remember because they can replace the rehabilitative moral model if practitioners are not careful. The deterrent and retributive subtypes have occurred in numerous state institutions to persons who are retarded or have mental health problems or are in correctional facilities.

Table 7.4
Health Models

	Moral	Wholistic Health
View of health	Behavior that is socially acceptable, functional and moral or good	A process of adapting to change which leads to adjustment and wholeness
Cause of nonhealth status	"Bad" behavior which is socially unacceptable, unfunctional and immoral was learned	Stress in such forms as physical illness, psychological maladjustment decision-making difficulties, isolation or purposelessness
Rationale for intervention by healers	"Bad" behavior can be unlearned and "good" can be learned	A person may achieve wholeness through use of individual resources and the resolve of others
Expected results A. Prognosis B. Goals	Good if subject and healer work together cooperatively; alter or change bad behavior to that which is socially acceptable	Good if individual resources and the resolve of others is sufficient to reduce or eliminate the stress; achieve a wholeness or internal unity (self-respect)
Practitioner's role A. Rights B. Duties	To be credited as knowledgeable about behavioral change; must be able to bring about changed behavior	Recognition as knowledgeable about stressors and their effect on health; relieve symptoms by locating stressors and select energies to reverse disease
Subject's role A. Rights B. Duties	Expects healer to restore person to society; must cooperate with efforts to change behavior	Healer will locate stressors and identify the energies to reverse the disease with subject's cooperation; cooperate and participate in the process toward regaining wholeness
Society's role A. Rights B. Duties	To defend itself from those who endanger others; provide facilities for behavioral change	Become informed about harmful stressors and resources of reducing, then provide assistance in identifying stressors and reducing their contribution to disease

Health as viewed by the moral model is demonstrated by behavior that is socially acceptable, functional, moral and good. Thus the emphasis is clearly on the social and cultural environments. Persons with mental health problems may be seen as candidates for the moral model's techniques, but many with physical conditions can be viewed as good candidates also since a person may be valued by acts alone (9). Nonhealth thus is "bad" behavior which is socially unacceptable, unfunctional and unmoral. Although both good and bad behavior is assumed to be learned as a child, the focus of intervention is based on the assumption that bad behavior can be unlearned and good behavior can be learned or relearned. Thus, the prognosis is good if the subject and healer work together cooperatively to attain the goal of altering or changing bad behavior to that which is socially acceptable.

The practitioners role (physician or psychologist) is to be credited as knowledge about behavior change and the duty is to be able to bring about changes in behavior. It is important to remember that the changes in behavior, however, are to be those which the individual agrees to change and not those which the healer decides to change. Otherwise, the meta model changes from organismic to mechanistic. The role of the healer is to guide change and not forcefully direct change. A subject expects that the healer will assist in returning the individual to society with a better repertoire of behaviors which society will accept. To be successful, the subject must cooperate with efforts to change behaviors. Society expects to be protected from persons who may be dangerous. Thus, its duty is to provide facilities for behavior change.

Programs of occupational therapy have been based on the moral or milieu model for many years. The problems however remain the same. One problem is that the goals must be clearly identified in terms of returning the person to society. Too often behavior change is directed to making the person function as a good patient or resident in the institution. Good behavior as an institutionalized person may not be good behavior as a community citizen. For example, in the institution the routine is often established, whereas in the community the person will have to establish an individual routine or function within a family routine. Both may be quite different from the institution. Another problem is the determination of exactly what behaviors will be most effective for an individual based on the social situation in which the person lives. It is easier to work for changes which are similar to those of the therapist because the changes are easier to recognize. For example, cooking American food is much different from cooking Oriental food. A therapist used to cooking American food may have difficulty assisting a person who wants to cook Oriental food but needs assistance in meal planning and preparation. Yet another problem is the change of behaviors which are socially acceptable in one aspect of society but not in another. For example, the use of and response to time can be an issue. Some subcultures in society tend not to follow the clock in terms of hours and minutes. They are more concerned with morning or evening. When such a person gets a job that requires getting to work at a particular time the conflict becomes apparent. Time watching is not acceptable in the subculture but is mandatory in the work culture. Thus changing behavior for one situation creates a conflict in another. Finally, some behavioral change projects remain too large to be effectively handled by the moral model. For example, autism in children, severe childhood schizophrenia and profoundly retarded persons seem to require such a large number of behavior changes that the intervention program becomes overwhelming in terms of energy, time and money. Either the change techniques must become more efficient or other models need to be tried instead of or in addition to the moral model.

WHOLISTIC MODEL

The wholistic or holistic model is based on the organismic and holistic models. It is based on the assumptions that the individual is an integrated whole with resources to promote personal health (10). Health is viewed as a process of adapting to change which leads to adjustment and wholeness. The cause of nonhealth is stress which may appear as physical illness, psychological maladjustment, difficulties in decision making, isolation or purposelessness (10). Intervention is designed to help the person reachieve wholeness through the use of individual resources and the resolve of others. The prognosis is good if individual resources and the resolve of others is sufficient to reduce or eliminate the stress in order to achieve the goal of wholeness and internal unity (self-respect).

The practitioner expects to be recognized as knowledgeable about stress and its effect on health. Duties include relieving symptoms by locating the sources of stress and identifying energies which can be used to reverse the disease and help the person who is stuck (sick) to get well. The subject expects the healer to locate the stressors and identify the resources for removing the disease. At the same time, the subject's duties are to cooperate and participate in the process of regaining wholeness. Society expects that the healers will inform citizens of harmful stressors and suggest the resources needed to reduce or avoid such stressors. The duty of society is to provide assistance in identifying stressors and to assist in reducing their contribution to disease.

Occupational therapists have not used this model to any great extent in literature to date. However, the model appears to have some real potential. One aspect of this potential is based on a commonly used statement that occupational therapy treats the whole person. Perhaps the grammar needs a little revision to clarify the assumption. If the statement were reworded so that occupational therapists treat the person *as a whole* the assumption fits into the wholistic model easily. The statement means that occupational therapists view the person as a totally integrated organism in which any disruption in one aspect of the organism causes disruption in other aspects. The most common sources of disruptions are problems in living according to occupational therapists.

In the wholistic model problems in living are caused by stresses. Practitioners attempt to work with the dis-eased person to relieve the stresses through a variety of techniques. Such flexible thinking appears compatible with the approaches in occupational therapy. Another aspect which should be appealing to occupational therapists is the view that the environment can be used as a resource which extends the potential resources of the person. Where other organismic models tend to view the environment as a challenge to overcome or fit into, the wholistic view sees the environment as something of a helper or friend which can facilitate the achievement of wholeness. Such a view may be useful in helping people accept adapted aids and equipment and in the removal of architectural barriers. When the environment is seen as a health resource rather than as a barrier, many possibilities exist to facilitate the transformation of a chronically disabled person into an abled person.

HEALTH DEVELOPMENT MODEL (Table 7.5)

The health development or developmental task model is based on the organismic and developmental models. Change is the result of internal forces which lead the individual toward a progression of steps to higher levels of development and growth. Health is viewed as the capacity to maintain normal or average developmental progression according to some prestated criteria such as a test, chart, or assumed pattern (11). Nonhealth depends on the degree of deviation from the expected level of development. Intervention is based on the professional ability in determining development process and skill in lessening the degree of deviation by specially designed programs. Intervention also is involved because when developmental stages or tasks occur on schedule, the individual experiences achievement, happiness and success in later tasks. When stages or tasks do not occur on schedule, the individual is unhappy, meets disapproval by society and has difficulty with later tasks (12). Prognosis is considered to be good if the deviation is slight but becomes progressively poorer as the degree of deviation increases. Thus, the goal is to decrease the amount of deviation from the norm.

The practitioner (physician, nurse, therapist) expects to be recognized as knowledgeable about normal developmental progression. Duties include determining if developmental deviation has occurred and if so to establish a program to correct the deviation. A subject expects to receive a developmental assessment, interpretation and a program if needed. In turn, the subject should be cooperative during the assessment and participate in the program if advised that one is needed. Society expects that deviations will be assessed and that those with extreme deviations will be segregated into special programs. Therefore, the duties are to provide services and programs for those with deviations, especially severe deviations. The definition of extreme or severe deviation varies according to the characteristics being measured and the social response to those characteristics.

Table 7.5
Health Models

	Health Development	Health Education and Prevention
View of health	The capacity to maintain a normal developmental progression	Influenced by heredity, physical environment, social conditions, health services, personal behavior
Cause of nonhealth status	Degree of deviation from expected development	Same as above
Rationale for intervention by healers	Deviations from normal developmental progress can be determined and lessened by special programs	Many disabilities can be prevented; many premature deaths can be delayed
Expected results A. Prognosis B. Goals	Good if deviation is slight, not good if deviation is great; decrease the amount of deviation from the norm	Good if individuals and communities act together; reduce preventable disability and reduce or delay premature death
Practitioner's role A. Rights B. Duties	Seen as knowledgable about normal developmental progression; determine if developmental deviation has occurred; establish a program of correction	To give medical advice, participate in planning health services; prescribe, diagnose, treat and rehabilitate
Subject's role A. Rights B. Duties	To receive a developmental assessment interpretation and program if needed; cooperate in the assessment	To receive quality health care; learn about health, use services appropriately, follow medical advice when given, participate in health service planning
Society's role A. Rights B. Duties	To have deviations assessed and to have persons with great deviations segregated for special programs; provide services and programs for deviant persons	Expect cooperation in determining the health needs of individuals and the community; coordinate health education and resources into effective action, plan to promote and improve the health of individuals and the community

Development as a measure of health has been a popular model for occupational therapists. Knowledge of development can be easily translated into a variety of assessment instruments. The instruments can provide objective quantifiable data. One of the problems with developmental measures of health is to find the developmental items which are most relevant to health. In other words, which aspects of behavior best reflect health? Is walking a sign of good health or simply an effective means of locomotion on two legs? What is the state of health for someone who never walked or is now unable to walk? A second problem is to differentiate between biological health as opposed to psychosocial health. The example of walking is useful again. Walking is not essential to biological health, but society tends to place a higher value on a person who walks independently. In turn the social value probably affects self concept so that a person views the self as more valuable if walking is possible. A third problem is to determine if a deviation is serious and will cause problems later. Is it true that children who do not creep on all fours will experience laterality and dominance problems later? Many predictions of consequences to later developmental health have been made without a sound rationale backed up by good research evidence. A fourth problem with the developmental health approach may be that it fails to identify alternate routes which may result in an acceptable outcome, even if the means do not follow the averages. The creeping example is useful again. Could scooting on one's bottom be an effective substitute for creeping? Perhaps neither is necessary. Again research evidence is not available. Fifth, assessment of health through development is like taking a snap shot. One only sees what happens to show up at a given time. Health is a dynamic process in a living organism. The snap shot assessment might not get the whole picture or may be true today but false tomorrow. Health needs to be assessed and programs provided which meet the dynamic quality of a changing process.

HEALTH EDUCATION AND PREVENTION MODEL

The health education and prevention model is based on the organismic and loosely on the humanistic model along with the general principles of education. Health education is defined as "a process with intellectual, psychological and social dimensions relating to activities that increase the abilities of people to make informed decisions affecting their personal, family, and community well-being" (13). The process is designed to facilitate learning and behavioral change in both health professionals and consumers. Health is viewed as influenced by the positive aspects of heredity, physical and social environments, health care services and personal behavior (14). Nonhealth is influenced by the negative aspects of the same four factors. The primary reasons for intervention through education are based on the knowledge that many disabilities can be prevented and that premature deaths can be prevented or delayed if people are informed and act on the information. Prognosis is considered good if individuals and communities act together toward the goals of reducing the incidence of preventable disability and reducing or delaying the incidence of premature death.

The role of the practitioner or physician remains similar to that under the traditional biomedical model. Rights include giving medical advice and participating in planning health care services. The duties are to prescribe, diagnose, treat and rehabilitate. The role of the subject or consumer, however, is much broader. The consumer expects to receive quality health care services. At the same time, the consumer should learn about many aspects of health, should learn to use health resources appropriately, should follow medical advice when given and should participate in health service planning. These duties are more comprehensive than in most other models. Society expects cooperation from both health care personnel and consumers in determining the health needs of individuals and the community. In turn, society's duties are to coordinate health education and resources into effective action plans to promote and improve the health of individuals and the community.

The health education and prevention model was traditionally practiced by public health nurses and by some public health officers. It became popular during the 1960s and 1970s as a base for national policy. Occupational therapy officially became aware of the model during that time. Through the use of the health education and prevention model occupational therapy can move from the clinic-based models to the community and into schools, health associations, businesses and homes of generally well people. The purpose is to provide information and education about the use of occupational activities and tasks to enrich lives, improve health and prevent some health problems from occurring. However, such a model requires much more than knowledge of assessment instruments and intervention strategies. The practitioner must understand how occupation works to maintain health as well as how occupation works in the restoration of health.

HIGH LEVEL WELLNESS MODEL (Table 7.6)

The high level wellness model is based on the organismic and the wholistic model. It is an extention of the wholistic health model. However, the high level wellness model does not use traditional medical treatment or personnel. Instead it uses a wide range of modalities to emphasize self responsibility for health and values the process of caregiving as well as the product (15). Health is achieved through high level wellness and is defined as an "integrated method of functioning which is oriented toward maximizing the potential of which the individual is capable" (16). Non-health is the result of inadequate integration which leads to misuse and misdirected energy which in turn reduces potential and capacity. The rationale for intervention is to assess health problem areas and provide programs which will promote health, wellness and wholeness. Prognosis depends on how soon the person becomes an expert on maximizing the

Table 7.6
Health Models

	High Level Wellness	Occupational Performance Adaptation through Occupation
View of health	Integrated method of functioning which is oriented toward maximizing the potential of which the individual is capable	Health is the ability to perform and integrate occupational areas into adaptive skills
Cause of nonhealth status	Inadequate integration which leads to misuse and misdirected energy which results in psychosomatic illness	Stress, trauma, chronicity, multifactors which result in occupational dysfunction and lack of integration of adaptive skills
Rationale for intervention by healers	Can provide assessment of health problem areas and provide programs which will promote health and wellness	Occupational performance can be learned, modified or relearned
Expected results A. Prognosis B. Goals	Depends on how well a person becomes an expert on maximizing self potential; help individual concentrate on moving to higher and higher levels of total fitness	Depends on active cooperation between practitioner and subject; optimize and integrate occupational performance with adaptive behavior of individual
Practitioner's role A. Rights B. Duties	Knowledge about self responsibility, nutrition, stress management, physical fitness and environment; to help a person take charge of life and to feel good about the self	Acknowledge to know about relationship of occupational performance to health; to assess occupational performance and plan/implement program to optimize occupational performance and integration
Subject's role A. Rights B. Duties	Be assessed and given programs to fit individual needs; to see the self as a growing changing person who can take charge	To be assessed and have program planned and implemented; to cooperate in providing information and to actively participate in development and implementation of program

Table 7.6—Continued

	High Level Wellness	Occupational Performance Adaptation through Occupation
Society's role A. Rights B. Duties	Have individuals contribute selves to progress, expansion and integration toward wellness; promote wellness of individuals families and communities	To be informed about the role of occupational performance in health; provide opportunities for service

potential of the self. The goal is to help the individual to move toward higher levels of total fitness (15).

The practitioner's role may be carried out by any number of professionals including physicians, psychologists, physical fitness experts, nutritionists and others. They are expected to be knowledgeable about self responsibility, nutrition, stress management, physical fitness and aspects of physical social and personal environments. Duties include helping a person take charge of life and to feel good about the self. Subjects expect to be assessed and given programs to fit individual needs. Their duty is to see the self as a growing changing person who can take charge of individual health. Society has a right to have individuals contribute knowledge and skill to the community so that progress, expansion and integration toward wellness can be made. Its duty is to promote the wellness of individuals, families and communities.

More than any of the other models, the high level wellness model seeks to focus on obtaining and maintaining health. In other words the object is to adopt a life-style that concentrates on increasing health. This concept is different from primary prevention which tries to halt the progression of disease because the prevention model is looking backwards at disease while the wellness model is looking forward to health. The aim of a practitioner using the wellness model must be to constantly seek resources which will improve health to a greater degree than presently exists. The aim for the client should be to become more aware of individual responsibility for personal progress. Occupational therapists have access to information in all of the areas currently being used to promote wellness. Occupational therapists have skills to help people plan their activities to balance work and play, to reduce stress and to take responsibility for individual action. Occupational therapists understand the basic concepts of physical and emotional fitness through the analyses of interests and activity selection. Occupational therapists know the importance of examining the interacting effects of physical, social and personal environments. Finally, occupational therapists can learn about nutritional qualities of foods as well as meal planning and preparation. Thus the tools are available to any occupational therapist who wishes to adjust the focus on obtaining greater health for clients rather than preventing disease.

OCCUPATIONAL PERFORMANCE MODEL

Occupational performance is based on the organismic, humanistic, wholistic, and systems models. It is based on the beliefs that humans can be responsible for health which involves all aspects of their biopsychosocial being and the interaction with the environment. Furthermore, there is a belief in the role of occupations as an aspect of health and in occupational performance as a means to support and gain health. Thus, health is based on a person's ability to perform and integrate the occupational areas of self maintenance, productivity and leisure into adaptive skills for interacting with the environment. Nonhealth is caused by such conditions as stress, trauma, chronicity and multiple factors which result in occupational dysfunction and lack of integration of adaptive skills. Intervention is therefore based on the rationale that occupational performance can be learned, modified or relearned.

Prognosis depends on the active cooperation between the practitioner and the subject. The goal is to optimize and integrate occupational performance within the person's repertoire of adaptive behavior. The practitioner who is an occupational therapist is acknowledged to know about the relationship of occupational performance to health and the role of occupational performance within the repertoire of adaptive skills. Duties include the assessment of occupational performance and the planning and implementation of programs to optimize occupational performance and integration. The subject or client expects to be assessed and to have a program planned and implemented if needed. In turn, the client's duties are to cooperate in providing information and to actively participate in the development and implementation of a program. Society expects to be informed about the role of occupational performance in health and adaptive behavior. Its duties include providing facilities for service. This model is described further in the last chapter.

REHABILITATION MODELS

The next two models represent the rehabilitation efforts which grew out of the federal legislation to provide education and retraining for employment. These models also had an impact on occupational therapy because early occupational therapy was concerned with employment and earning a living and because the objectives of vocational rehabilitation and occupational therapy have been related to returning the person to society as a functioning member.

The two typical rehabilitation models are summarized in Table 7.7 and are defined and described in the text which follows. Table 7.8 provides an additional comparison of the biomedical with the general concepts of social rehabilitation.

Table 7.7
Summary of Biorehabilitation and
Social Rehabilitation Models

	Biorehabilitation	Social Rehabilitation
View of health	Absence of effects of impairment and employment as a productive worker	Ability to perform social roles and daily activities
Cause of nonhealth status	Anatomical or physiological impairments and deviations due to pathological processes	Functional limitations in the ability to carry out daily activities and roles
Rationale for intervention by healers	Can correct or reduce effects of impairments, such as blindness, amputation or paralysis through surgery or special appliances	The effects of functional limitations and disability can be overcome through learning
Expected results A. Prognosis B. Goals	Depends on degree of impairment and treatment procedures available; returns the person to productive status and employment	Depends on person's willingness and motivation to learn; restore optimal functional reintegration into society
Practitioner's role A. Rights B. Duties	To determine best method of correcting or reducing impairment to diagnosis; assess degree of impairment and prescribe; plan treatment	Recognized as knowledgeable about learning, counseling, assess rehabilitation needs with subject, develop a training program
Subject's role A. Rights B. Duties	To be diagnosed assessed and treated; trained to follow treatment training program; and seek employment	To be assessed and provided with a program. Cooperate in assessment and participate in the training program to decrease dependency and deviancy to have person function at optimal level in spite of disability
Society's role A. Rights B. Duties	To decrease deviancy and to have impaired person returned to productive status; To provide medical and vocational training resources	Provide services to learn how to overcome functional limitations and achieve optimal functioning

Table 7.8
Comparison of Medical and Rehabilitation Models

	Medical Model	Rehabilitation Model
Person's role	Passive and dependent	Active and moving toward mastery and independence
Expectation	Rules are clear	Rules are ambivalent
View of person	Person is an object; valued in terms of life or death	Person is a human being with dignity and personal value
Duty	Has no responsibility for decision making	Expected to take up responsibility
Title	Patient status	Client status
Relation to others	Caretakers are strangers	Personnel become known and may become friends

BIOREHABILITATION MODEL

The biorehabilitation model is an extension of the biomedical model. It grew out of the early attempts in 1918 and 1920 to provide vocational rehabilitation which was and is designed to return people to useful employment and increase the manpower supply (17). Initially medical services were not covered, but with the 1943 vocational rehabilitation amendments, payment for medical and psychiatric services was included for the first time (17). Health is viewed as the absence of active pathology and impairment (18) and the ability to be employed as a productive worker. Thus, the causes of nonhealth are anatomical or physiological impairments or deviations due to pathological processes. Intervention is aimed at correcting or reducing the effects of the impairments, especially in those persons from whom the impairment is stable such as blindness, amputation or paralysis. Prognosis depends on the degree of impairment and treatment procedures available to correct or reduce the effects of impairment. The goal is to return the person to productive status and employment.

The practitioner who is a vocational counselor or physician expects to determine the best method of correcting or reducing the impairment. Duties include diagnosing the degree of impairment and prescribing a course of treatment which may include surgery, prosthetic devices and vocational retraining. The subject or trainee expects to be diagnosed/ assessed and to be treated or trained. Duties are to follow the treatment or training program and to seek gainful employment. Society expects to have the degree of deviancy reduced and to have the impaired person returned to productive status. In turn, it provides medical and vocational training resources to accomplish the objectives.

The term biorehabilitation was selected because it seemed to describe the close relation of this model to the biomedical model. Thus, many of the same problems exist in using the biorehabilitation model as a frame of reference for occupational therapy. Biorehabilitation is expected to be primarily a one time process in which the impairment is corrected or reduced to manageable proportions and the individual seeks and finds employment. Continuing services are not expected to be needed. Case files can be closed as having been successfully completed, *i.e.*, the person is successfully employed and no longer needs or expects assistance. This one time approach works for static conditions which might occur from polio, war injuries, amputation or industrial accidental blindness. Conditions such as mental illness, retardation and some cases of tuberculosis are less successful.

Another problem is the degree of role and social disruption which may occur. The model is not set up to accommodate the teaching of any occupational role except productive worker. Self maintenance and leisure roles are not included, and other role areas such as family and personal sexual are not considered. Thus, the best candidate for biorehabilitation has a static recognizable impairment, has a good work history and is able to adjust to changes in family and personal sexual roles without assistance from the biorehabilitation-oriented facility.

SOCIAL REHABILITATION MODEL

The social rehabilitation model based on a biopsychosocial model is much newer than the biorehabilitation model. In the hearings prior to the 1954 vocational amendments there was recognition that the dependent state of many people with residual disability was draining national resources (19). As a result more money was spent to support research, train personnel and construct facilities. Prior to the 1963 amendments, an even stronger statement was made which set the social rehabilitation model in place. Whitten, Director of the National Rehabilitation Association, emphasized that rehabilitation services should be available irrespective of the employment status and that "social rehabilitation would aim to restore a person to maximum usefulness to himself, his family and his community" (20). Thus, the 1963 vocational rehabilitation amendments were the first to include rehabilitation for other than employment potential.

Under the social rehabilitation model health is defined as the ability to perform social roles and daily activities (21). Nonhealth is defined in terms of functional limitations which compromise a person's ability to carry out daily activities and roles. The functional limitations are at least in part the result of the anatomical and physiological impairments. Rationale for intervention is that the learning counseling process can be used to overcome the effects of functional limitations. It follows then that the prognosis depends on the willingness or motivation to learn. The goal is to restore the person to an optimal functional reintegration into society.

The practitioner who is usually a vocational counselor is recognized as knowledgeable about the learning counseling process. Primary duties include assessing the rehabilitation needs with the subject and developing a training program. The subject or client expects to be assessed and provided with a training program. In turn the client is expected to cooperate in the assessment and participate in the training program. Society expects that social rehabilitation will decrease the level of dependency and degree of deviancy and will enable the person to function at an optimum level in spite of the disability. Its duties are to provide services which stress how to overcome functional limitations and achieve optimal functioning.

Although the social rehabilitation model appears to be similar to the concepts and goals of occupational therapists, methods and techniques do not seem to coordinate well with those of occupational therapy. One problem is the reliance on counseling and talking rather than on structured practice and doing to achieve functional skills. Where skills previously existed and need only to be reorganized counseling may be acceptable. However, where skills do not exist or must be relearned talking does not seem enough. Even when practice is permitted in work adjustment programs the prerequisite skills may be insufficient to meet the level demanded for acceptable performance. People who have lived in structured environments do not plan ahead to see the consequences of their actions. They never had to do so. Planning was someone else's job. Their job was to follow orders without regard for the consequences. Perhaps the most serious problem has been learning to define successful outcome in terms other than gainful employment. The result has been that vocational rehabilitation has been unable to implement the social rehabilitation model and falls back on the security of the biorehabilitation model and employability by default.

In summary, the ten health and two rehabilitation models represent a diversity of thinking that has been drawn from the two meta models and seven super models. The impact on occupational therapy has been as varied as the thinking. However, the models that seem to offer the best frame of reference for occupational therapy all come from the organismic meta model. Those from the mechanistic meta model such as the biomedical and public health models do not provide a workable frame of reference for occupational therapy because the philosophy is counter to the beliefs and values on which occupational therapy was founded. Most fundamental is the belief in internal locus of control or self responsibility which the mechanistic based models do not recognize. All of the organismic based models must make use of internal locus of control, although the degree varies from the physical developmental models in which self-control may be limited by heredity to the high level wellness model in which self-control is almost unlimited. This issue of locus of control has its greatest impact in health models in terms of the healer-subject roles. In the mechanistic based models, the healer maintains the balance of control and responsibility for health, whereas in the organismic models the client maintains the majority of the control and responsibility. Such contrasts influence the focus of intervention directly. Technically under the mechanistic models the healer issues orders and the subject follows them without question because the healer is knowledgeable and the subject is not, whereas in the organismic based models the healer is considered knowledgable but the use of the knowledge is as a consultant who offers advice which the subject actively chooses to follow, reject, or offer alternatives for review. In other words, more sharing of information is expected rather than a question and answer session.

In the same vein, the outcome is likewise affected. Under the mechanistic models the subject is not expected to learn from experience so that self-treatment or intervention might be implemented if the same health problem arises again. However, under the organismic models self learning and responsibility may be a primary goal as in the high level wellness model. Thus the differences in models are an important consideration to occupational therapists who develop models of practice for occupational therapy. By carefully reviewing the existing models the occupational therapists can select the aspects which best fit the fundamental assumptions of occupational therapy.

References

1. Siegler M, Osmond H: *Models of Madness, Models of Medicine.* New York, Macmillian, 1974, pp 16–18, 32, 131.
2. Engle GL: The need for a new medical model: a challenge for biomedicine. *Science* 196:130, 1977.
3. Reilly M: The educational process. *Am J Occup Ther* 3:299–307, 1969.
4. Mosey A: An alternative: the biopsychosocial model. *Am J Occup Ther* 28:137–140, 1974.
5. Gordon G: *Role of Theory and Illness: A Sociological Perspective.* New Haven, Conn, College and University Press, 1966, p 78.
6. Cogswell BE, Weir DD: A role in process: the development of medical professional's role in long term care of chronically diseased patients. *J Health Hum Behav* 5:95–103, 1964.
7. Wu R: *Behavior and Illness.* Englewood Cliffs, NJ, Prentice-Hall, 1973, p 184.
8. Heard C: Occupational role acquisition: a perspective on the chronically disabled. *Am J Occup Ther* 31:243–247, 1977.
9. Cunning J, Cumming E: *Ego and Milieu: Theory and Practice of Environmental Therapy.* New York, Atherton Press, 1962, pp 268–269.
10. Tubesing NO: *Whole Person Health Care: Philosophical Assumptions.* Hinsdale, Ill, Wholistic Health Centers, 1977.
11. Flapan D, Neubauer PB: Issued on assessing development. *J Am Acad Child Psychiatry* 9:669–687, 1970.
12. Havighurst RJ: *Developmental Tasks and Education,* 3rd ed. New York, McKay, 1972, p 2.
13. Ross HS, Mico PR: *Theory and Practice in Health Education.* Palo Alto, Calif, Mayfield, 1980, p 312.
14. Blum HL: *Expanding Health Care Horizons: From a General Systems Concept of Health to a National Health Policy.* Oakland, Calif, Third Party Associates, 1976, p 63.
15. Ardel DB: *High Level Wellness: An Alternative to Doctors, Drugs and Diseases.* New York, Bantam, 1977.
16. Dunn HL: *High-Level Wellness.* Arlington, Va, Beatty, 1961, p 4.
17. Straus R: Social change and the rehabilitation concept. In Sussman MB: *Sociology and*

Rehabilitation. Washington DC, American Sociological Assn., 1966, p 15.
18. Nagi SZ: Some conceptual issues in disability and rehabilitation. In Sussman MB: *Sociology and Rehabilitation.* Washington DC, American Sociological Assoc., 1966, pp 101–102.
19. Straus R: Social change and the rehabilitation concept. In Sussman MB: *Sociology and Rehabilitation.* Washington DC, American Sociological Assoc., 1966, p 19.
20. US House of Representatives, 87th Congress, 1st Session. *Special Education and Rehabilitation.* Hearings before the Sub Committee on Education of the Committee on Education and Labor August, 1961, p 128.
21. Nagi SZ: Some conceptual issues in disability and rehabilitation. In Sussman MB: *Sociology and Rehabilitation.* American Sociological Assoc., 1966, p 104.

CHAPTER 8

Occupational Therapy Models: Organization and Taxonomy

In reviewing the models of occupational therapy there appeared to be some clustering of models into related areas. Three principal areas seemed to evolve. There are (a) models on the acquisition and purpose of occupation, (b) models which describe some aspect of an occupation such as productivity or motor functions, and (c) models which outline the parameters of occupational therapy. Of the three models the second type, or descriptive models, is the most numerous. Therefore, the descriptive models have been further subdivided into three additional categories. The first is the subtypes of occupations category which includes self maintenance, productivity and leisure. The second category is the basic or common elements which include time and space, doing and action, and pattern and sequence. Finally, the third category is performance areas which is further divided into motor, sensory, cognitive, intrapersonal and interpersonal. The outline of model organization is presented in Table 8.1.

GENERIC MODELS

One type of generic models tended to focus on the process of acquiring occupation as a part of the human repertoire of behavior. Emphasis is

Table 8.1
Outline of Models in Occupational Therapy

1.00 Generic models
    1.10 Acquisition of occupations
    1.20 Purpose of occupations
2.00 Descriptive models
    2.10 Occupational areas
        2.11 Self maintenance
        2.12 Productivity
        2.13 Leisure
    2.20 Basic elements
        2.21 Time and space
        2.22 Action and doing
        2.23 Pattern and sequence
    2.30 Performance areas
        2.31 Motor
        2.32 Sensory
        2.33 Cognitive
        2.34 Intrapersonal
        2.35 Interpersonal
3.00 Parameter models

placed on learning processes, learning techniques and the role of the environment. The other type of generic model focused on the purpose or role of occupation in human behavior. Adaptation or adjustment is the principal theme. A more thorough discussion of the issues involved in acquisition and the role of occupation in human behavior is discussed in Chapter 16.

DESCRIPTIVE MODELS
Subdivisions of Occupations

There are three major subdivisions of occupation which can be identified. These are self maintenance, productivity and leisure.

SELF MAINTENANCE

Self maintenance includes those activities which are done routinely to maintain the person's health and well-being in the environment. Examples include self-care of the body, communication, locomotion, home management and economic resources. The major consideration for including an activity or task in this category is that the task is fundamental to individual physical and social survival. If the individual is unable to do the activity unaided, some modification will be needed or someone else will have to do the task for the individual. The activity cannot be left undone indefinitely or severe physical and social consequences will result. Of course some trade offs are common. In a household one person may provide the home management skills while another provides the economic resources. Other trade offs are possible. One person may wash another's hair in exchange for having a button sewn or a hemline fixed. On the other hand, children must rely on others to perform self maintenance tasks and may have few skills to trade off.

Some common features of self maintenance can be examined by this subdivision of occupation. These include locus of control, social norms, site of performance and common roles for self maintenance. The locus of control usually is the individual. Thus the importance of performing the activities independently unless trade offs are established. Social norms affect self maintenance primarily at the end point. That is, there are many acceptable ways to get self maintenance activities done, but the criteria for acceptable completion is more limited. For example, there are many ways to get dressed and groomed in the morning. One person may groom the hair first and put on the shoes last, while another may reverse the process. The order is not standardized in a social norm except perhaps within a given family. However, the end results will be socially evaluated and judged. Purple hair is sure to be noticed as is one green and one red shoe worn together.

Some self maintenance activities generally are performed out of sight of the public, such as dressing and hygiene. Putting on undergarments in public is not socially acceptable. Other self maintenance activities, such as eating, may be done either in public or private. Still others obviously are public, such as riding public transportation. On balance, however, most activities in self maintenance seem to have a more private component rather than public. Examples of specific roles include self caretaker, houseperson, breadwinner in everyday life. Some specialized roles which may be more temporary are baby-sitter or wet nurse. All of these roles have in common the emphasis of providing a means of accomplishing self maintenance activities.

PRODUCTIVITY

Productivity includes those activities which are done to enable a person to provide support to the self, family and society through the production of goods and services which will promote health and well-being. Examples include paid employment, volunteerism, hobbyism, amateurism and others for which payment is received in the form of money, goods or services. The critical dimensions are the economic value for society and a contribution of effort which is rewarded to the individual. Rewards include money, barter and recognition, such as praise or publicity.

Generally everyone is expected to contribute skills to the total effort of the society. In the past some people were not contributors because the assumption was made that they had nothing to offer. Such persons included the physically handicapped, blind, deaf and mentally retarded. Except in very severe cases of multiple handicapping conditions, such exclusion is unfounded. Other persons choose not to participate. These include persons who have few skills, have adequate economic resources or have retired. Children contribute by learning productive skills, taking part-time jobs or helping around the house or office.

In the area of productivity, locus of control usually is with others, especially if one is employed by others. Even a person who is self-employed finds that controls on business can be largely external. The individual is not able to change controls which are governed by rules and regulations as well as special customs. It follows then that productivity has many social norms. The age of first full-time job, dress codes, living area, and transportation used may all relate to social customs surrounding the job. The job also is closely related to self-identity. There is a tendency for people to give their names and occupation all in one sentence.

Today the most common site of performance is in a public setting. Most people, except homemakers and domestics, work outside of the home. Thus, productivity is a public performance in which the activity can be observed from beginning to end. A person can be evaluated for how the job is done as well as how well the steps within the job are done. Common roles as identified by the *Dictionary of Occupational Titles* are professional, technical, managerial, clerical, sales, service, agricultural, fishery, forestry, processing, machine trade, benchwork, structural work, transportation, packaging and handling, mineral extraction, utilities production, amusement and graphic arts.

LEISURE

Leisure activities are those which are done for enjoyment and renewal that the activity or task brings to the person, and which contributes to the promotion of health and well-being. Examples include hobbies, games, sports, or collections.

The major consideration for inclusion in this category is that the activity is not required and is chosen by the individual who determines what the outcome will be. Thus leisure activities may be done alone, with family or friends or in the community. Also some leisure activities are more easily adapted to solo or large group settings; the individual can decide whether to participate or not. Leisure activities are connected closely to the concept of intrinsic motivation because the reward system is not always evident. People may have a need to explore and master the environment that provides its own reward in satisfaction or achievement without any external control or reward. In other words, the person strings up a carrot and then goes after it because the chase is fun, not because the carrot is edible.

There is a flip side arrangement of productive and leisure activities. What is one person's work is another's play. Also, some people can play as they work while others seem to work at their play. A third group may not know how to play. Doing something just because its fun may be foreign to them. The idea that everything must be done for a purpose has overtaken the system to the point that "just for fun" does not occur as a possibility. Others have forgotten. They include retirees who did not develop or maintain leisure skills during their high productivity years. In retirement there is time and nothing to do because no one is directing the activity except the self which has forgotten how.

In terms of locus of control, leisure activities offer the widest choice. A person may direct all the individual activities or permit others to do the directing or just be passive and watch. The effect of social norms is less but may depend on the activity. Sports and games have rules which must be observed as well as minimal levels of acceptable performance to make the team. Even a city league softball team needs members who can hit the ball sometimes.

The site of performance is more variable. A person can pursue leisure activities in the home, yard, neighborhood, community or around the world; however, the site is related to the type of activity. Softball cannot be played inside most people's homes. Stamp collecting, on the other hand, is not a good outside hobby, especially when the wind blows. Thus, location must be considered in selecting a leisure activity.

Subdivision of Basic Elements

Occupations require time and space, involve action and doing and are accomplished in a pattern or sequence.

TIME

Models which use time as the major concept break the day or treatment period into subunits or chronological time. The activities or tasks done within the units of time are more or less interchangeable in relation to the time unit itself. The key factor is how long the activity is done and the resulting effect the length of time has on the person. If the time period is too long the person may become physically fatigued, may lose interest and motivation or may not have any time left for some other type of activity. A time period which is too short may have no measurable physical effect, may not capture any interest and may leave the person with "time on his hands" but no activity to do. Thus, time can be manipulated to achieve the desired effect. Time can be doled out in doses of so much for this activity and so much for that one. This concept of dosage is very useful in medical settings because time can be prescribed in a manner similar to dosages of drugs. As a result the physician can order so much time in minutes, for example, be devoted to strengthening the triceps or riding a bicycle jigsaw.

Time can also be used as a means of structuring the activities a person needs to do. The simplest way to structure time is to make a list of things/activities which need to be done, determine how much time is required to do them and establish a schedule in which to accomplish the activities. In such a fashion a job can be performed, studies can be completed and a number of errands accomplished.

Furthermore, time can be used to analyze the activities a person does and how much time is allotted to each activity or a group of activities. First, the person lists all the activities which are performed in a given time period, such as a week. Then the activities can be grouped into the same or similar activities. Finally, the amount of time can be summed for each activity or group. The summations in turn may be analyzed in an effort to determine if too much or too little time is spent doing a particular activity or group as opposed to doing something else. The result is an activity configuration which can be used to help a person make choices about how time will be spent, or should be spent, to accomplish a particular objective or goal.

SPACE

Models which use space as an organizing concept speak of several dimensions of space. The activities or tasks done within the various dimensions are generally quite different. Also, the use of space seems to change over the life-span so that acceptable use of space to a 2-year-old is not the same as that for a 35-year-old and changes again for a 70-year-old. Furthermore, the use of space varies according to different cultures. Some cultures permit humans to interact at very close range in public, even though the persons are not family members or spouses. In American culture such closeness in public is generally unacceptable and causes discomfort. It may even be interpreted as rude behavior.

Space includes the use and organization of both human and nonhuman objects. Nonhuman objects can be used to facilitate human function and interaction or hinder same. For example, objects in space can be organized within the range and easy reach of the upper extremities without having to stand on tip toes or bend over. Objects such as chairs can be arranged to facilitate conversation or discourage extended chit chat. In addition, the use of light, color, plants, aquariums, magazines and other items can be used to facilitate interaction and effect the sense of well-being in humans.

For persons with physical handicaps which require a wheelchair the use of space becomes a major facilitator or barrier to independent functioning. When the wheelchair cannot go through the bathroom door, independence in elimination may be lost. When the wheelchair will not fit under the table, the person may be denied the social interaction of the family at the dinner table. When stairs prevent the wheelchair from going outside, the person may be confined to the house and lose the opportunity to interact with neighbors and shop for goods.

SPACE AND TIME

Although time and space can be separate issues intellectually they become inseparable in actual performance. All activity occurs in a certain space and over a certain time period. Mastery over one dimension, such as time, but lack of mastery over the other is of questionable value. Adaptation requires a certain level of control over both simultaneously as well as longitudinally. Thus, any serious analysis of activity concerning one dimension should of necessity consider the other dimension in some way.

ACTION AND DOING

Action or doing is behavior of a person which is deliberate and intended to effect something to which it is directed, moving it to a condition which differs from its condition prior to being acted upon. Action involves, knowledge, motivation, purpose and movement. A person must have knowledge in order to provide the structure for action. An action or series of actions depends on knowing what to do and how to do it. Although most people are able to learn effective actions which result in achieving an objective, some people suffer from an inability to plan effectively. Their actions are deficient due to brain dysfunction or lack of opportunity to learn.

Motivation provides the energy for an action. Such energy may be derived from extrinsic or intrinsic sources. Extrinsic motivation is associated primarily with the reduction of physiologic or psychologic needs related to identifiable stimulus. Intrinsic motivation appears to be more independent of extrinsic rewards. Intrinsically motivated behavior is engaged in for its own sake. Examples include curiosity, exploration, manipulation, achievement, competence, mastery and self actualization.

In each case the "reduction" of need seems to come from doing something in and of itself without any objective, reward, or pay off. Whether some people have less intrinsic motivation or less opportunity to engage in such behavior is unclear.

Purpose is closely related to motivation because it is connected with goal directed behavior. Action or doing which has a purpose to the actor or doer seems to generate more activity and better learning than action which is meaningless. The key point is purpose to the actor or doer. What is purposeful to one person is nonsense to another. A purposeful activity includes action or doing which is significant or meaningful to the person engaged in the activity. Thus, the individual's standards of purpose must be evaluated before an activity is initiated. To perform an activity usually involves some form of motor movement. Except for cognitive processes which may not be translated into movement most behavior has a movement component. Movement can be difficult for those with problems of processing and integrating stimuli into a plan of response. Examples include dyspraxia, problems in muscle tone, or difficulties in coordinating body segments with each other.

In summary, action and doing are processes which permit the individual to impact upon the environment and the self. Action may be the result of inherent or learned behaviors.

PATTERN

Models which use pattern as a major organizing concept are based on the belief that behavior is a composite of traits or features which are characteristic of an individual. Role behavior is an example of such a composite. A person acknowledged to have a certain role is expected to behave or perform behaviors which are characteristic of an individual with that particular role. A housewife, for example, generally is expected to perform, and be able to perform, certain tasks such as cooking meals, washing clothes, and cleaning the house. A plumber is expected to be able to install plumbing equipment, repair broken pipes, and fix leaking faucets. Other types of individuals could be a father, baseball player, priest, baby-sitter, or president. In each case the title is the key to a pattern or cluster of role behaviors which society has attributed to the role and expects to see performed. When the role is not performed or is performed in a manner inconsistent with expectations, a person is subject to sanctions by society which may result in labeling, ostracism, or even institutionalization.

SEQUENCE

Models which use sequence as a major organizing concept are based on the assumption that performance results from a series or set of steps which occur in a certain order. Walking, for example, is assumed to be the end result of amphibian crawling, belly crawling, crawling on all fours, knee walking and finally walking on two feet. Furthermore, the act of walking itself is a sequence of substeps beginning with the heel strike on the left foot, moving the weight from the heel to the ball of the foot and pushing off with the toes, while at the same time the right foot has been moving through a swing phase from a posterior position to an anterior position in preparation for the right heel to strike. Thus, a sequence may be a series of steps leading up to an event or a series of steps within an event.

The sequence may be genetically determined, innately determined, or environmentally learned. Genetically determined sequences are based on the assumption that ontogeny recapitulates phylogeny and the phenotype recapitulates the genotype. In other words, the species such as homo sapiens repeat the sequence of locomotion which was established by the lower animals in the phyla scale, or the individual person (phenotype) repeats the pattern which is typical of people (genotype) in general. An innate sequence is usually considered to be preprogrammed as opposed to being learned. Innate sequences may be genetically determined or may be environmentally determined, but in either case the individual has no real control over the steps in the sequence or the outcome of the sequence. Learned sequences are those which a person acquires by repeating an action until the nervous system has mastered the tasks involved in the sequence. For example, a person learns to undress and then dress. There is a series of steps which should or could be followed in each case. Outer garments come off first and go on last, for example.

When the concept of sequence is applied to the treatment of patients or clients the sequence frequently becomes the plan. That is, the individual's performance is compared to the series of steps in the sequence to determine the level of performance or development. The level of performance is the last step the person can perform or has mastered. Treatment then begins with the next step and the next until the sequence is completed or the performance reaches a plateau.

Subdivisions of Performance Areas

Occupations require that at least one of five major areas be functional. These are: (a) motor, (b) sensory, (c) cognitive, (d) intrapersonal and (e) interpersonal.

MOTOR

The motor area of performance is evaluated to determine if the neuromuscular skeletal system is able to perform the basic movement skills a person needs to complete the occupational requirements. Motor skills are needed to enable a person to get food on the eating utensil and into the mouth. Motor skills are needed also to mount tires on a car and to bowl with friends. Examples of motor skills include strength, dexterity, coordination, speed, accuracy, reflexes and reactions, tolerance, developmental milestones (creep, walk, hop, jump, run), gestures, speech.

Motor skills are the primary output signals and responses which the person makes. Frequently it is impossible to know what a person is thinking or feeling until some motor response is made. It is difficult also to determine if an input or stimulus has been received by the brain until a motor act is initiated. The person with catatonic schizophrenia shows the problem of no motor or retarded response. Others may assume that the person is not listening and, therefore, does not hear what is said. As a consequence, the catatonic person can be ignored or humiliated without concern for individual dignity. People with motor handicaps may suffer similar indignities plus the added insult of being considered mentally retarded because the motor response if given may be delayed.

SENSORY

The sensory component of performance is evaluated to determine if the senses are able to function separately, in combination with each other, and with the motor area to permit efficient body action. Senses include vestibular, proprioception, kinesthesis, touch or tactile, vibration, pressure, pain, temperature, taste, smell, vision and hearing. Combinations of sensory input and interaction with the motor area facilitate cross model transfer, sensorimotor activity, perceptual motor development and sensory integration.

The sensory systems are the primary means of gaining information from the external and internal environments. If one or more senses is not functioning at all or functioning at a reduced level, the information into the brain may be affected. The impact depends on which sensory modality is involved, how the modality is malfunctioning, when and for how long the sense has been dysfunctional, and finally whether other senses can compensate and have been trained to do so.

COGNITION

The cognitive area is evaluated to determine if a person is able to use thinking and memory skills to facilitate the performance of various tasks. Examples of cognitive skills include orienting behavior, attention span, concept formation, comprehension, short- and long-term memory, and problem solving.

Cognitive skills appear to be most important in enabling a person to analyze previous behaviors and plan for future behaviors based on previous experience, current conditions and possible future events. Cognition also is highly related to learning. The ability to make verbal discrimination and generalizations, develop concepts, learn principles and apply decision-making strategies requires that opportunities to receive instruction, practice skills and evaluate feedback be provided.

People with lack of cognitive skills include those with limited general intelligence due to hereditary or acquired mental retardation. Also included are persons who have sufficient general intelligence but who lack opportunity to develop skills because of limited environments, such as institutions or low socioeconomic living conditions. Finally, some people may have difficulty learning from practice and experience because of feedforward or feedback problems in the nervous system.

INTRAPERSONAL

The intrapersonal area is assessed to determine the ability of a person to distinguish reality from nonreality and to cope with that reality. Examples of intrapersonal skills are feelings, emotions, self-image, self-control, defense mechanisms, object relations, reality testing and coping skills. The key element in intrapersonal skills is the person's ability to manage the self as an autonomous person. Such management skills result from experiencing and dealing with internal and external events so that the information can be used in subsequent situations. Opportunity to learn through experience which is guided by human and nonhuman objects is important to build the skills of interpersonal development.

INTERPERSONAL

The interpersonal areas of performance are measured to assess how well a person is able to relate to other humans. Examples can be divided into several subcategories. One includes dyad vs. group situations. Dyads are one to one settings such as two friends, a parent and child, husband and wife, two siblings, supervisor and employee, and others. Group situations are those in which three or more persons are involved. Examples of groups include a family unit, a classroom of children, a gang, a work crew, a bridge club, and others.

Another division can be made along role behaviors. Each person is assumed to occupy several roles over a life time and may occupy a number of roles simultaneously. Examples include child, spouse, worker, church member, home owner, foreman or team captain.

PARAMETERS MODELS

The third group of the models focuses primarily on aspects of the parameters of occupational therapy. These models may focus on the process of therapy such as approaches to assessment or intervention. Another area of focus is on program design in occupational therapy which examines the types of services occupational therapy might provide. Finally, such models may address the philosophy or assumptions on which occupational therapy is based.

In summary, the models of occupational therapy seem to fall generally into three groups: generic, descriptive or parameter. Of course some models fit into more than one category depending on how extensively the model has been developed. In such cases the model is described under the category which seemed to best fit the major thrust of the model.

TAXONOMIES

As the models were being organized some relationships became apparent. Since a taxonomy is based on a natural relationship the development of a classification scheme became an outgrowth of the initial organization of models for presentation. The three taxonomies presented are initial steps toward classifying the variables related to occupation and occupational therapy. There is no pretense to state the ultimate taxonomy for occupational therapy. Rather these taxonomies should be viewed as working drafts based on the sources available as this text was prepared. See Tables 8.2 to 8.4.

Table 8.2
Acquisition of Occupations Taxonomy

1.00 Occupational types
    1.10 Self maintenance
    1.20 Productivity
    1.30 Leisure
2.00 Learning environments
    2.10 Physical or inorganic
    2.20 Biopsychological or organic
    2.30 Sociocultural or superorganic
3.00 Learning processes
    3.10 Exploration
    3.20 Manipulation
    3.30 Competence or mastery
    3.40 Achievement
4.00 Teaching—learning technique
      (Note: Becomes basis for therapy methods)
    4.10 Trial and error
    4.20 Discriminative
    4.30 Demonstration/modeling
    4.40 Lecture/verbal directions
    4.50 Discussion
    4.60 Role playing or simulation
    4.70 Repetition and practice
    4.80 Problem solving
    4.90 Programmed
        linear
        branching
5.00 Learning types
    5.10 Knowledge-thought
    5.20 Skills/abilities
    5.30 Attitudes, norms, values,
6.00 Adaptational outcomes
    6.10 Adapt
    6.20 Nonadapt
    6.30 Maladapt

Table 8.3
Description of Occupations Taxonomy

1.00 Self maintenance
  1.10 Controlling elements
    1.11 Orientation
      1.111 Time
        1.1111 Past
        1.1112 Present
        1.1113 Future
        1.1114 Circadian
        1.1115 Diurnal
        1.1116 Clock
      1.211 Space
        1.2111 Horizontal
        1.2112 Coronal or frontal
        1.2113 Sagittal
        1.2114 Individual
        1.2115 Family
        1.2116 Community
        1.2117 Nation
        1.2118 World
        1.2119 Biosphere
    2.11 Activation (action and doing)
      2.111 Knowledge, skill and attitude
        2.1111 What
        2.1112 How
        2.1113 Why
        2.1114 Where
        2.1115 When
        2.1116 Who
        2.1117 How much
      2.211 Motivation
        2.2111 Extrinsic
        2.1112 Intrinsic
      2.311 Purpose
        2.3111 Individual need
        2.3113 Social goal
      2.411 Movement
        2.4111 Minimum
        2.4112 Moderate
        2.4113 Maximum
    3.11 Order (Pattern and sequence)
      3.111 Forward and backward
      3.112 Sideways-left/right
      3.113 Up and down
      3.114 Circular
      3.115 Fixed
      3.116 Flexible

Table 8.3—*Continued*

1.20 Performance areas
  1.21 Motor
    1.211 Coordination and dexterity
    1.212 Muscle strength
    1.213 Muscle tone
    1.214 Endurance/tolerance
    1.215 Gross skills
    1.216 Fine skills
    1.217 Range of motion
    1.218 Reflexes/reactions
    1.219 Adapted equipment
  1.22 Sensory
    1.221 Touch/tactile
      1.2211 Activity
      1.2212 Perception
      1.2213 Discrimination
      1.2214 Figure-ground
    1.222 Vestibular
    1.223 Proprioceptive/kinesthetic
    1.224 Taste
    1.225 Smell
    1.226 Pain/pressure
    1.227 Temperature
    1.228 Auditory
    1.229 Visual
    1.220 Sensorimotor
      1.2201 Perceptual motor
      1.2202 Sensory integrative
      1.2203 Cross model
  1.23 Cognitive
    1.231 Attending
    1.232 Comprehension
    1.233 Conceptualization
    1.234 Memory/retention
    1.235 Judgment/analysis
    1.236 Generalization
    1.237 Discrimination
  1.24 Intrapersonal
    1.241 Autonomy
    1.242 Coping
    1.243 Defense mechanism
    1.244 Object relations
    1.245 Reality testing
    1.246 Self-control
    1.247 Self concept
    1.248 Synthesis
  1.25 Intrapersonal
    1.251 Dyad
    1.252 Group
    1.253 Role
    1.254 Social

Table 8.3—*Continued*

1.30 Roles
    1.31 Self caretaker
        1.311 Hygiene
        1.312 Eating
        1.313 Dressing
        1.314 Grooming
        1.315 Miscellaneous
    1.32 Communication
        1.321 Understanding
        1.322 Speaking
        1.323 Writing
        1.324 Telephoning
        1.325 Typing
    1.33 Elevation and locomotion mobilizer
        1.331 Bed activities
        1.332 Sitting
        1.333 Standing
        1.334 Walking
        1.335 Climbing
        1.336 Use of private transportation
        1.337 Use of public transportation
    1.34 Home management—home manager
        1.341 Meal
        1.342 Beds
        1.343 Cleaning
        1.344 Clothes
        1.345 Budget
        1.346 Decorator and arranger
2.00 Productivity
    2.10 Controlling elements
        2.11 Orientation (see 1.11)
        2.12 Activation (see 1.12)
        2.13 Order (see 1.13)
    2.20 Performance areas
        2.21 Motor (see 1.21)
        2.22 Sensory (see 1.22)
        2.23 Cognitive (see 1.23)
        2.24 Intrapersonal (see 1.24)
        2.25 Interpersonal (see 1.25)
    2.30 Roles
        2.31 Homemaker—unpaid
        2.32 Child caretaker—unpaid
        2.33 Professional/junior member or officer—paid or unpaid
        2.34 Trainee/apprentice—paid or unpaid
        2.35 Regular schedule—paid (part-time or full-time)
        2.36 Irregular schedule—paid
        2.37 Self scheduled—paid or unpaid
        2.38 Volunteer—unpaid
        2.39 Unemployed or job seeking

Table 8.3—*Continued*

3.00 Leisure
    3.10 Controlling elements
        3.11 Orientation (see 1.11)
        3.12 Activation (see 1.12)
        3.13 Order (see 1.13)
    3.20 Performance areas
        3.21 Motor (see 1.21)
        3.22 Sensory (see 1.22)
        3.23 Cognitive (see 1.23)
        3.24 Intrapersonal (see 1.24)
        3.25 Interpersonal (see 1.25)
    3.30 Roles
        3.31 Games player
        3.32 Sports participant or observer
        3.33 Nature activities—nature lover (hiker, bird watcher, climber)
        3.34 Collector activities
        3.35 Craft activities—handicrafter (knitter, carver)
        3.36 Art and music activities—art or music lover
        3.37 Education, entertainment and cultural activities—attendee, presentor
        3.38 Volunteer activities—volunteer
        3.39 Organizational activities—member or officer

Table 8.4
Occupational Therapy Taxonomy

1.00 Philosophy and assumptions
    1.20 Of humans
    1.20 Of health and adaptation
    1.30 Of occupations
    1.40 Of occupational therapy
2.00 Process
    2.10 Results or outcomes
        2.11 Objectives
        2.12 Goals
    2.20 Assessment
        2.21 Observation
        2.22 Interview
        2.23 Testing
    2.30 Planning
        2.31 Therapist control
        2.32 Cooperative
    2.40 Intervention
        2.41 Media and modalities
            2.411
            2.412
            2.413 etc.
        2.42 Methods, techniques, approaches
            2.421
            2.422
            2.423 etc.
        2.43 Equipment
            2.431
            2.432
            2.433 etc.
        2.44 Prerequisite skills
            2.441
            2.442
            2.443 etc.
3.00 Types of programs
    3.10 Prevent
    3.20 Develop
    3.30 Remediate
    3.40 Adjust
    3.50 Maintenance

CHAPTER 9

Generic Models

Models grouped under the category of generic models were selected for this chapter because their major purpose seems to be to explain the overall philosophy of values and beliefs of occupational therapy. In generic models, the concepts are broadly defined and do not restrict the use of the model to one area of specialized practice or one area of performance. Furthermore, these generic models seem to address both the major strengths and weaknesses of occupational therapy as an applied profession.

OCCUPATIONAL BEHAVIOR
Frame of Reference

Occupational behavior is a model based on the organismic, humanistic, biopsychosocial and developmental models. The term "occupational behavior" first appeared in 1966 (1). Reilly was proposing some assumptions for a model of practice for occupational therapy in psychiatry based on the work of Adolph Meyer (2) who proposed a continuum of work, play, rest and sleep occupations. The model was used to determine whether the subject matter of occupational therapy in psychiatry should be included in the curriculum at the University of Southern California. The results of analysis were positive, and occupational behavior became a keystone in the curriculum design of the graduate program where it was expanded toward a generic model. In 1969 Reilly (3) outlined the theoretical framework of occupational behavior. Based on the idea that the task of occupational therapy is to prevent and reduce the incapacities resulting from illness, Reilly suggests that the frame of reference should be organized as it occurs in a developmental continuum of work and play and is acknowledged within the concept of occupational roles. The concept of achievement is based on the works of McClelland, White and Erickson. Developmental concepts are drawn from developmental psychology while role theory and socialization are borrowed from sociology.

Much of the actual work of developing and expanding the occupational behavior model has been done by Reilly's graduate students. Through graduate student theses the concepts have been explored, and evaluation instruments have been devised. Reilly herself has not contributed directly to the literature since 1974 when she authored a book on play (4) with several graduate student contributers.

Assumptions

The major assumptions of the occupational behavior model are as follows:

MAN

1. Needs are an indispensable part of human nature and imperatively demand satisfaction (from Fromm (5)).

2. Man has a need to master his environment, to alter and improve it (5).
3. There is a relationship between levels of aspiration or expectancy established in prior socialization and a current pattern of success or failure (3).
4. Man has a vital need for occupation (5).
5. Work is a physiologically conditioned need, and therefore a need to work is postulated as an imperative part of man's nature (5).

MAN AND HEALTH

1. Man, through the use of his hands as they are energized by mind and will, can influence the state of his own health (5).
2. There is a reservoir of sensitivity and skill in the hands of man which can be tapped for his health (5).
3. There is a rich adaptability and durability of the central nervous system which can be influenced by experience (5).

OCCUPATION

1. Society programs its members for occupational behavior through sequential experience in play, family living, school and recreation (1).
2. Occupational behavior is developmentally acquired (1).
3. Achievement has a developmental nature (3).
4. In the progress of growth the achievement drive generates such by-products as interests, abilities, skills, habits of competition and cooperation (3).
5. Achievement behavior can be facilitated and strengthened through play and work (3).
6. Play is the antecedent preparation area for work (3).
7. Adult social recreation pattern of behavior is a sublatent support to a work pattern (3).
8. Roles are learned in the process of socialization (3).
9. There are three role systems, masculine and feminine identification, group membership and occupational behavior (3).
10. Occupational roles include housewife, student, preschooler and retiree (3).

OCCUPATIONAL THERAPY

1. Occupational therapy is a milieu or a culture (1).
2. Occupational therapy's focus lies in the area of human productivity and creativity (5).
3. The task of occupational therapy is to prevent and reduce the incapacities resulting from illness (3).
4. The job of occupational therapy is to activate the residual adaptation forces within a patient (3).
5. Occupational therapy service should be directed toward biopsychosocial functioning of a disabled individual (3).
6. Occupational therapy should be directed toward patient achievement (3).

7. Occupational therapy should focus on a patient's ability to carry on the daily activities required by his social roles (3).
8. Occupational therapists should test and measure adaptive skills (3).

Concepts

The major concepts of the occupational behavior model are listed below and have been organized into the model shown in Figure 9.1.

1. *Occupational behavior*—that aspect of growth and development represented by the developmental continuum of play and work as they support competence, achievement and occupational role (6).
2. *Work*—the arena in which individuals endeavor to validate themselves (7).
3. *Play*—all forms of playful, recreative, leisure time activities (8).
4. *Motivation*—a mediating system, process or mechanism that attempts to account for the purposeful aspects of behavior (9).
5. *Intrinsic motivation*—refers to factors which are relatively independent of tissue need (hunger) and external agents with specific benefit or noxious effects/pain (10).
6. *Competence motive*—attempt to contact and master the environment (11).
7. *Achievement motive*—a motive based upon universal experiences with problem-solving tasks and which involves competition with a standard of excellence with respect to these tasks (9).
8. *Exploratory behavior*—behavior engaged in for its own sake (4).
9. *Competency*—sufficient or adequate behavior to meet the demands of the situation (12).
10. *Achievement*—a specified level of success, attainment or proficiency (13).
11. *Problem solving*—the process involved in discovering the correct sequence of alternatives leading to a goal or to an ideation solution (13).
12. *Decision making*—formulating a course of action with the intent to execute it (14).

Age	Process	Motive or Need	Biopsychosocial Behavior	Process	Occupational Behavior
Adult	Work	Achievement Motive	Achievement		Occupational Role(s)
↑	↑ Continuum →	↑	↑	Decision Making ↑ ↓ Problem Solving	↑
		Competency Motive ↑	Competence ↑		Occupational Choice ↑
Child	Play	Intrinsic Motive	Exploratory		Socialization and Learning

Figure 9.1.   Conceptual model of occupational behavior.

13. *Social behavior*—behavior molded and defined by the social institutions in the service of group needs (15).
14. *Occupational choice*—the series of developmental stages culminating in the selection of an occupation (16).
15. *Occupational role*—the attempt to assimilate oneself into an identified group that meets one's need for productivity, belonging and life-structuring activities (16).

The conceptual model shown in Figure 9.1 is based on the author's understanding of how the concepts should be organized. Reilly did not provide a working diagrammatic model in her published works. The key relationships seem to be the developmental progression of play and work into more complex systems of occupational behavior which terminates in the organization of roles. Acquisition of occupational behavior is accomplished through a series of motives or needs which urge the person toward certain behaviors (exploratory, competency and achievement) and are facilitated by the processes of problem solving and decision making.

Expected Results

As a result of intervention through the occupational behavior model a person may have:

1. learned, relearned or modified life skills (1)
2. increased decision-making skills (1)
3. increased sense of competency (1)
4. developed a balanced daily living pattern within the daily life space (1)
5. developed healthy adaptive behavior (1)
6. reduced the effects of incapacity and activated the residual adaptation forces (3).

Assessment Techniques

PROCESS OR PROCEDURES

The primary process or procedure used is the interview. The interview is used to gain such information as the following (6).

1. Learning and socialization in childhood roles
2. Exploration and the decision process around the issue of occupational choice
3. Patterns of achievement and failure and environmental conditions which appear to influence theses
4. Course of movement and solidification or lack of it in the period of adult occupational choice

ASSESSMENT AREAS

Examples of interviews include the occupational history, play assessment scales and interest checklists. Gray (17) suggests that therapists should be gathering data in the problem areas of self-care skills, motor skills, social skills, general work skills, specific work skills, use of time skills, play, recreational or leisure skills and decision-making skills.

Intervention Strategies

Matsutsuyu (16) records Reilly's ideas about intervention programs in occupational therapy as follows:

1. The program should reflect the developmental stages present in the acquisition of life skills.
2. The program should provide natural and legitimate decision-making areas for patients.
3. The program milieu must acknowledge competencies, arouse curiosity, deepen appreciation and demand behavior across the full spectrum of human abilities.
4. The program must have concerns for work, play and rest throughout the days, evenings and weekends, not just a single activity and fragment of time.
5. The program structure must provide opportunities for the practicing of life skills in a balanced pattern of daily living which takes into account individual interests and abilities and tailors events to age, sex and occupational roles.

An outline of intervention strategies is provided below.

Media
  Daily exercise
  Arts and crafts
  Sewing
  Cooking
  Recreation
  Social dancing
  Vocational skills
Methods
  Independent decision making
  Structured learning groups
Equipment
  No specific items mentioned
Prerequisite skills
  Play skills are prerequisite to work skills

Summary

Reilly's model of occupational behavior is based on Meyer's continuum of, and balance between, work, play, rest and sleep. The term occupational behavior is concerned primarily with the continuum of play and work. Thus, the word occupational is used to convey not only salaried employment but encompasses those activities that employ or occupy a person's time. In other words, Reilly is suggesting that occupational behavior, that is, the work-play continuum, is the basic concern of occupational therapy. Through the continuum a person learns the occupational roles needed to become competent in society. The model of occupational behavior was developed initially as a treatment approach for psychiatric patients. However, the model has been explored with children and can be applied to physically disabled persons.

ANALYSIS AND CRITIQUE OF THE OCCUPATIONAL BEHAVIOR MODEL

Frame of Reference

Occupational behavior appears to be based on a frame of reference which is highly consistent with the history of occupational therapy. Meyer provided the initial model for occupational therapy by organizing habits into a time frame. Other sources seem to be consistent. The use of White's competency model is consistent with the basic assumption of exerting an influence on the environment. Role theory and emphasis on moving away from the biomedical reductionist models also seem consistent with concern for social cultural influences in occupational behavior.

Clarity and Interrelatedness

Based on the literature published, the assumptions and concepts are not well defined and only partly interrelated. Although the graduate students have expanded greatly the original ideas, there remains no published comprehensive summary of the model. Instead it must be pieced together from a variety of sources. This lack of summarization makes the model difficult to understand fully and more difficult to teach students.

Uniqueness

The model is based on the work-play continuum which is called occupational behavior. Reilly (1) used the word "occupation" because she felt it acknowledged the economic nature of man. She felt that occupational therapists must become knowledgeable and responsible for maintaining and improving the economic skills and attitudes of clients so that each person would be able to assume an occupational role and fulfill economic needs. Such needs are not limited to gainful or paid employment (3, 4). Other occupational roles such as student, housekeeper, and volunteer also are included. Furthermore, she saw play as a primary means of learning occupational roles. Perhaps the one idea that is not emphasized enough is that a person may assume a number of occupational roles throughout a lifetime. For example, a person could be a student, a paid worker, a housekeeper, and a volunteer over the years. In some cases occupational roles can be assumed simultaneously such as housekeeper, paid worker and volunteer.

The uniqueness of the concept of occupational behavior appears to have two aspects. The first is the recognition of the occupational role as any creative or productive occupation and the second is the belief that play is the major rehearsal and practice arena for the development of occupational roles.

Research Guide

The model has been the catalyst for graduate student theses in the program at the University of Southern California. However, the lack of published work in a systematic organized manner probably is responsible for the lack of use by therapists other than those educated directly by

Reilly or her students. In spite of the current lack of specificity the model appears to have potential as a tool for furthering the study of occupation and occupational therapy.

Specialization

Occupational behavior has been classified as a generic model and fits the classification. The work-play continuum can be applied to any group of patients or clients which are seen commonly in occupational therapy today, with the possible exception of the older adult who is not discussed in the model. Clients with problems in physical or mental health can be assessed in terms of their work-play skills to see if skills have been learned and if the skills have been retained. Those with deficit or lost skills can be developed or relearned. Those with adequate skills can practice maintaining and increasing their work-play skills. Thus, specialization is possible with any age group or diagnostic label. Even persons with no diagnostic label such as the well or healthy person could learn about the normal development and maintenance of work-play skills and occupational roles.

Elaboration and Refinement

The model appears to permit considerable elaboration and refinement. Each of the major concepts can be elaborated and refined, such as work, play, work-play continuum, exploration, mastery, competence, occupational choice, occupational role and a variety of aspects of occupational preparation such as values, belief, habits, and skills which contribute to building occupational roles. In addition, the use of occupational therapy media and methods can be explored to determine which facilitate development and maintenance of occupational behavior.

Explanatory Usefulness

One of the difficulties with the lack of a summary presentation of the model is that of explaining the model to others. There are a few useful aspects, but a complete overview is difficult. The concept that play is preparation for work is a useful concept in explaining the use of tasks that appear to others to be child's play, recreational or leisure pursuits. Likewise, the concept of work-play continuum is useful to explain a progression of occupational skills. However, the relationship between occupation and health and vocational training and occupational therapy is still difficult to convey.

Commonality

Because the model of occupational behavior has not been systematically presented it is difficult to state for certain what the commonalities might be with other disciplines. Occupational behavior does have a relationship with vocational rehabilitation because there is a focus on occupation and skill development. There is a connection with education as well because of the teaching-learning techniques and career development curriculum. However, the relationship with physical therapy, nursing, social work, clinical psychology, and other activity therapies, such as art, music, dance and recreation, remains unclear. Thus, the occupational behavior model has not been useful in conveying the role of occupational therapy as a practice or applied discipline with other professional groups.

Practice Model Development

The model appears to provide an excellent base for practice model development. Reilly has outlined the ideas about program needs, which were summarized by Matsutsuyu and are included in the intervention strategy section. Students have outlined the programs in their publications of theses in the *American Journal of Occupational Therapy*.

A summary of the criteria used to evaluate the occupational behavior model appears in Table 9.1.

Critique of Model Application

1. REFLECTS THE REAL WORLD

Reilly's theory assumes that people have a basic need to explore, create and be productive. Furthermore, she suggests that play and work are part of a continuum in which play prepares a person for work by increasing problem-solving skills. What is unclear are the specific skills which are acquired in a person with adaptive behavior and which ones are missing in a person who is unable to adapt successfully to society and social expectations. Until the theory is better formulated, the degree to which the theory reflects the real world will be difficult to ascertain.

2. MODEL IS UNDERSTANDABLE

The assumptions and concepts and outcomes are understandable; however, they have been developed by several students each of whom has extended or expanded the model in his/her particular direction. Thus, it is difficult to get a cohesive picture of the model in total. No one who is really familiar with Reilly's ideas has taken the time to integrate the existing pieces of the model. The attempt in this chapter reflects published works only and may reflect the students' opinions more than Reilly's original ideas.

Table 9.1
Occupational Behavior Model Criteria Summary

Evaluation Criteria	Very Good	Moderately Good			Very Poor
		2	3	4	5
Frame of reference	x				
Clarity				x	
Uniqueness	x				
Research guide			x		
Specialization	x				
Elaboration	x				
Usefulness		x			
Commonality			x		
Practice models	x				

3. POWER TO PREDICT INDIVIDUAL BEHAVIOR

The model suggests that a child with deficient play skills will have deficient work skills unless corrective actions are taken. It also suggests that play and work skills can be lost when opportunity to practice the skills regularly is lost through disease, trauma or institutionalization. Again, the missing components are the specific skills. The model does not yet permit the pinpointing of critical skills or critical skills levels which must be maintained in order to allow a person to make adaptive behavioral responses in society.

4. PRACTICAL GUIDANCE

Occupational behavior as a model for practical guidance suggests that play skills are the critical behaviors which a person must acquire in order to function as an adaptive person in society. Therefore, the model should direct attention to the study, analysis and development of the effect play behavior has on all persons, but especially to those who are at risk of not learning or not maintaining play skills. The exact description of at risk persons has not been fully described. Some examples are those with chronic disease and those who are institutionalized for any length of time.

5. INTERNAL CONSISTENCY

The model of occupational behavior appears to be fairly consistent with itself. Considering the number of students who have developed thesis topics and subsequent publications based on some aspect of the model, it must have a consistent thread or the thread would be lost. However, because there is no official gathering together of thoughts developed by the students into a current statement, analysis of internal consistancy is difficult to accomplish.

6. ECONOMY

The final number of assumptions and mechanisms may be still an unknown factor since the model is not fully developed. At the present time, there does not seem to be an undue number of assumptions or mechanisms, considering the model is addressing the whole arena of occupational therapy practice. Furthermore, the concepts are developed from common terms and ideas. No elaborate mechanisms have been employed. However, this criterion must be reevaluated when and if there is more information provided.

7. STIMULATING NEW TECHNIQUES AND KNOWLEDGE

The model of occupational behavior has stimulated many research ideas for graduate students. Most of the research techniques have been borrowed from other disciplines, such as the case method and observation reports. However, the model has contributed considerably to the literature in occupational therapy. This contribution has been the hallmark of the model to date.

8. MODEL MAKES GOOD SENSE

The attempt to establish a model for occupational therapy which does not depend on other professions is a desirable goal. Using the concept of occupation as the core idea also is commendable. The lack of clarity between play/work and daily living tasks is a problem. Are daily living tasks incorporated within play and work or is there some difference? It is also unclear as to how the model of occupational behavior can be used in preventative and normal development. What developmental tasks are included in the work-play continuum which must occur to promote development, and what are the signs of high risk? As these questions are answered, the model should begin to make better sense.

9. CAUSATION

Occupational behavior is based on a needs concept of an inner motivational state which is activated through intrinsic motivation to explore and create. It appears that occupational behavior is based on a biopsychosocial being (material cause) which interacts with the physical and psychosocial environment (efficient) to develop and organize work-play skills into effective occupational roles (formal) for the purpose of achieving occupational behavior (final). Thus, causation is a personal or internal process which is consistent with the locus of control issue in the organismic model.

INTEGRATED THEORY OF OCCUPATIONAL THERAPY
Frame of Reference

The Integrated Theory of Occupational Therapy model is the result of a seminar held in 1967 to explore and integrate a mind-body theory in psychiatric occupational therapy. Concern for such a theory grew out of a series of workshops on object relations which had been held previous to the seminar. The purpose of the proposed theory was to create a "more meaningful frame of reference to facilitate the teaching and practice of occupational therapy" (18). As presented the model is quite incomplete. No expected results, assessment instruments or intervention strategies are included. Furthermore, the frame of reference is not well defined. Analysis of the conceptual models suggests that the developmental and psychoanalytic models are most prevalent, although wholistic and biopsychological concepts appear also. The influence of reductionism is apparent in the dualistic approach to the task.

Assumptions

The integrated model is based on the following assumptions (18).

MAN AND INTEGRATED BELIEFS

1. Man is a biogenetic organism.
2. Man develops, refines and maintains human activity through interrelatedness and interdependence of the maturational process and objects in the external world.
3. Man is a growing and interacting organism in the environment.

4. Man is a functioning whole who has:
   a. Static or structural aspects of a functional system in growth and interaction
   b. Dynamic process which ensue as a result of structural properties coming into contact with stimuli, *i.e.* the processes of interaction and growth
   c. The energy or the propelling force behind the evolution of structural dimensions and resultant dynamic processes which activate the process.
5. Man as a system is always in the process of change and becoming.
6. External influences, interpersonal, sociocultural factors and internal biogenetic factors are influential in man's prenatal state of development and in postnatal growth.
7. Idiosyncratic or atypical early maturation and development may be genetically built into the physiological structure of the person and become manifest as problems of adaptation, communication and interpersonal relations.
8. The way in which important people (the significant others) react to atypical development and the social and interpersonal habits and reactions which develop around these also influence development.
9. The environment feeds or deprives the infant of stimuli he needs for nurturance.
10. It is postulated that the organism needs stimulus encounters for survival.
11. Neurological development is from lower to higher centers, and ego growth is from rudimentary and undifferentiated activities to complex and defined functions.
12. Ego differentiation correlates with levels of neurological integrative functioning.

NEUROBEHAVIORAL ISSUES

1. Environmental stimuli are organized into meaningful patterns both from without and within. Examples include form, position in space, time, sequence and color.
2. The organism registers and responds primarily to those stimuli which are meaningful to it for survival.
3. The process of development seems to be directed toward organizing and patterning stimuli into gestalts.
4. Development proceeds toward increased differentiation and integration of those patterns which have meaning to both the inner and outer world of the child.
5. Perceptual-motor functioning is believed to approximate maturational levels or states of development.
6. Development is a dynamic process in time, involving continual interaction with the environment, and proceeds in more of a spiral than a straight line.

7. As the central nervous system matures functions of the lower centers are gradually incorporated and dominated by those of the higher centers.
8. The organism retains the ability to use ontogenetically earlier systems when stimulus encounters are unmanageable.
9. During overload the total capacity for response is reduced, that is, the organism cannot respond to any stimuli except those most critical for basic survival.
10. The higher centers appear to derive their capacities to function adequately from proper growth and development of the lower centers.
11. Stimulus encounters are made manageable by a process of incorporation into the conscious.
12. When stimulus encounters in the here and now overload the ability of the organism to respond at the cortical ego level then this structure is not available for utilization.
13. Responses are elicited at the level where meaningful integration occurs.

PSYCHOSOCIAL ISSUES

1. The ego has a rudimentary existence at birth but is not fully functioning until both consciousness and certain structural properties are developed.
2. The characteristic properties of a fully functioning ego are its abilities to:
   a. discriminate, make choices;
   b. adapt, maintain homeostasis, seek equilibrium;
   c. expand the self, reach for self actualization, drive for growth.
3. The prime function of the ego is to perceive and mediate between the realities of the external and the internal environment.
4. The ego must develop mechanisms for accurate and serviceable perception, motor control, self-preservation, assimilation, memory storage, affects, cognition and reconciliation of conflicting needs and demands.
5. The ego through maturity and differentiation evolves with increasing ability to engage the world by bringing internal and external forces into approximation.
6. Ego consolidation is achieved through a growth process involving practice, mastery and validation.
7. The ego is perceived as having innate energy available for its functions, and the procedure of stimulus intake is seen as a process of energy utilization.
8. In ego development, elements of stimulus intake are assigned either to the conscious functioning of the organism and expressed through ego maneuvers or they are assigned to the unconscious and stored.
9. Energy assigned to the conscious is believed to be free and available

for further use, while energy assigned to the unconscious is considered bound and can be used only if "won" from the unconscious.

10. Energy assignment is thought of as a process of maintaining homeostasis wherein the organism seeks to balance its encounters with the external environment.

OCCUPATIONAL THERAPY

1. Occupational therapy should attempt to restore higher levels of cortical ego functioning by meeting the integrative needs of the lower centers at their developmental level.
2. Therapeutic planning should be directed toward achieving increasingly greater differentiation and integration at the presenting level of integration.
3. Problems at the lower levels should be addressed before higher functions can be achieved.

Concepts

The following terms are defined.

Maturation—sequential change in time.
Objects—a dimension of identifiable mass in space.
Man—has an attendant mental and physical component.

The following terms are mentioned but are not defined: development, adaptation, interpersonal relationships, sociocultural factors, biogenetic factors, ego, differentiation, integration, perceptual-motor functioning, cortical-ego, discrimination, choice or selection, homeostasis, self actualization, drive for growth, assimilation, conscious, unconscious, ego consolidation, practice, mastery, and validation.

As stated previously the model does not include any discussion of expected results, assessment instruments or intervention strategies except those which are included within certain assumptions.

Summary

The integrated theory of occupational therapy model is an attempt to put together the two divergent frames of reference which are known in practice as psychiatric and physical disabilities occupational therapy. Psychiatric occupational therapy has been influenced by the psychosocial concerns of the psychoanalysis and behavioral models, while physical disabilities have been influenced by the neurobehavioral issues of the developmental and systems models. Both have suffered from the influences of the biomedical model in the practice arena which created the two separate practice areas in the first place. Specifically the mind and body dualism tends to suggest that acquisition and maintenance of function of the body is different and serves a different goal than that of the mind. This dualistic approach is augmented by the use of different terminologies which appear in organismic and mechanistic meta models and between super models of the organismic classification.

The model of integration is an attempt to relate the internal and

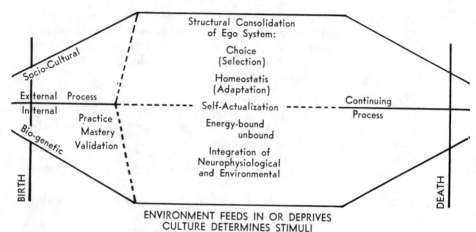

Figure 9.2. Model of integration. (Reproduced with permission from J. Mazer (18). © 1968, *The American Journal of Occupational Therapy*.)

external environments by proposing a continual process from birth to death of interaction between biogenetic and cultural factors (Fig. 9.2). The ego is consolidated into a working unit through (a) choice of whether stimulus intake goes to the conscious or unconscious, (b) use of homeostasis as an adaptive mechanism, (c) achievement of self actualization (d) amount of bound or unbound energy and (e) integration of neurophysiological and environmental elements. The process of ego consolidation is achieved through practice, mastery and validation. The environment and culture also influence ego consolidation by controlling whether stimuli are received and the type of stimuli received.

Table 9.2 illustrates that development is conceived as occurring in four major phases in the perceptual motor (sensory integration) literature. Table 9.3 shows a comparison of terms used to describe perceptual motor and psychosocial levels of development and symbol formation. Basically, the perceptual motor literature used the same terms to describe level state or phase and to describe symbol formation, whereas psychosocial literature uses five terms to describe levels of development and four terms to describe the development of symbol formation.

ANALYSIS AND CRITIQUE OF THE INTEGRATED THEORY MODEL
Frame of Reference

With the exception of Rene Spitz and A. J. Ayres none of the works or ideas is documented. Reference is made to cognitive perceptual motor development, neurobehavioral language, psychosocial development and ego functioning. Concepts include maturation, object relations, stages, discrimination, homeostasis and self actualization. It is evident that the models of development and psychoanalysis were used in part as frames of reference. Perhaps the models and concepts were more fully identified at the seminar but were not recorded in the summary. Nevertheless, the

Table 9.2
Approximate Sequence of Perceptual-Motor Development[a]

Phase I: Sensorimotor	Phase II: Integration of Body Scheme and Postural Bilaterality	Phase III: Discrimination	Phase IV: Abstract Thinking
Tactile perception	Body scheme development	Discriminative multisensory perception	Reading
Activation of vestibular mechanisms	Integration of function of the two sides of the body	Fine motor planning skills	Writing
Proprioception from muscles and related structures	Equilibrium skills and postural flexibility	Establishment of laterality	Number concepts
Visual perception	Gross motor planning skills		Ability to conceptualize
Auditory discrimination	Simple perception of form and space		Abstract thinking
Gustatory	Auditory perception		
Olfactory			

[a] Adapted from A. J. Ayres: Perceptual Motor Training for Children. *In Approaches to the Treatment of Patients with Neuromuscular Dysfunction*, Manual IV, WFOT Conference, 1962. Dubuque, Iowa, WC Brown Book Co, 1964. From reference 18, © 1968, *The American Journal of Occupational Therapy*.)

Table 9.3
Comparison of Terminologies between Perceptual Motor and Psychosocial Literature[a]

Levels	I	II	III	IV
Perceptual motor	Sensorimotor	Integration of body scheme	Discrimination	Abstract thinking
Psychosocial	Oral	Anal	Oedipal and latency	Adolescence
Symbol formation				
Perceptual motor	Sensorimotor	Integration of body scheme	Discrimination	Abstract thinking
Psychosocial	Pattern	Sign	Representation	Symbol

[a] Adapted from reference 18.

printed version is somewhat difficult to analyze with any degree of certainty.

Clarity

The assumptions are identified in some detail, although the impact on health and illness is not well defined. Also, of the several concepts mentioned, only three are defined. In some cases the concepts are not even used within a sentence structure which might provide some clue as to how the terms were being used. Because of the scant attention paid to concept definition, it is difficult to determine the relevance of the concepts to occupational therapy from the model itself. The author of the article points to the significance of such definitions, however, by stating that half of the week long conference was spent in defining concepts. It is regretable that the efforts were not recorded.

Uniqueness

The integrated model is useful in pointing out the concern of occupational therapists for the mind and body as integral systems of a functional whole. Concern for wholism is not unique to occupational therapy, but it is in contrast to the parts approach of the biomedical model. The model helps to point out that an occupational therapist cannot practice just physical disability occupational therapy or psychosocial occupational therapy. Such a division is consistent with biomedical practice but not with wholistic practice. Occupational therapists must understand the philosophy of practice as well as the techniques of practice.

Research Guide

As an integrated approach suggests, there is a continuum between mind and body as well as a developmental process. Research could clarify the relationship between physical, cognitive and social development. Another project could clarify the use of objects as facilitators to the three areas of development. A third project could be to illustrate the role of occupational therapy in increasing the amount of ego-free energy. An additional project is to explore how occupational therapy can help an individual make effective use of ego-free energy for mastery of the environment. A fifth project is to determine the relationship of stress to development, differentiation and integration of the mind and body. Finally a project could suggest how occupational therapy curricula can facilitate the integration of the mind-body issue to encourage monadic rather than dualistic thinking in occupational therapy students.

Specialization

Perhaps the significance of the integrated model is to warn against overspecialization without a firm understanding of the basic philosophy of occupational therapy. The participants apparently struggle with vocabularies developed from other disciplines which were not integrated sufficiently into the occupational therapy philosophy. Specialists must be careful that concepts borrowed from other disciplines are integrated into the occupational therapy language so that specialization of practice does not lead to division of the profession.

Elaboration and Refinement

According to the written summary of the seminar the participants wanted to put together an integrated theory of assumptions and concepts for occupational therapy. A major point of elaboration would have been to build an integrated philosophy before the theory-building process was attempted. The mind-body dichotomy is a philosophical issue, not a theoretical issue. A theory must be based on either monadism or dualism. It cannot use both. Philosophy issues should be settled before a theory or model of practice is begun. However, a model depicting philosophical differences could be useful to clarify a frame of reference based on one or the other philosophical opinions.

Refinement would be useful to continue the process of examining parallel vocabularies and concepts. An integrated vocabulary should facilitate model building and the development of theories for practice.

Explanatory Usefulness

As an explantory tool to others the integrated model is of limited use. It does not really explain the purpose of occupational therapy or even the process of development used as a frame of reference for occupational therapy practice. The primary usefulness of the model is as an internal guide to the struggle of creating a unified model or theory of occupational therapy as a professional and as a practice discipline.

Commonality

Probably the point of commonality with other professions is illustrated in the discription of the struggle to create the model. Other professions have had similar problems. Nursing has been perhaps most active in publishing its efforts at model and theory building, but other professions have had similar problems. Nevertheless, the integrated model is not particularly helpful in establishing areas of commonality in practice between disciplines.

Practice

The integrated model should be useful in building practice models in two ways. One is a negative example. Do not fail to clarify the philosophy and define the concepts. The other example is more positive. A developmental approach can be useful in explaining how function occurred during normal growth and how dysfunction can be alleviated through occupational therapy practice.

A summary of the integrated model critique is provided in Table 9.4.

HUMAN DEVELOPMENT THROUGH OCCUPATION—CLARK
Frame of Reference

The human development through occupation model appeared in 1979 and is based on an analysis and synthesis of four existing models according to the author (19). These are the adaptive performance, bio-

Table 9.4
Integrated Theory of Occupational Therapy Criteria Summary

Evaluation Criteria	Very Good 1	Moderately Good 2	3	4	Very Poor 5
Frame of reference				X	
Clarity			X		
Uniqueness			X		
Research guide			X		
Specialization			X		
Elaboration			X		
Usefulness				X	
Commonality				X	
Practice model			X		

development, facilitating growth and development and occupational behavior models. Adaptive performance is viewed as an integration of Fidler and Fidler and Mosey's models of "doing as being" and "recapitulation of ontogenesis" both of which stress the role of adaptive skill performance in learning to meet the requirements of daily life. Biodevelopment is used to describe the works of Ayres and others. It includes the variety of sensory integrative, neurodevelopmental, neurobehavioral and kinesiological theories and models. Facilitating growth and development is based on the work of Llorens, which focuses on the horizontal and longitudinal aspects of development in the physical, social and psychological parameters. The occupational behavior model is the work of Reilly and her students which examines the behaviors of work and play as the primary activities that occupy human time, energy, interest and attention. The model is discussed at the beginning of this chapter. The other models mentioned are discussed in later chapters.

Clark analyzes the four frameworks according to the art and science factors related to occupational therapy. Under the art of occupational therapy she reviews the focus of intervention, state of function, state of dysfunction and actions of the four frameworks (Table 9.5). The science of occupational therapy is examined through the types of research methods and validation procedures which are identified with the theoretical models.

Assumptions

Clark has identified the following assumptions:

VIEW OF MAN (20)

1. Man is an adaptive creator.
2. Human adaptation is distinguished by man's capacity to purposefully effect his own world of self, culture and environment.
3. The unique richness of this purposefully creative function is the product of two biological characteristics:
   a. the ability of the human brain to formulate and symbolize concepts

Table 9.5
Analysis of Four Theoretical Frameworks for Occupational Therapy[a]

Theory	Focus of Intervention	Art of Occupational Therapy			Science of Occupational Therapy: Research Validation
		State of Function	State of Dysfunction	Actions	
Adaptive performance Fidler and Mosey	Adaptive skills of doing Self-care Intrinsic gratification Service to others	Balance between skills and subskills promotes competence and efficacy	Imbalance due to influence of internal processes or external environment causes subskill deficits and problems of doing	Identify levels of functions in skills and subskills Provide shared learning experiences in life-work situations Promote subskill development	Descriptive/analytical criterion-referenced measurements Program plans
Biodevelopment Ayres, Rood, Bobath, King, Moore, Huss, Farber, Fiorentino	Developmental sequence of human biological processes	Integrative use of biological processes promotes adaptive skills Conceptualization Manipulation Socialization	Impairment of ability to process and act upon information received from the environment	Identify process deficits Use developmentally sequenced sensory motor activities, special techniques and equipment to normalize biological process	Descriptive/experimental Norm-referenced measurements Standardized measurement Program plan
Facilitating growth and development Llorens	Physical, social, and psychological parameters of human life roles, tasks, and relationships	Mastery of tasks and relationships necessary to engage in life roles	Stress, trauma, or disease affect performance or achievement of necessary behaviors	Role of change agent Controlled use of purposeful activity to stimulate role behaviors Developmental analysis of problems	Quasi-experimental Descriptive/analytical criterion-referenced measurements Standardized measurements Program plans Program modalities
Occupational behavior Reilly	Acquisition and performance of work and play behaviors	Self-directed achievement of role requirements	Internal and/or external forces impair capacity for participation and adaptation	Promote exploration and competency of role requirements through identification and development of functions, habits, skills, and task performance	Descriptive/analytical criterion-reference measurements Program plans

[a] Adapted from P. N. Clark (19). © 1979, *The American Journal of Occupational Therapy*.

  b. the ability of the human hands to translate concepts into action.
4. Man's awareness of these (creative) abilities primes the will for purposeful activities.
5. Man spends most of his time occupied in certain types of purposeful activities.
6. There is a recognized sequence to the emergence and primary engagement of such occupying activities.
7. Play is the anticipator and facilitator of subsequent goal-directed activities.
8. The behaviors acquired through playful exploration of the self, culture and environment serve as the bridge to adult competence and creative achievement.
9. Work provides the economic function of man in his world and the healthy state of man.

VIEW OF HEALTH (20)

1. Man's ability to direct and effect his own purpose in life can be seen as a most unique and primary indicator of his general well-being or health.
2. Man maintains health through a flexible balance of work, play and self maintenance activities which develop and change throughout the life-span.
3. In the healthy state, the individual is able to adapt and achieve a satisfactory life, function adequately in chosen personal, sexual, and occupational roles and enjoy a sense of well-being.
4. Healthy performance of roles is influenced by four major factors—biological endowment, maturation, cultural requirements and personal requirements.
5. Physiological characteristics account for a foundation of sensory integrative, motor and cognitive functions that permit the development of adaptive skills.
6. The interrelation between the individual and culture, physical space, and other environmental elements becomes increasingly complex throughout the life-span.
7. The individual must learn to effect a satisfying balance between meeting internal needs and adapting to external influences.
8. The human processes that develop through the interaction of internal and external forces provide a foundation of psychological and social functions.

VIEW OF THE PROFESSION (20)

1. Occupational therapy provides services that facilitate man's achievement of health through occupation in purposeful activities.
2. Occupational therapy must be relevant to the time, cultures and environments of the consumer's health needs.
3. The therapist's role is to assist the client with those adaptation processes necessary to promote a balanced, satisfying and productive life-style.

4. Occupational therapy must be directly related to each client's mastery of occupational roles.

Concepts (20)

Purposeful activities—the goal-directed use of a person's resources, time, energy, interest and attention.

Self maintenance—includes self-care, sleep, rest, recreation, and other activities directed toward preservation of the self and the species and the preparation for play and work.

Play—includes sensorimotor exploration and symbolic activities, such as drawing, dramatics, and games.

Work—includes education, vocational and home management activities.

Role performance—involves the use of selected purposeful activities, including the various skills, habits, tasks and relationships acquired through the acculturation of the individual.

Biological endowment—includes the various body systems, functions and genetic capacities which provide the individual with the potential to develop and learn a variety of skills.

Maturation—the hierarchical (change) of the basic (biological) components as the individual grows and accommodates to changing environments, assimilating new experiences and learning.

Cultural, spatial and temporal requirements—the elements that influence task performance.

Personal requirements—not defined, similar to above concept.

Occupational therapy—an applied health science concerned with the quality and satisfaction of daily living from birth to death.

The concepts of self maintenance, play and work are organized into a conceptual model as shown in Figure 9.3. The terms self-direction, productivity and purpose are not defined but appear to be outcomes or goals for the person to attain through the organization of self maintenance, play and work.

Expected Results

The following goals are listed in the reference text but do not agree with those in Figure 9.4 from the same article. The discrepancy is not explained. Also the goals tend to be stated as program goals and not as consumer goals. In other words, the lead statement is worded as the "program is designed to enable all consumers through the . . . " rather than the "consumer will be able to . . . " The difference is in generality vs. specificity in relation to the individual consumer. A well designed program may not meet an individual consumer's needs. An individualized program must meet the consumer's needs. Clark's stated results (20) are the following.

1. The *development* and *maintenance* of functions and skills necessary for performance of desired and/or required activities.
2. *Prevention* of inadequate development, deterioration, and/or loss of

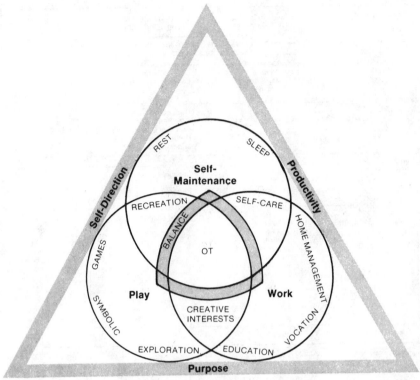

Figure 9.3. Conceptual model of the philosophy of practice. (Reproduced with permission from P. N. Clark (20), © 1979, *The American Journal of Occupational Therapy.*)

those functions necessary to engage in play, work, and the various self maintenance activities.

3. *Remediation* or rehabilitation of dysfunction that impairs acceptable performance of daily activities.

4. *Facilitation* of the consumer's adaptive capacity to influence and change their own health stage of life.

5. *Collaboration*, communication and cooperation in the planning and achievement of goals with the client and significant others in the client's life, including family and other service providers.

Assessment Instruments (20)

Clark has divided the assessment phase into four areas. These are:

1. General performance screening which involves the initial contact between the therapist and client to determine whether a client has problems in play, work, and/or self maintenance behaviors.

2. Basic assessment methods which include (a) observation within an uncontrived activity performance situation, (b) interview using care-

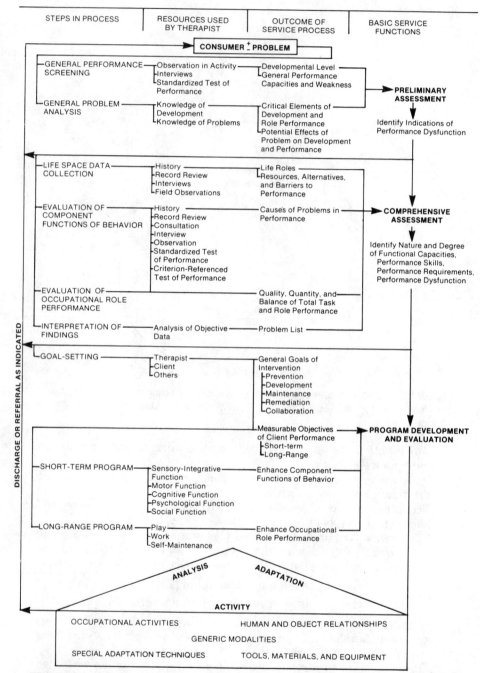

Figure 9.4. Conceptual model of the occupational therapy process. (Reproduced with permission from P. N. Clark (20), © 1979, *The American Journal of Occupational Therapy*.)

fully structured, open ended questions, unbiased observing, listening, and feedback, and (c) performance-based screening test to identify developmental level, general performance capacities, and weaknesses.
3. General problem analysis which is a thought process used by the therapist to guide preliminary planning.
4. Comprehensive assessment including:
   a. Life space data collection—thorough history taking, interviews and field observations from which the therapist defines the client's life roles and environmental, cultural and performance requirements.
   b. Evaluation of component functions of behavior—through standardized and criterion referenced tests of performance, functional capacity is evaluated to determine why a client has performance problems.
   c. Evaluation of occupational role performance—through the same techniques listed above, the therapist measures the client's abilities to perform specific activities required in daily self maintenance, work and play roles.

Intervention Strategies (20)
MEDIA AND MODALITIES
Clark lists occupational activities from work, play and self maintenance, relationships both human and object, tools, materials, and equipment, generic modalities, and special adaptations.

METHODS AND TECHNIQUES
Clark suggests the following.
a. Adaptive techniques, such as modification of activities to the position of the body or work surface
b. Simple to complex progression which is a method of manipulating the activity process
c. Step by step progress which is another method of manipulating the activity process
d. Changing expectation by altering the expectation of the client or significant others for independence in a specific task
e. Short-term program methods which are directed toward improving basic capacities of the five component functions of sensory-integrative, motor, cognitive, psychological and social function
f. Long-term programs which are concerned with promoting acceptable performance in required role activities related to play work and self maintenance

No equipment needs or prerequisite skills are stated.

Summary
The human development through occupation model is an example of a composite model which unites and is derived from four theoretical frameworks including adaptive skill, biodevelopment, facilitation of

growth and development and occupational behavior. The influence of the adaptive performance concept is most evident in the philosophy of practice and in the language of the conceptual model. Sequencing of program objectives and methods is based on the biodevelopment model. The basic structure of the assessment and planning process is organized from the Llorens model of growth and development. Finally the assumptions, concepts and designated categories of occupational activities that serve as the focus for intervention are drawn from the occupational behavior model as is illustrated in Figure 9.4.

The intervention process itself is concerned with the development, integration, adaptation, competence and initiative in task performance. Therefore, therapy is directed toward providing opportunity to enhance the individual's preparedness to deal with the requirements of daily living. Intervention strategies are the activities of daily living in the broadest sense. The processes of activity analysis and adaptation are the core functions of the occupational therapist. Together, these tools and processes of the discipline enable therapists to enhance the most human of abilities in their clients. Clark has summarized the model of practice in Figure 9.4.

ANALYSIS AND CRITIQUE OF THE HUMAN DEVELOPMENT THROUGH OCCUPATION MODEL
Frame of Reference

The unique aspect of this model is that the frame of reference is drawn from other occupational therapy models. Thus many of the core assumptions and concepts about occupational therapy are emphasized and reemphasized. Such a focus on occupational therapy models presents an opportunity to reflect on the central themes of occupational therapy as seen by the combined model builders.

Clarity

Although the selection of assumptions seems to summarize the philosophy of the four frameworks or models there are several concepts which are not described. These include adaptation, development, developmental task and occupation or activity. In the conceptual model of the occupational therapy process (Fig. 9.4) no definitions are provided for the terms balance, productivity or self-direction. In addition, the text does not address the relationship between self, productivity and purpose to self maintenance, work and play, although the model suggests a relationship. Are the former functional outcomes, or goals, of the latter? If so, what is the relationship of either to balance, which appears in the first ring around the center in Figure 9.3? Furthermore, in the analysis of the four models integration and mastery are listed as functions, yet they do not appear in the model.

Another problem is the failure to provide or account for a developmental process. Clearly development is a key concept to the composite model and to all four frameworks, yet no statements are made as to what developmental stages or levels actually occur. Only the four types of developmental change agents are mentioned.

These problems illustrate the difficulties in building a composite model. A composite model which selectively picks and chooses parts of the original model and ignores others leaves the reader wondering why certain parts were used but not others. A composite model should account for all major aspects of the original models by deliberate inclusion or a statement of rationale for exclusion.

Uniqueness

The uniqueness of the model is the attempt to unify four existing frameworks. Basicly the idea is a good one. The summary table (9.5) can be further uncluttered so that the key words are even more apparent (see Table 9.6). Such an analysis illustrates some repetitive themes. These are development, performance and active directed learning. Other possible similarities exist. For example, is it possible that balance and integration are the flip side of the coin to mastery and achievement? Thus the functions are really addressing the goal of creating a functionally adapted person who can meet the demands of the external environment and the needs of the internal (self) environment. If the goal is the functional adaptation, then differences in intervention are a matter of focus rather than being real indivisible differences. Further analysis could provide additional information about the unique aspects of occupational therapy which are common to all occupational therapy models.

Research Guide

The analysis provided in the section on Uniqueness should provide suggestions for research projects. Descriptive analysis could identify further the common themes among the occupational therapy models. Comparative techniques might illustrate where results and effects are similar or different. Finally, experimental designs might indicate which model is most useful with certain types of real or potential problems.

Specialization

A composite model can be very useful to anyone who specializes because the composite should indicate the most generic or common aspects of occupational therapy. If the model for specialization includes and addresses the generic aspects there should be less chance that specialization will cause the practitioner to stray from the practice of occupational therapy into another discipline. Thus, a good composite model should be useful to occupational therapists who specialize or limit their practice to certain selected populations.

Elaboration or Refinement

The primary direction of a composite model is usually toward refinement and remodeling. In other words, the composite model is based on a task of analyzing similarities and differences through the process of comparing and contrasting the various elements of the models against a

Table 9.6
Comparison of Occupational Therapy Models

Theory	Focus of Intervention	State of Function (Result)	State of Dysfunction (Effect and Cause)	Action
Adaptive performance Fidler and Mosey	Adaptive skills	Balance	Effect is imbalance Cause is internal or external environmental processes	Identify skill levels Promote subskill development Use learning experiences
Biodevelopment Ayres, Rood Bobath	Sensorimotor development	Integration	Effect is dysintegration Cause is impaired ability to process and act upon information from environment	Identify deficits Promote sensorimotor development Use learning experiences
Facilitating growth and development Llorens	Biopsychosocial development	Mastery of tasks	Effect is failure to master Causes are stress, trauma, disease	Identify developmental problem Promote needed behavior Use purposeful learning activity
Occupational behavior Reilly	Work-play acquisition and performance	Achievement of roles	Effect is failure to achieve Cause is internal and external forces which impair capacity	Identify development problems Promote exploration and competency Use learning experiences

set of issues or criteria. Table 9.5 shows the process of comparing and contrasting. However, the analysis of similarities and differences was incomplete. The common concerns were not identified completely and integrated successfully into one model. Thus the task remains available to others to try.

Explanatory Usefulness

The potential of a composite model to be useful in explaining occupational therapy to others is good because the most central or common aspects should emerge. Although the model of human development through occupation is incomplete as stated in previous sections of the critique the tasks of analyzing and synthesizing the major aspects of occupational therapy is a goal which should be pursued. An explanation of occupational therapy based on the composite similarities should be a useful communication vehicle.

Commonalities

The commonalities with other professions have been mentioned in the model as presented. Specific identification and relevance were not addressed since the explanation was aimed at occupational therapists themselves. Some of the areas of commonality are the concern for growth and development issues which lead to developmental delay, the concern for identifying effective intervention methods and programs and the concern for identifying useful research strategies. Many disciplines relate to these issues.

Practice Models

Application of a composite model to the practice of occupational therapy should provide the means to identify the central or common themes for assessment instruments and intervention strategies. The model of human development through occupation has identified the major assessment procedures used in occupational therapy. These are observation, interview and testing. However, in the process model (Fig. 9.4) examples of assessments rather than generic categories are listed which tend to muddy rather than clarify the role of assessment in occupational therapy.

Within the intervention process the model of human development through occupation provides some media and modalities, but the five items listed probably are not inclusive. Occupational therapy continues to have a problem in identifying its legitimate media and modalities. A summary of the human development through occupation model critique is provided in Table 9.7.

HUMAN OCCUPATION—KIELHOFNER

Frame of Reference

Kielhofner has based his model of human occupation primarily on the works of Reilly and the theory of occupational behavior. Other sources include the systems theory of Bertalanffy and Boulding, Bruner's analysis

Table 9.7
Human Development Through Occupation Criteria Summary

Evaluation Criteria	Very Good 1	Moderately Good 2	3	4	Very Poor 5
Frame of reference	x				
Clarity				x	
Uniqueness			x		
Research guide			x		
Specialization			x		
Elaboration			x		
Usefulness			x		
Commonality			x		
Practice model			x		

of play, Neff, Ginsberg, Super and Herzberg's theories of work, White's theory of competence, Buehler's stages of human development, and Clausen's concept of benign and vicious cycles.

The model of human occupation was published as a series of articles in 1980. It represents a third generation model in occupational therapy. Human occupation is based on the occupational behavior which is in turn drawn from the time-binding model of Adolf Meyer and the habit-training model of E. C. Slagle. As a third generation model human occupation has the unique distinction of being in a class by itself at the present time.

Assumptions

The model of human occupation has a number of assumptions which are as follows.

SYSTEMS

1. An open system exists in an environment (21).
2. An open system interacts with the environment by the process of input, output, throughput and feedback (21).
3. An open system is preserved through constant change (21).
4. The basic process that underlies change is a cycle (23).
5. Self-transformation of an open system is always hierarchical (23).
6. Adaptive change in a system is hierarchical in the direction of increased complexity and differentiation (23).
7. Trajectory of change is influenced by the internal characteristics of the system and the interaction with the environment (23).
8. The balance between successes and failures is a direct result of the match between the systems capacities environment (23).
9. No system can be evaluated or understood in isolation from its particular environment (23).
10. An environmental change is the surest way to effect permanent organization change in an open system (23).
11. Benign and vicious cycles provide a means of evaluating the quality

and results of a given trajectory and facilitates analysis of its features to guide planning for change (23).

12. Benign and vicious cycles involve both internal beliefs and external objective successes and failures (23).
13. A change in the system must begin with the volitional (conscious) subsystem (23).

MAN

1. Man is an open system, and his occupation is the output of that system (21).
2. Man creates his physical and symbolic environment at the time he learns to act competently in it (21).
3. Man, through the use of his hands as they are energized by mind and will, can influence the state of his health (from Reilly (5)).
4. There is a hierarchy for the organization of motives from exploration, and competency to achievement (22).
5. The nature of exploration is optimal for generating skills (22).
6. The motive of competency is optimal for organizing habits (22).
7. The motive of achievement is optimal for acquiring competent role behavior (22).

OCCUPATION AS A WORK-PLAY CONTINUUM

1. Occupation (work and play) is a central aspect of the human experience and is the essence of human existence (21).
2. Human occupation arises out of an innate spontaneous urge to explore and master the environment (21).
3. Temporality is a universal property of occupation (22).
4. The patterns of change in the human system are largely patterns of change in human occupation (21).
5. Society and culture are built upon and require human occupation for their maintenance (21).
6. The social organization of the human species is such that occupation mainly includes actions that exist on a continuum of play and work (22).
7. Play energizes change: work maintains the individual and the social group (22).
8. Within play, man organizes his behavior and initiates change in the self and society (22).
9. Play supports the work routine by recreating or regenerating energy to support the worker role (22).
10. Within work, man is productive for himself and maintains himself through self-care (22).
11. Within work, man is also productive for the social group and maintains the group through his labor (22).
12. Work has been the dominant feature of the human struggle for personal and group survival and the building of culture (22).
13. Work has a stabilizing effect on the daily life pattern (22).

14. Work is a principal factor in self-identity (22).

OCCUPATION AS A DEVELOPMENTAL CONTINUUM

1. There is a hierarchy of human occupations from volition and habituation to performance (21).
2. The performance subsystem is critical to the overall adaptation of the system and constrains the higher level subsystem (21).
3. The ontogenesis of occupation occurs throughout a life-long series of experiences which are shaped by internal choices and external social demands and expectations (22).
4. Since both play and work originate from the same global tendency toward exploration and mastery, they interrelate throughout the life-span (22).
5. The skill-building and rule-generating activity of play prepare the child for the student role and the adult world of work (22).
6. In childhood play the volitional subsystem is differentiated and organized, early habit structures are developed and organization of action into skills occurs (22).
7. The primary energizing force of adolescence is the urge to develop competence in adult roles (22).
8. The adolescent faces increased responsibilities and must shift from external control and dependence on parents to internal control and mature interdependence with others (22).
9. Adolescent play is characterized by devotion of time to personal hobbies, group games and social events (22).
10. Occupational choice is the major transition of occupational behavior that bridges the continuum from childhood play to adult work (22).
11. Occupational choice occurs in three periods: fantasy, tentative and realistic (22).
12. The adult period of life is characterized by the drive for achievement and is organized around procreative and/or productive roles (22).
13. The adult must achieve a sense of efficacy and the concomitant habits and skills for work role performance (22).
14. The exploratory phase reappears in the preparation for old age and retirement (22).
15. Successfully retired individuals can serve as role model for those in midlife (22).
16. In old age the model changes from active mastery to passive mastery (22).
17. The basic drive toward curiosity and effectance continue through adulthood to old age (22).
18. Successful retirement revolves around the ability to transfer to a daily life pattern in which leisure replaces work as a primary source of satisfaction (22).

OCCUPATIONAL THERAPY

1. Occupational therapy is founded on the idea that by engaging in occupation designed as therapy, man can restore, increase and maintain his ability as an occupational creature (24).
2. Occupational therapy taps a most powerful adaptive response: the ability to find challenge and meaning in one's daily undertakings, one's occupations (21).
3. Occupational therapy must embody the characteristics of purposefulness, challenge, accomplishment and satisfaction through occupation (24).
4. Occupational therapy should be conceptualized as an organizing process (24).
5. Occupational therapy should serve as an environment that can begin to present demands for performance and elicit the enactment of responses that can result in positive feedback (23).
6. Occupational therapy should begin at the lowest level of motivation in the volition subsystem, exploration, and the lowest level of behavior organization, skill (23).
7. Occupational therapy should be directed toward enabling man to fulfill his unmet need for occupation and the rich and varied stimuli that solving life problems provides him (24).

Concepts

Environment—the physical, social and cultural setting in which the system operates, such as external objects, people and events (21).

Human occupation—the interaction of the system (man) with the environment (21).

Systems terminology (see Fig. 9.5)

Output—consists of the mental, physical and social aspects of occupation (21). It includes both information and action (22).

Input—information that comes into the system from the environment (21).

Throughput—the internal organization process (21).

Hierarchy—refers to laws that explain how a system is organized along a continuum of increased complexity over time (22).

Occupations hierarchy (see Fig. 9.6)

Volition—the highest level of human occupation which governs the lower subsystems and consists of innate and acquired urges to act toward exploration and mastery (motivational structures). Action is freely and consciously chosen (21).

Habituation—the middle level of human occupation which includes the components that arrange behavior into patterns of action. Represents automatic and routine behavior (21).

Performance—the lowest level of human occupation which consists of the basic capacities for action (skills). Governs small patterns of skilled action (21).

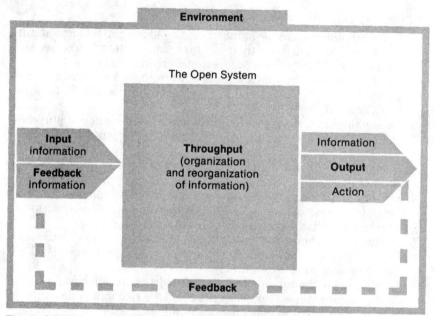

Figure 9.5. The open system. (Reproduced with permission from G. Kielhofner and J. P. Burke (21), © 1980, *The American Journal of Occupational Therapy*.)

Hierarchy of products (see Fig. 9.7)

Personal causation—refers to the image of the self as a competent or incompetent actor (21).

Valued goals—commitments to action based on pleasure associated with past experiences and future possibilities. They reflect the external realities of society and culture (21).

Interests—preferences for action based on pleasure associated with past experience and future possibilities. They reflect the unique aspects of occupations (21).

Internalized roles—the entire set of required behaviors that go along with occupying a position in a social group (21).

Habits—automatic routines which repeat certain actions. They structure the use of time to achieve more efficacy in daily occupational performance (21).

Skills—consist of flexibly organized and interrelated component actions that lead to the accomplishment of a purpose or goal under variable environmental conditions (21).

Occupational role—refers to the productive roles that determine the bulk of daily routines and thus organize most of the behavior within the system (21).

Rules—contain information about how to interact successfully with the environmnt to achieve certain ends (21).

Pawn—a person who does not believe he is in control and does not actively see environmental challenges that would allow mastery (21).

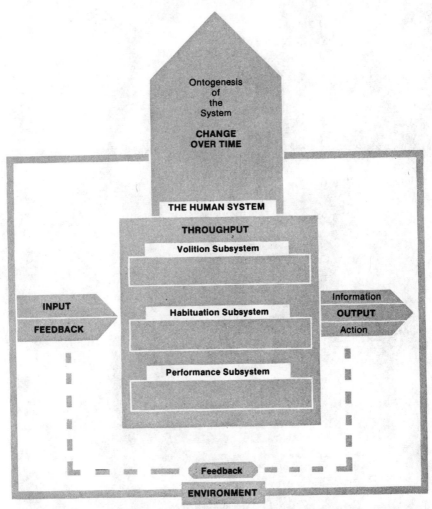

Figure 9.6. The system and its environment. (Reproduced with permission from G. Kielhofner and J. P. Burke (21), © 1980, *The American Journal of Occupational Therapy*.)

Origin—a person who sees himself in control, strives to explore and master the environment and seeks out challenges (21).
Trajectory—the directional change of a system (23).
Innate characteristics—the urge toward exploration and mastery of the environment (23).
Learned characteristics—those performances and abilities that result from experience (23).
Benign cycle—one that results in a trajectory that supports adaptation (23).
Vicious cycle—one in which the system does not satisfy its own internal

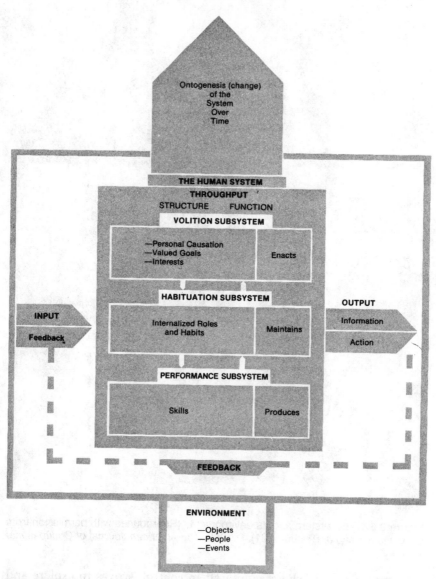

Figure 9.7. A model of human occupation. (Reproduced with permission from G. Kielhofner and J. P. Burke (21), © 1980, *The American Journal of Occupational Therapy*.)

urge to explore and master and does not fulfill the demands of society (23).

Adaptation—includes meeting environmental requirements and yields personal satisfaction (23).

Expected Results

According to the model of human occupation the client should gain through occupational therapy intervention some or all of the following:

1. Increased skills and skill action.
2. Developed habits and routines.
3. Developed and organized the behaviors involved in role behavior.
4. Identified interests.
5. Acted on goals.
6. Increased sense of competence and personal causation.
7. Increased ability to problem solve and make decisions.

These results are based on the author's interpretation of the volition, habituation and performance subsystem products and outcomes. Results are not well defined or delineated by Kielhofner.

Assessment Instruments (24)

The major areas to be evaluated are the components of the volitional, habituation and performance subsystems. These include personal causation, values, interests, internalized roles, habits, and social, cognitive and physical skills. The information may be collected through observation or interview using a variety of instruments. Examples are given in Table 9.8.

After the data are collected it should be evaluated to determine if a benign or vicious cycle exists. The interpretation is based on the person's history of experience, environmental circumstances and internal makeup (24).

Intervention Strategies

The intervention strategies are not well developed in the model as yet. Table 9.9 provides an outline of intervention based on the author's analysis of examples given for treatment (24).

Summary

The structure and content of the human occupation model are based on the open systems and developmental models. Interaction of an open system with the environment is achieved through the process of input, output, throughput and feedback. The innate features of the human occupation system are proposed to be the basic urge to explore and master the world which is expressed through work and play.

The human occupation model proposes three subsystems each of which serve a different purpose. First is the volition subsystem which guides the choices of action through personal causation, valued goals and interest. Second is the habituation subsystem which is composed of habits and internalized roles. Habits and roles function to maintain action. Third is the performance system which functions to produce action through skills such as social, cognitive and physical.

The process of ontogenesis is proposed to describe the change in the system over time. Change in the system is the result of the interaction

Table 9.8
Assessment Outline[a]

Subsystem	Example	Test Example
Skills	Movement	Reflex and motor assessments
	Perception	Visual perception test
	Coordination	Mechanical ability test
	Symbolic function	Decision-making inventory
	Self-care skills	ADL checklist
Habits	Self-care habits	ADL interview
	Chores—household	Interview
	Time management	Time and activities inventory
	Tool use	Observation
Roles	Family member	Interview
	Player	Occupational history
	Student	Adolescent role assessment
	Preworker	
	Worker	
	Home manager	
Interests	Use of free time	Interest checklist
	Leisure activities	Play history
		Interview
Values	Use of free time	Interest checklist
	Leisure activities	Play history
		Interview
Personal causation	Self-control	Observation

[a] Adapted from S. H. Cubie and K. Kaplan: *American Journal of Occupational Therapy* 36:646, 1982.

of the three subsystems to produce motives. These motives are first, exploration then competency and finally achievement. Exploration produces skills, competency produces habits and achievement produces roles. In each stage of life, childhood, adolescence, adulthood and aging, the process of change which occurs through the subsystems is repeated in order to organize behavior and to meet environmental demands (see Fig. 9.8). The same process is necessary to learn to cope with disability.

Occupational therapy can be useful in the transition from one stage to another to help the person acquire new interests, valued goals and habits. Finally, occupational therapy may help the person reorganize the system to facilitate adaptation to the environment and restore a normal course of occupational ontogenesis. Occupational therapists assess the quality of the change in terms of the trajectory or direction of the behavioral cycle. In the benign cycle the individual is determined to be competently performing the occupational requirements of the environment and is satisfied with the performance. In a vicious cycle, neither the external demands nor internal satisfaction is being met.

According to Kielhofner *et al.* (24), the model serves to guide treatment by (a) identifying critical concepts that should be attended to in evalua-

Table 9.9
Outline of Intervention Strategies

Media and modalities
  Games
  Arts and crafts
  Social and cultural events
  Play
  Meal preparation
Methods, techniques or approaches
  Structured play
  Recommendations to join organized groups such as scouts, education courses
    or volunteer organizations
  Job hunting and interview techniques
  Problem-solving and decision-making situations
  Time organization and management
  Work efficiency and energy conservation techniques
  Leisure activity planning
Equipment
  Assistive devices
  Adapted equipment
  Tools for crafts
Prerequisite skills
  See examples under the skills section in Table 9.8

tion, (b) proposing how behavior is organized and thus providing a framework for identifying disorganization of behavior, (c) positing a sequence of change that characterizes adaptation and can be used to organize therapy, (d) proposing the concept of career with stages of change in human occupation which serves as a standard in assessment, and (e) providing an exploration of function and dysfunction in the concept of benign and vicious cycles, which allow for explanation of a system's failure to adapt and serves as a guide for planning the reorganization of the system in therapy toward a benign cycle.

CRITIQUE AND ANALYSIS OF THE HUMAN OCCUPATION MODEL
Frame of Reference

The frame of reference is based on values and beliefs which are consistent with occupational therapy and have been used as the basis for other models. The human occupation model actually is an expansion and elaboration of occupational behavior model by Reilly.

Clarity

In general the assumptions are much more complete than in Reilly's model, except in the area of health as it relates to man and occupation. The only item is drawn directly from Reilly. No expansion or additions are offered. Most of the concepts are explained more adequately than in Reilly's model, but such terms as problem solving, purposefulness, satisfaction, and productivity remain unclear.

The Balance of Work and Play

	Work Yields	Relationship of Play & Work	Play Yields	Waking Hours Occupied By Work & Play
CHILDHOOD	Productive behaviors are practiced through chores and in school.	**Exploration** Skills for productivity are acquired and work roles explored through imitation and imagination.	Reality is explored via curiosity for rules of competent action.	Time spent in play
ADOLESCENCE	The work role is practiced and the commitment process of occupational choice takes place.	**Competency** Personal and interpersonal competency are developed in a matrix of co-operation yielding habits of sportsmanship & craftsmanship.	Competent behavior is learned and experienced in games, personal hobbies, and social events.	
ADULTHOOD	There is entry into worker roles with the requirement of establishing and maintaining a productive and self-satisfying career.	**Achievement** Play supports the worker roles by providing an arena of retreat and rejuvenation. Exploration in novel situations allows the ongoing development of new competency for work.	Relaxation and recreation support the worker role. Exploration of novel situations allows new roles to be taken on.	Time spent in work
OLD AGE	Retirement brings reduced expectations for productivity and personal capacities for productive action are waning.	**Exploration** Retirement leisure signals that the productive obligation to society has been fulfilled. Past work has earned for the person the right to leisure. Leisure replaces work as the major source of life satisfaction.	Play allows the exploration of past achievements and the unknown future, and maintenance of competence through leisure pursuit of interests.	

Figure 9.8. The balance and interrelationship of work and play during the lifespan. (Reproduced with permission from G. Kielhofner (22), © 1980, *The American Journal of Occupational Therapy*.)

The major problem occurs when the systems model and developmental model are combined but not integrated. Thus, the concepts are not clear in terms of an age, stage or level. For example, at what age does the occupations hierarchy develop and change? Does the function change? How does the need or motive and output categories relate to the occupations hierarchy? In addition, no information is provided about a terminal goal. It is also unclear what need or motive operates the volitional system, and what the output of the performance and volitional systems are. Furthermore Michelman (25) has suggested that exploration and manipulation can be differentiated as aspects of play. Manipulation satisfies tactile and emotional impulses or needs, while exploration permits the experimentation with materials to discover their potentials. Perhaps manipulation should be added as a concept. These concerns are summarized in Figure 9.9

The problems expressed in the previous paragraph illustrate the difficulty in model building when two different models and their techniques, systems and development, are used to put together a single model. Concepts which fit well in one model technique become incomplete or inadequate when used in another modeling technique. Model building is hard work.

Uniqueness

The human occupation model continues the assumption that occupation is the central core of occupational therapy as an area of study as well as an applied discipline. Using a systems model complemented by a developmental model, the human occupation model presents the hierarchy of occupational subsystems, functions and motivations. Therapy becomes, therefore, a process of identifying the real or potential problem areas and providing a correctional program beginning at the lowest level of difficulty and progressing upward to the higher levels. Although these ideas were present in the occupational behavior model, they are much better described in the human occupation model and thus facilitate the documentation of the unique service of occupational therapy as well as the unique assumption.

Research Guide

The human occupation model should provide an excellent model for guiding research. The hierarchy and developmental processes should be confirmed and the structural element in the subsystems should be expanded to provide better information on which to develop assessment instruments and propose intervention strategies.

Specialization

There appears to be no problem in using the human occupation model in various areas of specialization. The model uses a developmental continuum which includes all age groups. The addition of aging is an improvement over Reilly's model. Diagnostic group specialization is not a problem, since the focus is on occupational roles and not on signs and symptoms.

Age	Occupations Heirarchy	Input	Structures	Functions	Need or Motive	Output	Terminal Goal
Aging	? Volition	Information from the physical social cultural environment and feedback	? Interests Valued goals Personal causation	? Enacts	Exploration (Mastery of occupations)	Leisure (Self-care work-play functional independence)	? (Adaptive behavior)
Adult	Habituation		Roles	(Develops) Maintains	Achievement	Occupational roles	?
Adolescence			Habits		Competency	Occupational choice	?
Child	Performance		Skills Motor Sensory Cognitive Intrapersonal Interpersonal	Produces	Exploration and (Manipulation)	(Occupational preparations)	?

Figure 9.9. Overview of problems in the occupations model. Items in parentheses added by author as possible items.

Elaboration and Refinement

The model provides many opportunities for elaboration and refinement. There is a need to expand the assessment and intervention areas and to refine the concepts so that the model ties together as a practice-oriented approach.

Explanatory Usefulness

The concept of a hierarchy of subsystems which supports occupational behavior is perhaps the most useful explanatory idea. Such an idea expands the explanation of occupations as the central aspect of occupational therapy by illustrating the skills, habits and roles that are necessary to develop and maintain occupational behavior. Further, the model suggests how values, interests and personal causation influence the selection of and participation in specific occupational behaviors.

Commonality

The hierarchy of subsystems is recognizable to any professional group which has used the systems approach to build models. Skills and routine habits are behaviors which are recognizable to most professions. For example, nurses and physical therapists are familiar with self-care activities. They may not, however, think about the importance of maintaining self-care routines as well as maintaining self-care skills as individual units. Educators and vocational counselors are concerned with occupations. They also may be unaware of the need to develop occupational roles starting with player, chore doer and family member in order to provide the preparatory skills and habits to support an occupational choice.

Practice Models

The model should provide excellent material for developing better practice approaches, such as assessing and identifying patterns of occupational dysfunction or developing specific techniques which are cost-effective in helping people learn or redevelop skills, habits, interests or values. A summary of the analysis and critique appears in Table 9.10.

ADAPTIVE RESPONSES—KING

Frame of Reference

Adaptation as a frame of reference is based on the works of Konrad Lorenz, Niko Tinbergen and Rene Dubos, all of whom are biologists concerned with the role of adaptation in species and individual survival. Individual adaptation in relation to activity is based on the work of Abraham Maslow in motivation and needs, the work of J. P. Zubek in sensory deprivation and the work of Hans Selye on stress. King's model of adaptive responses was presented as the Eleanor Clarke Slagle lectureship in 1978. Although the model is designed to provide a framework for practice, no assessment strategies are mentioned, and only an incomplete list of intervention strategies is given. Thus the model is incomplete at this time, but does provide the initial steps on which to build a practice model(s) and thus is included in the review of generic models.

Table 9.10
Model of Human Occupations
Criteria Summary

Evaluation Criteria	Very Good 1	Moderately Good		Very Poor 5
		2	3	4	
Frame of reference	x				
Clarity		x			
Uniqueness	x				
Research guide			x[a]		
Specialization	x				
Elaboration	x				
Usefulness	x				
Commonality	x				
Practice model	x				

[a] Model too new for adequate evaluation.

Assumptions

VIEW OF MAN AS AN INDIVIDUAL ADAPTOR (26)

1. Adaptation demands of the individual a positive or active response as opposed to a passive or inactive response.
2. Adaptation is called forth by the demands of the environment and the challenge of the individual to make an adaptive response.
3. Adaptive responses are most efficiently organized subcortically below the conscious level.
4. Adaptive responses are self reinforcing, and each response serves as a stimulus for more complex environmental challenges.
5. Sensory input is the raw material for adaptation at any age.
6. The negative effects of sensory deprivation on the maintenance of adaptive responses are cumulative.
7. Loss of sensory input or inability to deal with the stress of change can reduce the effectiveness of adaptive responses and cause disadaptation or maladaptation.
8. Changes within the person demand that the individual alter habitual responses.
9. Adaptation (after stress) means the possibility of actualizing potential that would otherwise be wasted.

VIEW OF THE PROFESSION (26)

1. Occupational therapy deals with purposeful behavior: with people doing.
2. Purposeful behavior is inextricably woven into the total fabric of human function, including biochemical, psychological, social, economic, or ecological man.
3. The adaptive process constitutes the core of occupational therapy.
4. The specific attributes of adaptation are also the significant and characteristic attributes of occupational therapy.

5. The basic characteristics of an activity used in occupational therapy are:
   a. It requires an active response by the client.
   b. It responds to specific environmental demands, such as needs, tasks and goals.
   c. Its effects are organized most efficiently below the level of consciousness.
   d. It is self reinforcing, with each successful adaptation serving as a stimulus for the next more complex environmental challenge.
6. In purposeful activity, the activity itself is an end, as well as being a part or means to a larger end. Therapy or adaptation, thus, is the result of double motivation.
7. Unless the organism is completely exhausted, activity of some sort is much more appropriate to dissipate stress than too much rest.
8. Facilitating adaptive development that is sensory integrated improves coping behaviors.
9. Activity helps to metabolize stress hormones and thus increases the client's feeling of well-being.

Concepts

Evolutionary adaptation—refers to changes in the structure or function of an organism or any of its parts, that result from the process of natural selection.

Individual adaptation—refers to adjustments made by the individual that primarily enhance personal rather than species survival and secondarily contribute to actualization of personal potential.

Double motivation—motivation of the activity itself and motivation toward health or an adaptive goal.

Purposeful behavior—that which people are doing or engaged in during most of their working years.

Purposeful activity—tasks, including crafts, or other goal-directed activities, such as play that focuses attention on the object or outcome.

Disadaptation—failure of organization and response.

Maladaptation—sensory data is organized incorrectly, and therefore the response is inappropriate.

Stress management or stress reduction therapy—making available to patients, purposeful, goal-directed activities that allow the patient to make an adaptive response to stress.

Adaptational therapy—the use of physical and mental activities to dissipate accumulated tensions which result from stress hormones and their physiological effects.

Adaptive process—the means which are involved in man's active acquisition of knowledge and techniques.

Adaptive response—eliciting goal-directed or purposeful behavior.

Occupational therapy—consists of structuring the surroundings, materials and demands, of the environment in such a way as to call forth a specific adaptive response.

Expected Results

King primarily emphazises the importance of assisting the client to make adaptive responses which meet the individual's needs and the environmental demands.

Assessment Techniques

None are mentioned.

Intervention Strategies

The use of crafts and play are the only two media mentioned. Under methods, King discusses the use of adaptive responses, developmental learning sequences and stress-reducing activity in some detail. Adaptive equipment, work simplification, splinting, sensory integration and development of strength and skill are mentioned. Equipment and prerequisite skills are not discussed.

ANALYSIS AND CRITIQUE OF THE ADAPTIVE RESPONSE MODEL
Frame of Reference

The frame of reference appears to be consistent with the values and beliefs of occupational therapy. Information is drawn from some of the key people in the area of adaptation. However, the concept of adaptive response is only one of many related concepts in the area of human adaptation. Others include adaptive levels, adaptive mechanisms, adaptive modes, and a variety of problems in adaptive behavior. Models of occupational therapy will need to address these other issues as well.

Clarity

King's explanation of an adaptive response is useful primarily in evaluating a given medium, task or activity. If the response from the client is an active one which is goal-directed, facilitates integration and is self reinforcing, then the medium, task or activity qualifies as eliciting an adaptive response which facilitates mastery. These concepts are organized into a model (see Fig. 9.10).

King does not specify whether the adaptive responses are innate or learned. Assuming that adaptive responses are learned, King does not state how they are learned. Dubos (27) suggests that creative responses require making deliberate choices. His term "creative responses" sounds similar to King's adaptive response. A creative response is described as goal-oriented and involving the conscious participation of the organism as a whole. Assuming that the concepts are similar, the process of making choices implies learning through problem solving and decision making. Thus, adaptation in general and adaptive response behavior specifically is learned rather than being innate. The issue of innate vs. learned is important because innate behavior appears to be difficult to modify or change, whereas learned behavior appears to be more amenable to modification or change through the efforts of therapy, for example.

King also does not specify why adaptive responses are needed. Klein-

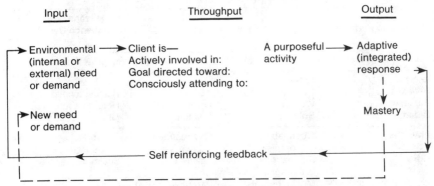

Figure 9.10.   A systems model of an adaptive process.

man and Buckley (28) suggest that adaptive responses are a part of a continuum. The adaptive continuum is a range or hierarchy of responses which increases in the degree or level of consciousness, duration and complexity (see Figs. 9.11 and 9.12) Adaptive responses are preceded by homeostatic reactions which are externally evoked and are involuntary responses. Dubos (27) says that such adaptive mechanisms are better suited to conditions of the past than to those of the present. For the most part homeostatic reactions are unconscious and innate.

After the adaptive responses come adaptive skills which involve a combination and repetition of a variety of adaptive responses. Finally there are adaptive patterns which represent a constellation of skills that contribute to an adaptive life-style. These four levels have been identified further in Table 9.11.

In addition, King does not specify when or where adaptive responses are needed. According to Dubos such responses are needed when and wherever a homeostatic response is inadequate. Homeostatic responses are likely to be inadequate to meet many sociocultural demands and may be inadequate to meet some physical demands. As an example, Dubos suggests the problem of a physical agent or situation which is a product of modern technology such as an odorless gas or toxic, man-produced chemical. Adaptive responses are more likely to be adequate in meeting such social and physical problems because the individual can consciously decide on the direction of personal health instead of leaving it to chance.

Finally, at some point it may be necessary to answer the question as to how many adaptive responses or adaptive skills are needed. The answer depends on the terminal outcome or goal. Is the terminal outcome to be functional independence, achievement, autonomy, mastery, competence or some thing else? It is important to remember that goal-directed behavior can be interpreted four ways. These are (a) individual goals, (b) medical goals, (c) social goals and (d) therapist goals. Although congruence of the four would be ideal, the reality may be something less. Table 9.12 outlines the factors which may produce a problem, adjustments

Capacity to Perform	Performance		Constellations of Performance Over Time
Homeostatic Reactions►Adaptive Responses ►	Adaptive Skills ►		Adaptive Patterns
(e.g.) Reflexes Blushing Breathing	(e.g.) Catching a ball Wedging clay Solving a puzzle	(e.g.) ADL Driving a car Reading	(e.g.) Raising a child Holding a job Going to college
Physician Nurse Physical therapist	Occupational therapist Recreational therapist Music therapist	Occupational therapist Teacher Parent surrogate	Vocational counselor Social worker Clinical psychologist

Figure 9.11. Adaptation continuum. (Reproduced with permission from B. L. Kleinman and B. L. Buckley (28), © 1982, *The American Journal of Occupational Therapy*.)

which can be made through occupational therapy and possible goal selection.

Uniqueness

Adaptive response as a concept is presented by King as a unique aspect of occupational therapy. However Kleinman and Buckley (28) pointed out that other therapists, such as music, recreation, drama, art or dance therapists, could be considered to be promoting, developing, increasing or maintaining adaptive responses. These therapies are not included, however, under the category of adaptive skill. In other words, occupational therapists are concerned with both aspects of performance, while other professionals are concerned with one or the other aspects of performance (Table 9.13). Still other professions are concerned with the capacity to perform or the constellation of performance over time. Further differentiation within the adaptive skills subcategory can be made by stating that occupational therapists work primarily with abnormal or at risk populations and not as much with normal populations which are served by teachers or child care workers. Further differentiation within the adaptive response category can be made between those professions that use only one medium or modality and occupational therapists who use multiple media and modalities.

Research Guide

The concept of adaptive responses should be useful in sorting out which media or techniques belong in occupational therapy. The four criteria of an adaptive response can be used as a guide for evaluation and a guide for modification wherever a modality or technique could be applied passively but can be adapted to permit more active participation.

Other research questions suggested by Kleinman and Buckley are:

1. How can the organizing effect of purposeful activity be described and measured?

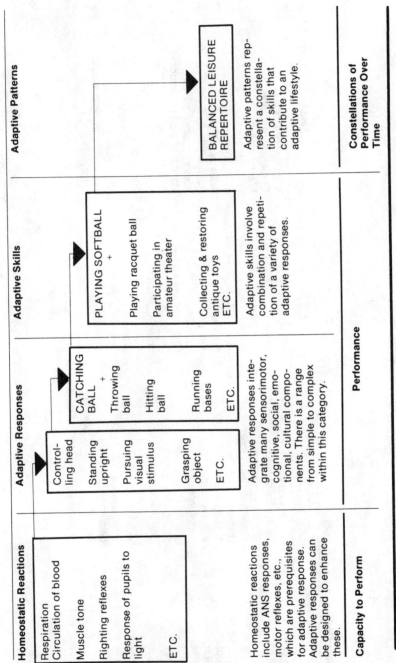

Figure 9.12. Adaptation continuum: Example. (Reproduced with permission from B. L. Kleinman and B. L. Buckley (28), © 1982, *The American Journal of Occupational Therapy*.)

Table 9.11
Adaptive Continuum[a]

Homeostatic Reactions	Adaptive Responses	Adaptive Skills	Adaptive Patterns
Reflexes	Performance areas	Automatic behavior	Vocation practiced
Reactions	Motor responses	Chaining	Employment status
Tone	Sensory responses	Routines	Marital status
Respiration	Cognitive responses	Habits	Parental status
(involuntary)	Intrapersonal	Roles	Religious affiliation
Heart beat	responses	Rituals	Political affiliation
Digestion	Interpersonal	Values	Racial affiliation
Circulation	responses	Attitudes	Socioeconomic status
Temperature		Rote memory	Place and type of residence
control	Occupational areas:		Sibling status
	Self maintenance	Combined behavior	Health status
	responses	ADLs	Age status
	Productivity	Work	Educational status
	responses	Play/recreation	Life-style
	Leisure responses		Community service status
			Family affiliation

[a] Adapted from B. L. Kleinman and B. L. Buckley: *American Journal of Occupational Therapy* 26:17, 1982.

Table 9.12
Adaptation Factors Related to Outcome or Goal Attainment Through Occupational Therapy[a]

Forces or Potential Problems	Adjustment Modifications Use in Occupational Therapy	Outcomes or Goals
Physical environment Biopsychological environment Sociocultural environment	Physical modifications a. Use adapted equipment b. Eliminate architectual barriers c. Redecorate, rearrange, remodel existing structure Biopsychological modifications a. Change old or learn new skills, habits, roles, values b. Learn to plan and organize, problem solve, make decisions c. Invent, construct, create new ideas or things Sociocultural modifications a. Change or modify customs or norms b. Start or participate in social groups	Survival Function independently or autonomously Become competent Achieve mastery Develop adequate self concept Conserve energy, time or space Improve the quality of life Meet individual needs Meet sociocultural demands Meet environmental situations

[a] Adapted from J. F. Murphy: *Theoretical Issues in Professional Nursing.* New York, Appleton Century Crofts, 1971, p. 51.

Table 9.13
Professional Roles in the Adaptive Continuum[a]

Capacity to Perform:	Performance		Constellation of Performance Over Time:
Homeostatic Reactions	Adaptive Responses	Adaptive Skills	Adaptive Patterns
Physician	Occupational therapist	Occupational therapist	Vocational counselor
Nurse	Recreational therapist	Teacher	Social worker
Physical therapist	Music therapist	Child care worker	Clinical psychologist
Medical technologist	Art therapist		
Radiologic technologist	Drama therapist		
	Dance therapist		

[a] Adapted from B. L. Kleinman and B. L. Buckley (28).

2. What precisely is the mechanism that produces the beneficial effect of specific adaptive responses?
3. Are there other consistent qualifiers of adaptive responses than those King identified?
4. Are there states of the individual that are consistently conducive to adaptive responses?
5. What is the key to the self reinforcing mechanism that perpetuates the response?
6. What is the relationship between attention and interest and the fatigue factor?
7. What is the nature or kind of disadaptive or maladaptive response?
8. What is the relationship of stress to adaptive responses?

Specialization

The model of adaptive responses as presented by King should be useful to practitioners in terms of analyzing media and methods to be sure that the essence of occupational therapy is maintained. The expanded model of the adaptive continuum developed by Kleinman and Buckley should be useful in delineating the tasks and outcomes which occupational therapists attempt to achieve. All occupational therapists should find such information useful, regardless of the specialized nature of the individual therapist's practice.

Elaboration and Refinement

King referred to two types of adaptation in her article: evolutionary and individual. Actually there are three types of biological adaptation of which two relate to individuals. According to Lasker (29) the three types are evolutionary events, individual growth and behavioral and physical change. The concept of adaptive responses can be elaborated by analyzing the two types of individual adaptation. One type relates to growth and the other relates to behavior and physiological changes within the person. A summary of levels, modes, characteristics, effects and examples is provided in Table 9.14. The important points to elaborate are the use of adaptive responses in facilitating plasticity as long-term, not reversible change and acclimatization as a short-term, reversible change. The question not answered by the information is whether adaptive responses work in the same way for both or whether the processes are different.

Refinement is needed in the concepts of disadaptation or maladaptation. Specifically there is a need to examine the types and causes of poor adaptation. Again the focus is primarily on individual adaptation. Thus environment can be used as a central point of orientation. Tables 9.15 and 9.16 list some of the possible types and causes of problems in adaptation. The examples are drawn from the literature on low stimulus situation, role stress, and cultural change. No attempt has been made to make the examples comprehensive but only to provide a framework for discussion.

Table 9.14
Types of Biological Adaptation[a]

	Evolutionary Events (Species)	Individual Growth (Individual)	Behavioral and Physiological Changes (Individual)
Levels	Selection of genotype	Ontogenetic modification	Physiological and behavioral events
Modes	Selection	Plasticity	Acclimatization
Characteristics of modes	Defines inherent capacities—not reversible	Occurs during the growth period—not reversible	Occurs throughout life; is reversible
Effect	Changes in gene pool produce change in structure and function	Change and modification occur during growth and development	Change and modification occur through short-term periods
Examples	Genetic change Cultural change Biochemical change	Maturation Enlargement Differentiation of function	Adjustment to: Altitude Heat and cold Nutrition Learning situations?

[a] Adapted from G. W. Lasker (29).

Table 9.15
Examples of Possible Types and Causes of Problems in Individual Adaptation

Types of Adaptational Problems	Physical Causes	Biopsychological Causes	Sociocultural Causes
Breakdown	Earthquake Sudden catastrophe	Trauma Acute disease Total immobilization	Move to a new culture Total loss of support system
Reduction	Famine Increasing catastrophe	Chronic disease Aging Partial immobilization	Insufficient change within person to meet new demands or needs
Loss	Seasonal crop failure Technological change	Disease or trauma affecting specific body system Change in motivation	Failure to use known skills Lack of alternative skills
Inadequate/incomplete	Partial continuous famine Inadequate shelter	Sensory or perceptual distortion	Adherence to old values or beliefs
Failure to learn	Incompatible with life unless protected by others	Failure to discriminate or generalize	Lack of opportunity Lack of role model
Maladaptive	Incompatible with life	Hereditary, congenital disease Sensory deprivation Distorted reality	Inappropriate role model and social skill development

Table 9.16
Working Definitions of Adaptational Problems

Breakdown	Person has been successful in initiating adaptive responses and appropriate coping mechanisms but suddenly is unable to respond or cope with demands from the environment.
Reduction	Person has been successful in initiating adaptive response and using appropriate coping mechanisms but gradually is less able to respond or cope with demands from the environment.
Loss	Person has been successful in initiating adaptive responses and using appropriate coping mechanisms but now is unable to respond to or cope with some specific demands but can respond to and cope with other demands.
Inadequate/ incomplete	Person is partially able to initiate some adaptive responses and use some appropriate coping mechanisms, but either the response is inadequate to the situation or the coping mechanism is incomplete.
Failure to learn	Person has not learned to initiate a repertoire of adaptive responses and does not know which coping mechanisms are appropriate in given situation and thus cannot respond to or cope with demands from the environment in specific or general situations. Also cannot meet individual needs.
Maladaptive	Person initiates responses which are not adaptive and uses inappropriate coping mechanisms and does not respond to or cope with demands from the environment in an effective or acceptable manner in specific or general situations.

Table 9.17
Adaptive Response Model Criteria Summary

Evaluation Criteria	Very Good 1	Moderately Good			Very Poor 5
		2	3	4	
Frame of reference	x				
Clarity			o[a]	x	
Uniqueness		o	x		
Research guide		o	x		
Specialization	x				
Elaboration		o	x		
Explanation		o	x		
Commonality	x				
Practice model			x		

[a] With data from B. L. Kleinman and B. L. Buckley (28) included.

Explanatory Usefulness

The concept of adaptive responses by itself may be difficult for many to understand. Explanation with the adaptive continuum proposed by Kleinman and Buckley (28) should be more helpful in explaining occupational therapy to others. However, adaptive responses and the adaptive process are highly abstract constructs. Explanations need to be based on more concrete concepts and examples. Such ideas as learning through doing or accomplishing a goal are easier to grasp. The use of adaptive responses is more helpful to occupational therapists than to others in furthering the development and understanding of occupational therapy.

Commonality

The term "adaptive responses" is not a particularly common one in other professions. However the term "adaptation" is known widely. Nurses, for example, discuss adaptation at some length. Roy (30) has proposed a model on adaptation for nursing. Thus, as a general goal, adaptation probably is well known and can provide a common thread to other disciplines. Perhaps more effort should be made to include the concept of individual adaptation as a general outcome or goal of occupational therapy in presentation and articles addressed to other disciplines. At the same time, however, the term "adaptive response" will require more careful explanation to avoid potential confusion.

Practice

Adaptive response as a concept in practice should be useful in evaluating all media and methods. As such the concept can be included in a variety of practice models. Thus the major role of adaptive response in theory building is as one of several concepts. On the other hand, the concept of an adaptive continuum could be used as a major organizing idea with a model or theory. Further analysis of disadaptive or maladaptive behavior could enlarge the role of adaptation and adaptive response in occupational therapy practice. A summary of the adaptive response model is provided in Table 9.17.

References

1. Reilly M: A psychiatric occupational therapy program as a teaching model. *Am J Occup Ther* 20:61–67, 1966.
2. Meyer A: Philosophy of occupation therapy. *Arch Occup Ther* 1:6,1922.
3. Reilly M: The education process. *Am J Occup Ther* 23:299–307, 1969.
4. Reilly M: *Play as Exploratory Learning.* Beverly Hills, Calif, Sage, 1974.
5. Reilly M: Occupational therapy can be one of the great ideas of 20th century medicine. *Am J Occup Ther* 16:1–9, 1962.
6. Woodside H: Dimensions of the occupational behaviour model. *Can J Occup Ther* 43:11, 1976.
7. Shannon PD: Work adjustment and the adolescent soldier. *Am J Occup Ther* 24:112, 1970.
8. Shannon, PD: The work-play model: a basis for occupational therapy programming in psychiatry. *Am J Occup Ther* 24:215, 1970.
9. Florey, L: Intrinsic motivation: the dynamics of occupational therapy theory. *Am J Occup Ther* 23:322, 1969.
10. Florey, L: An approach to play and play development. *Am J Occup Ther* 25:275, 1971.
11. Wolman, BB: *Dictionary of Behavior Science.* New York, Van Nostrand Reinhold, 1973.
12. White, R: The urge toward competence. *Am J Occup Ther* 25:273, 1973.
13. Chaplin, JP: *Dictionary of Psychology,* rev ed: New York, Dell, 1975.
14. English, HB, English, AC: *A Comprehensive Dictionary of Psychological and Psychoanalytical Terms.* New York, McKay, 1958.
15. Moorhead, L: The occupational history. *Am J Occup Ther* 23:329, 1969.
16. Matsutsuyu, J: Occupational behavior—a perspective on work and play. *Am J Occup Ther* 25:292, 1971.

17. Gray M: Effect of hospitalization on work play behavior. *Am J Occup Ther* 26:180–185, 1972.
18. Mazer J (Ed): Toward an integrated theory of occupational therapy. *Am J Occup Ther* 22:451–456, 1968.
19. Clark PN: Human development through occupation: theoretical frameworks in contemporary occupational therapy practice, part 1. *Am J Occup Ther* 33:505–514, 1979.
20. Clark, PN: Human development through occupation: a philosophy and conceptual model for practice, part 2. *Am J Occup Ther* 33:577–585, 1979.
21. Kielhofner, G, Burke, JP: A model of human occupation. Part I. Conceptual framework and content. *Am J of Occup Ther* 34:572–581, 1980.
22. Kielhofner, G: A model of human occupation. Part II. Ontogenesis from the perspective of temporal adaptation. *Am J of Occup Ther* 34:657–666, 1980.
23. Kielhofner, G: A model of human occupation. Part III. Benign and vicious cycles. *Am J of Occup Ther* 34:731–734, 1980.
24. Kielhofner, G, Burke, JP, Igi, CH: A model of human occupation. Part IV. Assessment and intervention. *Am J Occup Ther* 34:777–88, 1980.
25. Michelman, S: The importance of creative play. *Am J Occup Ther* 25:289, 1971.
26. King, LJ: Toward a science of adaptive responses. *Am J Occup Ther* 32:429–437, 1978.
27. Dubos R: Health and creative adaptation. *Hum Nature* 1:74–82, 1978.
28. Kleinman, BL, Buckley BL: Some implications of a science of adaptive responses. *Am J Occup Ther* 36:15–19, 1982.
29. Lasker GW: Human biological adaptability. *Science* 166:1480–1486, 1969.
30. Roy C: *Introduction to Nursing: An Adaptation Model.* Englewood Cliffs, NJ, Prentice Hall, 1976.

CHAPTER 10

Descriptive Models: Basic Elements

TIME MODELS
Philosophy of Occupation Therapy Model—Meyer
FRAME OF REFERENCE

Dr. Meyer believed that many persons suffering from mental disorders had problems in organizing and performing the habits of daily living (1). He felt a program that would organize daily life patterns would be helpful. However, he found that the idea of putting patients to work was viewed as a means of relieving employees and saving administrators money. Neither of these were part of his idea of treatment. In occupation workers (early occupational therapists) he found the type of person who could organize work and play for the benefit of patients by structuring time (2).

Meyer found also that the philosophy of the 1900s did not concur with his values of work and time. He was encouraged to see the rise of energetics "application of work" and behaviorism with its emphasis on performance replace the interests of thought, reason and fancy which he considered to be a step to action but not the same as actual performance based in reality.

Meyer does not state the sources of all of his ideas. Some are mentioned in passing. These are a Professor Ostwald, a scientist of energetics, Pierre Janet, an early neurologist; Herbert Hall, an early supporter of occupational therapy; Cassimer J. Keyser and Alfred Korzybski, philosophers, who were interested in time binding as a human activity. Perhaps more important was Meyer's own skill of observation in his own work as an alienist. Alienists were part-time pathologists and part-time psychiatrists in the state hospitals. Later Meyer developed a theory of psychiatry called psychobiology which stressed the holistic functioning of the individual within the person's environment (3). His work on history taking as an assessment tool is recognized today.

ASSUMPTIONS

All assumptions are from reference 2.

Assumptions about Man

1. The whole of human organization has its shape in a kind of rhythm.
2. The body is a live organism pulsating with its rhythm of rest and activity.
3. Man is an organism that maintains and balances itself in the world of reality and actuality by being in active life and active use.
4. There are values of reality and actuality.
5. Man must be able to balance work, play, rest and sleep.
6. Balance is attained by actual doing, actual practice.

Assumptions about Time

1. Man has the capacity to use time with foresight based on a corresponding appreciation of the past and of the present.
2. The great feature of man is his sense of time, with foresight built on a sound view of the past and the present.
3. Mental life is the integrator of time.
4. The human organism uses, lives and acts its time in harmony with its own nature and the nature about it.
5. Man learns to organize time, and he does it in terms of doing things.
6. There is a development of the valuation of time and work.
7. Human ideas (should) include religious valuation of actual time and its meaning in wholesome rhythms.
8. Time comes and comes and only waits to become an opportunity used.
9. The proper use of time in some helpful and gratifying activity appears to be a fundamental issue in the treatment of any neuropsychiatric patient.

Assumptions about Occupation and Performance

1. There should be a blending of work and pleasure.
2. The best of reality and actuality is real performance.
3. Performance is its own judge and regulator and therefore the most dependable and influential part of life.
4. Performance and completion are the backbone and essence of realization of reality.
5. Personality is fundamentally determined by performance.
6. It is the use that we make of ourselves that gives the ultimate stamp to our every organ.
7. Man today has lost the capacity and pride of workmanship and has substituted for it a measure in terms of money.
8. Work and play, ambition and satisfaction (should not) lose their natural contact with the natural rhythms of appetite and gratification, vision and performance, and finishable cycles of completion of work and play and rest and sleep.

Assumptions about Health

1. Many diseases are largely problems in adaptation.
2. Psychiatrists recognize the need for adaptation and the value of work as a help in the problems of adaptation.
3. Mental problems are problems of living and not merely diseases of a structural and toxic nature or constitutional disorder.
4. Habit deterioration presents a serious problem.
5. The systematic engagement of interest and concern about the actual use of time and work is an obligation and necessity in dealing with habit deterioration.

Assumptions about Occupational Therapy

1. Occupational therapy takes resourcefulness and an ability to respect at the same time the native capacities and interests of the patient.

2. Occupational therapy which tries to do justice to special human needs can serve as the center of a great gain for the normal as well as the sick.
3. Occupational therapy should be concerned with awakening a full meaning of time as the biggest wonder and asset of our lives.
4. Occupational therapy should be concerned with the valuation of opportunity and performance as the greatest measure of time.

CONCEPTS (2)

Occupation—should be free, pleasant, profitable, including recreation and any form of helpful enjoyment

Rhythm—includes heartbeat, night and day, sleep and waking hours, hunger and gratification, *i.e.*, work, play, rest and sleep

Performance—the complete full-fledged activity which disposes of the situation. Into this executive ability go all the preliminary point-steps which serve in an orienting and activating capacity, including sensing, feeling, thinking, planning, imagining and habit resources

Habit—essential fabric of the creative resources of the organism. The doing of things forms the basic structure of mental life

Habit formation—a process that applies to every item of human behavior

Disorganization of habits—the deterioration of the learned but fundamental ways of meeting life

Time—not defined, involves the use of past, present and future as well as the 24-hour day in organized habits of work, rest, play and sleep

Appreciation of time—not defined, involves being aware of the relationship of work and time

Balance—not defined, involves maintaining the rhythms and cyles of life such as work, play, rest and sleep or hunger and its gratification

Opportunity—not defined, involves giving chances and allowing for choice as opposed to prescribing for patients

Reality—not defined, involves actual doing and performance as opposed to thought or feeling

Adaptation—not defined, involves being able to perform in society and to have organized habits

Achievement, pride or pleasure in—not defined, involves completion and pleasure in doing work or occupation

Doing, practice—the opposite of thought, feeling and fantasy

EXPECTED RESULTS (INCENTIVES)

1. A pleasure in achievement.
2. A real pleasure in the use and activity of one's hands and muscles.
3. A happy appreciation of time.
4. Obtain performance wherever it has failed to come spontaneously.
5. Give satisfaction of completion.

ASSESSMENT TECHNIQUES

None are mentioned.

INTERVENTION STRATEGIES

1. Media and modalities

   Those mentioned include raffia, bookbinding, metalwork and leatherwork.
2. Methods, techniques and approaches

   a. Select simple tasks not requiring too big movements and uncontrollable excitement.

   b. Produce things that are finished in one or a few sittings and yet have an independent emotional value.

   c. Give opportunities rather than prescription

3 & 4. Equipment needed and prerequisite skills are not discussed.

SUMMARY

Meyer felt that time should be organized to create a balance of work, play, rest and sleep for patients suffering from disorganized habits (Fig. 10.1). He stated that time was to be valued because it provided a natural wholesome rhythm to life and could be measured in terms of opportunity to perform an actual performance. Opportunity was important because it permitted planning and creation as opposed to prescription. Performance was important according to Meyer because actual doing, completing, and achieving were based in reality as opposed to dreams and fantasy (Fig. 10.2). Meyer's ideas provided the first model of practice in occupational therapy.

Habit Training Model—Slagle

FRAME OF REFERENCE

Habit training was based on Meyer's concept of organizing work, play, rest and sleep as a means of treatment for schizophrenic patients with disorganized habits. The idea also is supported by work of William James (4), a psychologist who felt that "habit diminishes the conscious attention with which our acts are performed." In other words, habits become automatic. Thus, the training program for patients was aimed at reestab-

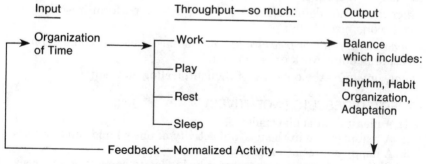

Figure 10.1. Model of time organization.

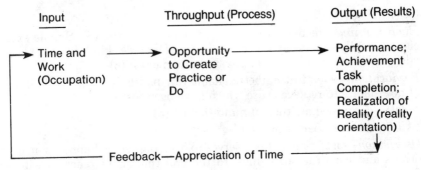

Figure 10.2. Time and work occupation model.

lishing an automatic or habit-forming schedule of activities including occupation and leisure recreation.

ASSUMPTIONS ABOUT HABIT TRAINING

1. Reeducation follows the same growth and development as normal education (5).
2. There is no general habit or general form common to all mankind, only individual habit and memory (5).
3. Regression of habits, interest, coordination and attention generally goes back to the period of life of the patient in which he or she was comfortable and happy (5).
4. We are all creatures of habit (5).
5. The key to the program is motivation (5).
6. Habit training is the first step in therapeutic, economic and social reconstruction (5).
7. In habit training, "directed activity" is a fundamental and basic principle (6).
8. For the most part, our lives are made up of habit reactions (7).
9. In habit training, it is necessary to build on the habit of attention (7).

ASSUMPTIONS ABOUT OCCUPATIONAL THERAPY

1. Occupational therapy should be emphasized as early as possible to forestall a deteriorating habit (6).
2. Programs for both mental and nervous patients must incorporate work, play and entertainment essentials (6).
3. Both in work and play there must be an outlet for physical energy; therefore, a balance program means much in the way of play and exercise (6).
4. Habit training is the first step in a program which also includes Kindergarten and Occupational Center (curative workshop) (7).
5. Occupational therapy program includes habit training, ward classes and occupational centers (8).

CONCEPTS

Habit training—reeducation in decent habits of living (5). Simple exercises carefully supervised and often repeated includes kindergarten methods, graded exercise, manual, physical and mental (8)

Reeducation—substituting better habit (for bad habits) or the building of new habits to replace those which have been lost (5).

Ideals—continued attitude of mind (habit) (5)

Skill—a habit of performance (5)

Occupation—used remediately, serves to overcome some habits, to modify others and construct new ones, to the end that habit reaction will be favorable to the restoration and maintenance of health (7)

EXPECTED RESULTS

1. The reclamation and rehabilitation of the patient
   a. To return the patient to the community if possible or
   b. To make him a more acceptable member of the hospital community (5)
2. Resulting economic advantages
   a. The patient becomes less destructive and untidy. The saving on clothes destroyed and laundry.
   b. Requires less care and supervision (5)
3. To arouse confidence and interest (6)
4. To help reestablish courage (6)
5. To round out the old mental order of things (6)

ASSESSMENT TECHNIQUES

Assessment is accomplished by a review of the person's chart and observation. The following items are considered good indicators for success in habit training (5).

1. Patients should not be over 35 years of age. Younger patients are more easily adjusted to new types of work.
2. Psychosis should not be of more than 15 years duration from date of onset.
3. Patients should be in reasonably good physical health, although malnutrition, unless caused by chronic disease, need not bar patient from class.
4. History of patient should show that fair grade of intelligence was present before psychosis (this would exclude defectives).
5. Patient should understand and speak English.
6. Patients who are mute, but appear to understand simple orders, can be included.
7. Patients with vicious tendencies, those who require tube feeding, should be excluded.
8. Patients who wet and soil are not be be excluded unless these features are due to organic or physical defect, or unless these habits

exist to such a degree as to become constantly annoying to others in the class.
9. Patients with active delusions and hallucinations of a persecutory nature should be excluded. Such patients generally resist attention, scold and upset the morale of the class. Simple hebephrenic types offer the greater possibilities of improvement by habit training.

Reassessment occurs in about 6 months. If no change has been observed then the person is discharged from the group and another is selected.

INTERVENTION STRATEGIES
1. Media and modalities—the following are taught in the Syllabus (5).
   a. Scrapbook cover
   b. Paper beads
   c. Knitting
   d. Rake knitting
   e. String and card work
   f. Knotting and netting
   g. Raffia baskets
   h. Hooked rugs
   i. Braid weave rug
   j. Braided rug
   k. Figure of eight rug
   l. Basketry
   m. Woodwork
2. Methods
   a. The primary method is the 24-hour schedule which includes work, play, rest and sleep in organized sequences (Tables 10.1 and 10.2).
   b. Within the schedule a graded program of activity can be included to accommodate changes in responsiveness and ability.
3. Equipment and mechanics—it is recommended that a separate building be used for the group of about 20 patients. The environment should be "normal, cheerful home atmosphere" (5).
4. Prerequisite skills—outlined in the initial assessment criteria.

SUMMARY
According to Slagle, the ultimate plan and purpose of habit training "is to establish a well balanced day in which work, games, and recreation play such an important part that gradually the substitution of a new interest in life will crowd out many fixed ideas and will establish a normal attitude of mind" (9). Habit training is based on the belief that habits form the major portion of human behavior and health and that they are learned and can be relearned. In practice, persons with disorganized habits are placed in a group where the schedule of events is planned for each 24 hours in a repetitive but not monotonous pattern. The program

Table 10.1
The Twenty-four Hour Schedule[a]

9:30–11:30 a.m.: Have patients go to toilet; glass of water. Class work, occupational therapist and attendant on duty:
  Cutting out pictures.
  Making scrapbook.
  Spool knitting.
  Knit wash-rags and rugs.
  Crochet very simple fillet patterns.
  Crochet rugs and face cloths.
  Crochet shoe strings.
  Simple raffia work, as baskets, napkin rings, picture frames, etc.
  Tear and sew carpet rags.
  Color pictures with colored crayons.
  Braid carpet for rugs.
  Simple patch work.
  Plain sewing and mending.
  Several patients may be able to perform the same kind of work. It may be necessary to choose some particular kind of work from the above list for certain patients. The thing to do is to get them interested in some form of useful employment, and gradually advance them to more complicated tasks.

11:30–11:45 a.m.: Putting up work; each patient assisting. A box or paper bag with each patient's name on it should be provided.

11:45–12 noon: Prepare patients for dinner. Have them go to toilet, wash their hands and faces, clean their nails and tidy hair.

12:00–12:30 p.m.: Dinner.

12:30–1:15 p.m.: Scrub teeth (those able). Rest in ward.

1:15–2:30 p.m.: Toothbrush drill, consisting of the usual movements with toothbrushes in the practice of brushing teeth. Each patient should have her own toothbrush. This can be kept in box or bag.

2:30–3 p.m.: Have patients go to lavatory and drink a glass of water; empty bladder. Tidy up and go out on lawn.

3–3:30 p.m.: Physical instructor on duty. Simple gymnastic exercises on lawn. In inclement weather on porch, or open ward windows and put patients through exercises in ward.

3:30–4:30 p.m.: Folk dancing or games, tossing bean bag, catching ball, throwing rings, etc.

4:30–5 p.m.: Nurse on duty. Take patients to toilet. Rest. Make tidy for supper.

5–5:30 p.m.: Supper.

5:30–8 p.m.: Music in ward, gramophone, piano, dancing; singing if possible.

8 p.m.: Take patients to toilet. Brush teeth and hair. Retire.

11 and 2 p.m.: Toilet for bed-wetters.

For the Better Grade of Patients

1:30 p.m.: Wednesday afternoons, moving pictures; also attend other afternoons when special pictures are shown.

2 p.m.: Monday afternoons. Community singing in assembly.

3 p.m.: Alternate Thursday afternoons. Vaudeville show when given.

2 p.m.: Tuesday afternoon. Dancing, assembly hall.

Monday and Thursday mornings. Bathing.

[a] Reprinted from E. C. Slagle: *Journal of Mental Science* 80:643, 1934, with permission from *The British Journal of Psychiatry*.

Table 10.2
Habit-Training Schedule for Juvenile Cottages[a]

6:30–7 a.m.: Rising hour. Wash, comb hair, toilet, teach patients to clean teeth, to use mouth wash occasionally and to dress properly. Pride in personal appearance must be stimulated. Patients to drink a glass of water before breakfast. Put beds in order and tidy up room.
7–7:45 a.m.: Breakfast.
7:45–9 a.m.: Toilet, get ready for school, put clothes in order.
9–10:15 a.m.: School. Simple academic ungraded school work.
10:15–10:30 a.m.: Toilet and get ready for physical training.
10:30–11:20 a.m.: Folk dancing, exercises, etc.
11:20–11:45 a.m.: Outdoor games and recreation; free play.
11:45–12 noon: Toilet; get ready for dinner; glass of water.
12–12:30 p.m.: Dinner.
12:30–1:30 p.m.: Toilet. Rest 30 minutes. Get ready for afternoon school.
1:30–3 p.m.: School. Simple handwork, adapted to fit individual children's needs; variety is especially essential. Glass of water.
3–3:15 p.m.: Toilet.
3:15–4:20 p.m.: Exercises, outside games, etc.
4:20–4:45 p.m.: Make beds; get dormitory ready.
4:45–5 p.m.: Toilet; get ready for supper. Glass of water.
5–5:45 p.m.: Singing, free play. Get ready for bed. Toilet.
7 p.m.: Bed.
Each child has definite duties assigned, according to individual abilities.

[a] Reprinted from E. C. Slagle: *Journal of Mental Science* 80:644, 1934, with permission from *The British Journal of Psychiatry.*

of habit training was the first of a three part program which included ward occupations and an occupational center.

Temporal Adaptation—Kielhofner

FRAME OF REFERENCE

Kielhofner has drawn upon the work of Meyer and Slagle as a base for developing further the concept of time as a basic element in the use of occupation and application of occupational therapy to assist people in overcoming problems of living. Summarizing the influence of Meyer and Slagle, Kielhofner states that the occupational therapy "received the proposition that in the richness of man's daily routines and his purposeful use of time, there was both health-maintaining and health-regenerating potential" (10).

ASSUMPTIONS

Temporal adaptation also draws upon the occupational behavior model of Reilly. Thus, there are similarities of assumptions and concepts with Kielhofner's human occupation model. They are repeated to provide a better understanding of the temporal adaptation model as a basic element in the process and practice of occupational therapy.

Kielhofner has stated seven propositions which he feels can be used to generate approaches to the evaluation and treatment in occupational therapy based on the concept of time (10). These are:

1. Each person bears a temporal frame of reference that is culturally constituted.
   a. A temporal frame of reference is maintained and transmitted in the form of norms and values.
   b. In American society, the notion of time is that of straight line or path extending into the future.
   c. The American culture values time as a commodity which can be bought, sold, saved (positive value) or wasted (negative value).
   d. The American culture uses time as something that can be sectioned off into segments which are to be filled with activities.
   e. American sense of time is expressed in scheduled events, orderliness and punctuality.
   f. Random behavior that lacks a pattern of organization is not functional in the mainstream of American society.
2. A unique temporal frame of reference is accumulated through learning and socializing experiences that begin in childhood.
   a. There are three levels of social learning, related to time: technical, informal and formal.
   b. Children learn time concepts through teaching, modeling, precept and admonition.
   c. Children learn how and when to behave at certain times and what to expect of time.
3. There is a natural temporal order to daily living organized around the life space activities of self maintenance, work and play.
   a. There is a natural rhythm in the organization of daily life around life space.
   b. Life space is assigned to activities that represent a social order, determining appropriate time for role behavior.
   c. Daily life can be divided into three life spaces, existence, subsistence and discretionary time.
   d. Recreation and leisure comprise dual aspects of play in adult life.
   e. Homeostasis describes the biological health of the organism while balance in daily life describes the conditions for psychosocial health.
4. Society requires its members to organize their use of time according to ascribed social roles.
   a. Individual daily patterns must be organized around occupational roles.
   b. Life spaces are filled according to the occupational roles in which they are assigned.
   c. Within the daily routine an individual's life space may be divided between several occupational roles.
   d. Adaptation requires individuals to use their time in a manner that supports their roles.
   e. The organization of time around one's roles is not static, and occupational roles change and overlap within a lifetime.

    f. Taking on a new role requires a new strategy for organizing one's time.

    g. When role change is abruptly forced upon an individual through an incurred disability, developing new temporal skills is a critical factor in adapting to the disability.

5. An individual's use of time is a function of internalized values, interests and goals.

    a. Values are established by an internal order of what comes first and how much time will be allotted to various activities.

    b. The individual's values set priorities of actions, and the consequences create a personal valence that is ultimately translated into a life-style.

    c. Interests sustain action and serve to maintain commitment over time.

    d. Values and interest yield automatic goal setting and consequent adjustment and organization of daily patterns of time use.

    e. The process (of goal setting and organizing daily patterns) is necessary for ordering daily life.

    f. An individual must be able to identify and execute appropriate actions for goal attainment.

    g. Lack of goals or goal setting leads to frustration or helplessness.

    h. Problems arise when an individual cannot identify and carry out proper sequences of activities that lead to successful goal attainment.

6. Habits are the basic structures by which daily behavior is ordered in time and psychosocial health is maintained.

    a. All that is familiar, routine and predictable in daily life bears a relationship to habit.

    b. Habit structures an individual's daily life.

    c. Habits are the products of one conscious choices which have been organized into unconscious routines.

    d. Habits affect actions related to values and interests cemented over time in daily patterns.

    e. Habits contribute to adaptation by organizing societal requirements for competence.

    f. Habits assure that skills are used in an adaptive manner.

7. Temporal dysfunction may exist in relationship to categories of pathology.

    a. Temporal dysfunction may occur as an integral part of some mental illness or as a consequence of imposed physical disability.

    b. Some problems include disorientation in time, distortions of the preception of time, and disorganization of time.

    c. Disorientation is associated with amentia, senility or psychotic disorder.

    d. Distortions of the perception of time occur in some cases of mental illness.

    e. Disorganization of time is associated with nonfulfillment of social roles, a subjective sense of helplessness and incompetence in mental illness.

f. In physical disability, disorganization is associated with an inability to maintain the pace of life and to find new meaningful activities and roles to replace old ones.

CONCEPTS

Temporal adaptation—is the integration of an entire spectrum of activities, the organization of which supports health on an ongoing daily life basis

Temporal dysfunction—refers to problems that arise in this daily life organization

Technical time—learning to tell time and comprehend the division into seconds, minutes and hours

Informal time—learning the activities and mannerism of daily life associated with acting in time

Formal time—learning the expectations and prohibitions of traditions and values associated with time

Existence time—life space spent for eating, sleeping, personal hygiene, and other aspects of self maintenance

Subsistence time—life space devoted to working

Discretionary time—life space reserved for recreation and leisure

Recreation—is the period of time when man is made ready for the next cycle of work through relaxation

Leisure—is earned time made possible by the satisfying performance of work

Health—consists of the proper balance of life spaces that is both satisfying to individuals and appropriate for their roles within society. It comprises an interrelated balance of self maintenance, work and play

Balance—an interdependence of life spaces and their relationship to both internal interests, and goals and external demands of the environment

Occupational behavior—the sum total of man's activity within the life spaces

Values—commitments to action that organize an individual's use of time

Interests—state of readiness for choices and actions

Goals—represent strategies toward the fulfillment of values and interests

Habits—are instantaneous, automatic choices of time made throughout the day

Disorientation in time—person does not know the day, month or year

Distortions of time—not defined, concerned with speeding up or slowing down of the passage of time

Disorganization of time—person is unable to organize time or function at the pace of time to fulfill social roles

EXPECTED RESULTS

1. Identify and pursue short-term objectives toward an overall goal.
2. Maintain a satisfying daily schedule that balances work, play and self maintenance.
3. Organize time around the necessary role of being a worker or other occupational role.
4. Reconstruct the self image through successful experiences in areas related to past interests.
5. Explore new activities to develop interest.
6. Reconstruct daily routine to accommodate different life spaces.
7. Refocus career goals to a viable and acceptable objective.

ASSESSMENT INSTRUMENTS—GUIDELINES

1. Collect information on several variables.
2. Consider internal constraints on time as revealed in the nature of patient's physical, mental or emotional disability.
3. Consider the external factors influencing time use, such as the patient's roles, family expectations, cultural background, and demands of time and physical space.

INSTRUMENTS

No examples given.

INTERVENTION STRATEGIES

Not stated.

SUMMARY

The model of temporal adaptation is an attempt to update the concept of time, rhythm and balance of Meyer and the habit structuring of Slagle. Temporal adaptation includes some current assumptions about the significance of time to American culture, how time is learned, how it is organized, how it is used in society and how it is used by individuals in society (Fig. 10.3). The model also addressed the role of time in maintaining health and the impact of time in certain problems of health (Fig. 10.4).

Because time is a basic element of human existence, the significance of time is pervasive in the acquisition and performance of occupation. The actual significance of problems in time management should not be overlooked in the application of occupational therapy to individual problems.

Temporal Adaptation Practice Model—Neville

FRAME OF REFERENCE

Neville (11) has provided an example of practice model in temporal adaptation based generally on Kielhofner's concept of temporal adaptation. She was interested particularly in time distortions and their effect on future time perspectives and adaptation. The assumptions and concepts were not altered.

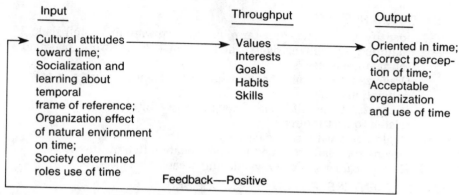

Figure 10.3. Model of temporal adaptation.

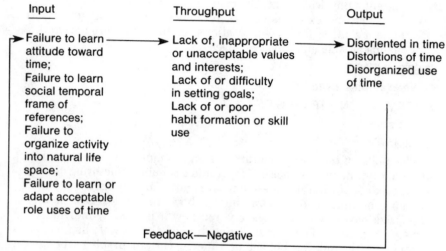

Figure 10.4. Model of temporal dysfunction.

EXPECTED RESULTS

1. Indicate how time is spent outside the hospital.
2. Classify activities in relation to work, play and self-care.
3. Identify a need for change.
4. Formulate goals for oneself.
5. Organize these goals into priorities.
6. Formulate specific activities to accomplish these goals.
7. Begin working on these activities.

ASSESSMENT INSTRUMENTS

An activity history is used as part of the initial evaluation in occupational therapy, but the name or example was not provided.

IMPLEMENTATION

1. Media
   a. Vocational tests
   b. Work evaluation
   c. Leisure activities
2. Methods
   a. Planned activity followed by discussion
      1. "Pie of life"—circle divided into 24 sections representing hours. Patients were instructed to fill in each section as to how time was spent prior to hospital and to code and count number of hours spend in each activity. Discussion involved stating satisfaction with how time was spent or what changes the individual wanted to make.
      2. Laken's (12) steps to time management were used to emphasize goal setting.
   b. Suggested activities
      1. Time questionnaires
      2. Story completions
      3. Future biographies
   c. Suggested programs: Modules on work, leisure and self-care
3. Equipment—not stated
4. Prerequisite skills—not stated

SUMMARY

The patient who is assigned to the time management group is selected according to intake information which indicated difficulty in managing leisure and work time before hospitalization. The first task is to complete a "pie of life" which is a circle divided into 24 equal sections corresponding to the 24 hours in a day. Each patient is instructed to fill in the pie by accounting for a day's activity prior to hospitalization. Different types of activities are color-coded on the pie, counted into hours and then recorded. Upon completion of the pie, the patient is asked to indicate if the time was spent satisfactorily or if there are changes the patient would like to make in the use of time. Based on the changes which are identified, goals are established and activities initiated.

Neville suggests further that the entire occupational therapy program could be structured around the use of time and activity modules. Evaluations and intervention methods could include time questionnaires, story completions and future autobiographies. Programs could be developed according to self-care, work and leisure models. Patients would attend those modules which were major problem areas in their time management profile. Figure 10.5 outlines the summary of literature findings upon which Neville based her practice model.

Analysis and Critique of Time Element Models

FRAME OF REFERENCE

The general frames of reference in this section appear to be consistent with the philosophy of occupational therapy. Time is the basic element

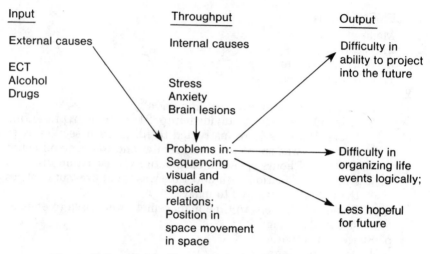

Figure 10.5.   Model of temporal dysfunction in the future mode.

which provides both a structure of organization and permits a structure to be organized by humans. All humans must adapt to time in terms of natural rhythms and can adapt time to the individual through the development of a balanced program of self maintenance and work and play.

CLARITY

Models, assumptions and concepts are culturally based. So are professions and professional practices. Meyer's philosphy and Slagle's application both illustrate the cultural and professional change. The practice of psychiatry proposed by Meyer was replaced by psychoanalysis. While Meyer studied the past to better plan for the future, psychoanalysis uses the past as the future. While Slagle saw many seriously depressed people in need of habit training through occupational therapy and nursing, the nurses increasingly organized the schedule without occupational therapists' assistance. Also, because scheduling a program for each person admitted became more routine the amount of regression was reduced. Thus, the use of habit training declined, and the philosophy on which it was based was overtaken by another set of ideas commonly known as dynamic psychiatry.

With the renewed interest in humanism and wholism the relationship of humans to work and time once more began to surface as issues related to overall health and wellness. Although many concepts have been retained and expanded in Kielhofner revitalization, some of Meyer's thoughts have been rearranged. The most significant is the concept of self maintenance in place of rest and sleep. Self maintenance is a more comprehensive term and seems to improve the comprehension of the model, since time can be divided into three definable categories of life space. Another modification is the division of adult play into recreation and leisure. Furthermore, Kielhofner has suggested there may be three types of what Meyer referred to as disorganized habits and Kielhofner calls temporal dysfunction: namely, disorientation, distortion and disorganization.

Both Meyer and Kielhofner, however, failed to organize their concepts into a description or model so that the relationship between the concepts could be understood. Figures 1 to 4 attempt to provide a basic framework, but some information is lacking. For example, do the three areas of self maintenance, work and play develop simultaneously and equally or does one occur first and account for more time in the life space and then the others develop? The same question applies to planning an intervention program. Where should the emphasis be placed first, or should all three areas be emphasized equally and simultaneously? Without a model to suggest the interrelations of concepts such decisions are difficult to make. Figure 10.6 is a hypothetical view of the interrelation between the three life spaces over the life-span.

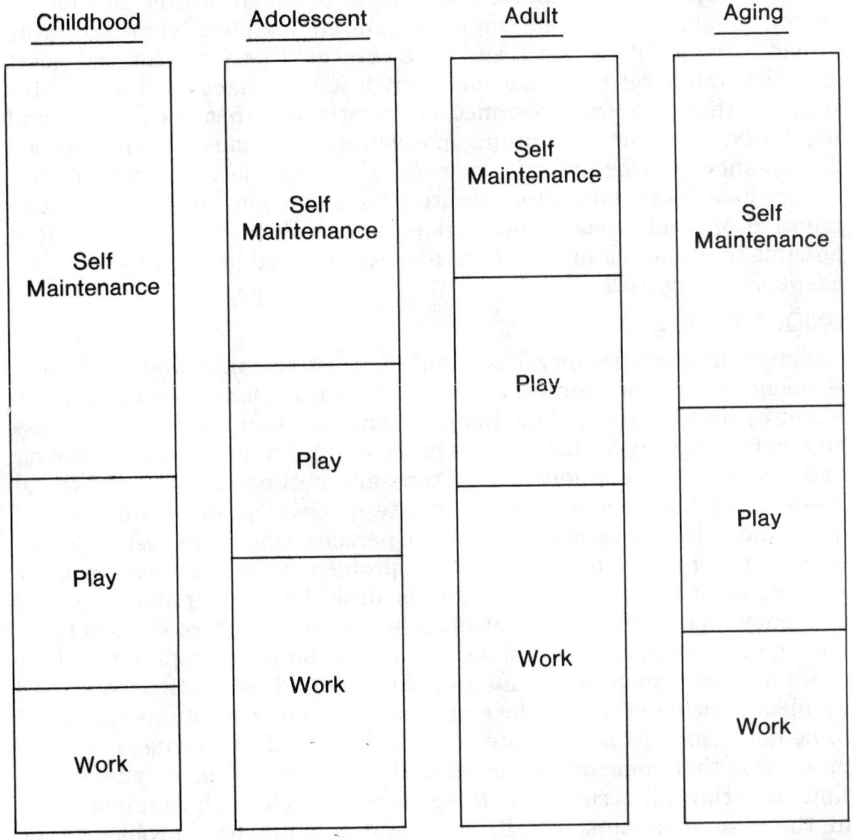

Average amount of time spent in self maintenance play and work.
A hypothetical model.

Figure 10.6. Model of development and change in the use of time for life space tasks.

Furthermore, both Meyer and Kielhofner have failed to include some concepts at all. For example, what about time threshold? Barash (13) suggests that a time threshold is the point in time in which a person's behavior changes from organized to disorganized. This concept may be similar to what is called loss of attention span, although attention span usually involves focusing on a specific task as opposed to coping effectively with the total situation.

Another related concept is time spanning. Time spanning is the ability to sustain controlled behavior and is assumed to increase gradually in skill with age. Thus, time should be structured in short intervals for children and increased intervals for adolescents and adults. The task of the time manager is to regulate daily activity in such a manner as to help the person achieve a better ability to cope with time spanning. Time spanning appears to be the basic concept of habit training or time management. Both time threshold and time spanning are subconcepts to temporal tolerance. Temporal tolerance is the span of time to which a person is able to respond in an organized manner. Time spanning provides the ability or skill, and time threshold provides the end point at which temporal tolerance has been lost or exhausted. Barash (13) suggests that temporal tolerance is learned and that consistency and regularity, frequency, duration, motivation, and capacity are aspects. Consistency provides repetition, regularity sets the time interval, frequency establishes how often, duration fixes how long, motivation determines effort and capacity indicates potential. With these concepts it is possible to propose a model of the process involved in learning temporal adaptation (Fig. 10.7).

UNIQUENESS

Time and work, temporal adaptation, habit training, and time management all have as a central concept the organization of occupation into a unit or units of time. Time management has been studied in business and manufacturing for many years in an attempt to increase productivity and efficiency. The uniqueness of time and occupation in occupational therapy has been the attempt to create or develop an organization of occupation, activities and tasks with persons who have lost or never learned to organize occupation. The problem is not to become more productive or efficient but to learn a basic level of productivity and efficiency. Occupational therapists encounter at least three kinds of time-managing problems. One problem is having too few occupational skills to fill up a day, such as is sometimes experienced by a retiree. A second problem is being unable to face or deal with the occupations that need to be done, such as is encountered by a depressed housewife. The third problem is that some occupational skills consume too much energy and time to permit all occupations to be accomplished, such as might occur in the case of a person with quadriplegia. For these problems, the interrelated concepts of temporal adaptation, temporal dysfunction and time management seem to provide a unique base for occupational therapists.

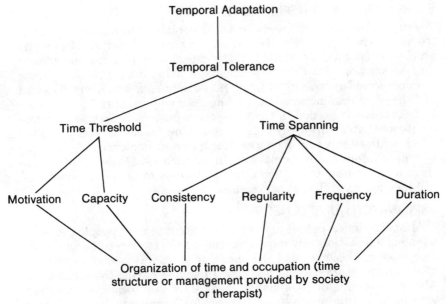

Figure 10.7.   Temporal adaptive process model.

RESEARCH GUIDE

Temporal adaptation, temporal dysfunction and time management should provide many opportunities for research efforts. Some possible questions have been mentioned already:

1. What is the developmental sequence of self maintenance, work and play tasks?
2. Which tasks should occur first in a management program?

Other questions to which research could be directed are:

1. What are the techniques of temporal adaptation over the life-span?
2. How does the balance or rhythm of life space change with time?
3. What is the relationship of temporal adaptation to personal values of health and occupational role performance?
4. Are there crisis periods in the life-span when temporal dysfunction is more likely to occur?
5. Can temporal dysfunction be predicted and prevented?

SPECIALIZATION

If time is a basic element in the classification system of occupational therapy, then the study of temporal adaptation and use of time management techniques should be useful in maintaining the essence of occupational therapy in any specialization area. Perhaps the biggest problem is to remember how many occupational therapy tasks make some use of time and time sequences.

ELABORATION AND REFINEMENT

Temporal adaptation needs to be elaborated into a more complete model in which the concepts are interrelated and the developmental process is expanded. In particular, the impact of culture and subcultures may be valuable. How many problems in living among minorities, for example, could be traced to temporal adjustments which are different and therefore dysfunctional in the American cultural norm?

Refinement is needed in the application process. Assessment instruments and intervention strategies need to be developed and published which address aspects of temporal adaptation. For example, how can technical, informal and formal learning of time be assessed? Since these three levels appear to develop different focuses of temporal adaptation will they require different management techniques?

EXPLANATORY USEFULNESS

Although time is certainly a familiar concept to most people the use of temporal adaptation may require special efforts to succeed as an explanatory tool for occupational therapy. Our society is geared to thinking about getting more done in less time or simply having too much to do. Also, the learning of time management skills is a socialization process with little institutional support, except for learning to tell clock time. Many people may not think of time management as a useful skill because they must do "what comes naturally." The idea that time management and temporal adaptation should or could be formally taught in therapy to help people with physical and emotional problems may seem strange. Neville (11) probably received some typical responses when her patients refused to respond as to how they spent their time or stated that the responses were too personal. The use of time, temporal adaptation and time management can be used to describe occupational therapy, but they must be employed carefully to avoid further confusion. The problem of explaining occupational therapy remains the same, that is, how to explain something so basic and simple that it becomes complex.

COMMONALITY

Again time is a common theme, but the focus on temporal adaptation for persons with disoriented, distorted or disorganized time problems is unique to occupational therapy. Teachers know about teaching clock time, vocational counselors know about rates of productivity and time schedules or daily logs are included in many time management books. The difference as Meyer said is in the doing and practice of self maintenance and play tasks as well as productivity. Other professions may have difficulty following the complete concept of time as used in occupational therapy.

PRACTICE MODEL DEVELOPMENT

There are many possible practice theories which could be evolved out of time and temporal adaptation. However, there may be a need to better understand how time concepts affect life-span development and to develop assessment instruments to evaluate the effect of time on the individual.

Green (14) has provided a model of time development in relation to the self which could be useful in studying the effect of time on life-span development. The 11 stages are summarized briefly in Table 10.3. An assessment instrument could be constructed from the developmental continuum. Other assessment instruments could be developed based on practices related to time, such as wearing a watch or setting an alarm clock. Attitudes toward time could be assessed, such as whether the person feels guilty if late for an appointment or finds there is too much leisure time.

Knapp (15) has developed scales for evaluating time practice and time attitudes which could be used as reference. Another area of assessment is temporal orientation to determine past, future, and present orientation. Braley and Freed (16) have developed a Q-sort which addresses temporal adaptation. Such tests in addition to the time log and activity history could provide a better focus for intervention planning.

Time models are summarized in Table 10.4.

SPACE MODELS

FRAME OF REFERENCE

There seems to be two different perspectives on the study of space and its effect on human activity. One view is concerned with how space affects cognitive and perceptual development. The other view is concerned with how space is valued in terms of exploration, social interaction, privacy and security. Developmental psychologists have contributed to the first view, especially Jean Piaget, whereas environmental psychologists have been interested in the second view.

There has been surprisingly little interest in the development of spatial concepts and relationships in the models of occupational therapy. In fact, there are no models devoted totally to the development of spatial information. The model of spatial-temporal adaptation by Gilfoyle and Grady comes the closest. Some attention has been directed to the effect of the environment *on* the individual but not on individual adaptation *to* space.

Because only one model exists in the spatial category of models, the author has suggested some assumptions and concepts which might be useful in developing spatial models and can be used to critique the model that does exist. The assumptions are drawn from Kielhofner's temporal adaptation model (10) on the premise that spatial development and adaptation may be influenced by similar mechanisms and may be subject to similar types of problems. The concepts are those identified by Liben (17) and Pick and Lockman (18) as relevant to the study of spatial development and adaptation. Concepts related to spatial dysfunction are based on those of temporal dysfunction by Kielhofner.

ASSUMPTIONS

1. Each person has a spatial frame of reference that is culturally constituted.

Table 10.3
Temporal Stages in the Development of the Self[a]

I. Permanance of objects and persons (during year 1)

The infant's first time problem is permanance or the continued existence of objects and persons. Security of the self depends on the development of permanance. If early experience indicates an untrustworthy or capricious environment, anxiety may result which foreshortens the future time sense.

II. Clock time (1–3 yr)

This adjustment is based upon the establishment of routines for eating, sleeping, and toilet training. Clock time is arbitrary and external which necessitates some reorganization of subjective time and increases the sense of cultural time. Maladjustment may occur if children are forced to conform to meticulous schedules too early.

III. Restriction time (3–5 yr)

At this age, the child finds that there are times which can be used to expand personal interest and times which require one to stop, obey and accept a dependent status. The child's view of time tends to be associated with the type of discipline received.

IV. Causal sequences (6–11 yr)

This age is exploring larger and larger casual chains or sequences in the time units necessary for accomplishment of tasks through trying, doing, reality seeking and muscle flexing. The child begins to use a systematic approach and orderly method for reaching goals.

V. Personal time (12–15 yr)

The problem is the acceptance of the configuration of the self through assessment of capacities and inadequacies; through the process of self-assessment and assessment of others the person forms a conscious self-image.

VI. Mutual time (15–25 yr)

The problem is the search for intimate compatibility with another person for the purpose of completely sharing time and experience. Sharing time with someone else accelerates one's self-development.

VII. Alternatives in time (18–25 yrs)

The point is a choice point. The individual can decide to continue in the societal mold, reject it or join others to try to make changes. A person decides what leisure activities to pursue as well as work patterns. The past and future can be weighed in terms of the present.

VIII. The use of time (25–40 yrs)

This is a period of convergence between external or objective time and subjective time; reality commitment to job, marriage, children and property focuses the use of time toward establishing and securing these goals.

IX. Reconsidered time (40–50 yrs)

This is a period of reevaluation of life's course. Doubts surface as to the value of decisions made, stations won or the direction of states.

X. Foreshortened future (50–60 yrs)

The person realizes that the body has only so much energy. The push forward still exists to achieve goals and to appreciate them, but there is an awareness that time is running out.

XI. Rich past (65 plus)

The main temporal problem is the division of the inner life between concentrating on the present and pursuing the past. Crucial decisions are worked through again in search or self-justification.

[a] Based on H. B. Green (14).

Table 10.4
Time Models Criteria Summary

Evaluation Criteria	Very Good 1	Moderately Good		Very Poor 5
		2	3	4	
Frame of reference	x			
Clarity			x	
Uniqueness		x		
Research guide	x			
Specialization		x		
Elaboration/refinement		x		
Explanation		x		
Commonality		x		
Practice model		x		

2. A unique spatial frame of reference is accumulated through experiential learning and socializing that begins in childhood.
3. There is a natural spacial order to daily living organized around the life activities of self maintenance, productivity and leisure.
4. Society requires its members to organize their use of space according to prescribed social roles.
5. An individual's use of space is a function of internalized values, interests and goals.
6. Habits are the basic structures by which daily behavior is ordered in space and biopsychosocial health is maintained.
7. Specific dysfunction may exist in relation to categories of pathology.

CONCEPTS (17)

Absolute space—a framework that exists independently of anything contained within it and is irrelevant of the observer's perspective

Relative space—an expression of a set of relationships among objects

Place—a small portion of the earth's surface identified by a name

Location—the scene of action

Psychological space—any space which is attributed to the mind and would not exist if minds did not exist

Physical space—any space attributed to the external world independent of the existence of minds

Origins of psychological space
   a. Empiricist position—development of psychological space is hypothesized to be derived directly from experience with physical space.
   b. Nativisit position—development of psychological space is thought to be determined by the inherited endowment of the organism.
   c. Constructivist position—development of psychological space is actively constructed by the individual, although inherited and experiential factors interact or produce these constructions

Functions of a psychological space
   a. Mystic or expressive space—locations and directions are emotionally charged and ordered on a sacred-profane dimension with no

separation between things and places or between subject and object

b. Sensory or representative space—what is represented and labeled through language is space as it "is" in the empirical-perceptual world as in the extension or arrangement of individual objects

c. Conceptual or scientific space—laws or rules of arrangement and order that function in space which is constituted through science and abstracted beyond the empirical world

Spatial behavior—sensorimotor activity in the environment, such as manipulation of objects in space or the locomotion of the self through the environment

Practical space—concerns the capacity to act in space (Piaget)

Conceptual space—concerns the capacity to represent space by drawing, map reading or making a model (Piaget)

Type of spatial representation

a. Spatial products—refers to the external products that represent space in some way such as sketch maps, miniature models or verbal descriptions

b. Spatial thought—refers to thinking that concerns or makes use of space in some way which includes knowledge, reflection, spatial problem solving and spatial imagery

c. Spatial storage—refers to any information about space contained in the neurophysiological structures except cognition

Contents of spatial representation

a. Environmental cognition—the knowledge or information a person has about space that enables the individual to maneuver the environment

b. Spatial abstraction—the notions a person has about space, including projective relationships, alternative and conflicting frames of reference and continuity of space

Spatially coordinated behaviors

a. Body-body relations—spatial adjustment of one body part with respect to another, such as getting the thumb to the mouth or participating in gymnastics

b. Body-object relations—spatial adjustment of the body or body part with respect to an object or objects, such as learning to throw a ball or a skilled juggling

c. Object-object relations—spatial adjustment of complex tasks, such as handsewing, intricate stritches in a homemade garment or activity involved in object manipulation and locomotion

Spatial frame of reference

a. Egocentric—defines spatial positions in relation to loci on the body

b. Allocentric or geocentric—defines spatial positions in relation to loci external to the person

Properties of spatial information

a. Reversibility—knowing how to go from A to B implies knowing how to go from B to A

   b. Transivity—knowing how to go from A to B to C implies knowing how to get from A to C

   c. Detour ability—knowing how to go from A to B by some route implies being able to go from A to B by other routes

Topic features of space

   a. Proximity—the "nearby-ness" of elements belonging to some perceptual field (Piaget)

   b. Separation—dissociation or segregation of elements

   c. Order or succession—occurs when two separate elements are arranged one before the other

   d. Enclosure—that which is surrounded or inside

   e. Continuity—without interruption or change in related elements

Spatial adaptation—the integration and organization of activities in space which support health on an ongoing daily life space

Spatial dysfunction—refers to problems that arise in daily life organization related to spatial behavior or spatial representation

   a. Disorientation in space—person does not know or recognize familiar space and cannot maneuver through familiar space without getting lost or confused

   b. Distortions of space—person has difficulty with the perceptual or sensory representations of space

   c. Disorganization of space—person is unable to organize activity and function in a space or does not organize and function in ways that fulfill role expectations

Spatiotemporal Adaptation Model—Gilfoyle and Grady

FRAME OF REFERENCE

   The spatiotemporal adaptation model by Gilfoyle and Grady (19) is based on the developmental systems and biopsychosocial models. The developmental aspects are based on the milestones of development which Arnold Gesell established and the sequence of learning established by Jean Piaget. Systems concepts are used to describe the adaptational process and the effects of stress. Biopsychosocial concepts are incorporated to broaden the model beyond the substantial neurophysiological base. Specifically, I. J. Gordon's concept of "self system" is included (20). Treatment concepts have been borrowed from Bertha Bobath, Mary Fiorentino and A. Jean Ayres.

ASSUMPTIONS

   All assumptions are from the book *Children Adapt* (19) or the chapter in *Willard and Spackman's Occupational Therapy* (21) by Gilfoyle and Grady.

Assumptions about Man

   1. Movement puts a child in relationship with his surroundings so that through his relationship the child can have an effect upon his environment as well as be affected by his environment.

2. Through the adaptation of movement life survives and protects, experiences, develops and expresses.

3. Movement provides experiences for interaction and perception of the environment including the self, objects, object relationships, movement of objects in space and of the effect of self-movement upon objects.

4. Movement promotes mental and social development through the expression of thoughts and ideas.

5. Through the relationship of movement and environment, the child adapts.

6. Movement and adaptation are viewed in terms of a single whole that is set to work as a system of relationships which promotes purposeful experience.

7. Human adaptation is a dynamic organized process of expanding a child's repertoire of behavior.

8. Adaptation evolves from the transactional process between a person and the environment.

9. The adaptation process of sensorimotor-sensory (SMS) integration is dependent upon the interaction between nervous system maturation and previously acquired behavior with environmental experiences.

10. The adaptation process is hierarchical with increasingly higher levels of behavior gradually emerging from the lower level behaviors as a result of continual environmental interaction.

11. The integration of higher level behavior influences and increases the maturity of the lower level behaviors.

12. Development is a function of nervous system maturation which occurs through a process of adaptation.

13. Maturation is dependent upon the child's attention to and active participation with events in the environment.

14. Adaptation is dependent upon attention to and active participation with purposeful events of the environment.

15. Purposeful events (behaviors and activities) provide meaningful experiences for enhancement of maturation by directing a higher level of adaptive response.

16. Adaptation spirals through primitive, transitional and mature phases of development occur at the same time within different body segments.

17. Each child becomes unique by creating an entirely individualistic and complex "self system" derived from all the factors that contribute to development.

18. Through development a child seeks to expand his environment and pursue his quest for autonomy and competence.

19. Autonomy and competence depend upon his ability to move about the environment as he engages in goal-directed, purposeful experiences.

20. Competency and autonomy serve as an internal motivator to encourage the child to extend "self" and seek a variety of experiences.
21. Environmental experiences may present situations of spatiotemporal stress.
22. Lower level SMS behaviors will emerge during the adaptational process when the environmental demands exceed the functional capacities of a child.
23. During normal developmental progressions, a child will adapt with more primitive behaviors:
    a. when adapting to new experiences
    b. when the SMS integrative process is temporarily altered, and
    c. during the transitional phases of the developmental progressions.
24. Spatiotemporal distress provokes dysfunction when the adaptational process is interrupted or incomplete resulting in maladaptation.

Assumptions about Health and Dysfunction

1. The child with impaired movement experiences dysfunction in performance and develops purposeless behaviors and activities.
2. Dysfunctional performance has an effect upon the total developmental process, ultimately resulting in developmental deviations and/or disabilities.
3. A developmental deviation occurs if lower level behaviors persist and are not modified by the adaptational process.
4. Any factor affecting the developmental process (heredity, environment or state of health) may interrupt or delay the sequence and rate of growth, maturation and development.
5. The interruption or delay results in an inability to effectively interact and adapt behaviors and activities.
6. Immature, primitive or pathological behaviors accompany dysfunctional performance and in turn further affect the adaptational process.

Assumptions about Occupational Therapy

1. A child with dysfunctional performance can benefit from a (re)habilitation process designed to develop within the individual a more effective way of functioning.
2. (Re) habilitation is based upon the process of adapting purposeful behavior and activities to performance skills.
3. The unique contribution of occupational therapy is the facilitation of purposeful activities to be adapted by the person for acquisition of performance skills, self-care, work, play, recreation and leisure activities.
4. Occupational therapy assumes that a child's active participation

with purposeful activity is meaningful to the nervous system to facilitate maturation and development.

5. The child's cortical attention is directed toward the end result, and the subcortical attention is directed to the process.

CONCEPTS (19)

Spatiotemporal adaptation—the continuous, ongoing state or act of adjusting those bodily processes required to function within a given space and at a given time

Space (spatial)— refers to the area surrounding an individual, including the supporting surface for the body, the gravitational and three-dimensional space surrounding the body and the space occupied by the body or by other persons or objects within the area

Time (temporal)—the duration, regulation, memory and sequence of a person's actions, body movements or movements of other persons or objects within the area

Spatial dimensions—encompasses the environment in which a person exists and functions

Temporal dimensions—encompasses the sequencing (planning) and timing (processing) of actions in relation to stationary or moving objects

Growth—the biological/structural changes of the body (*i.e.,* skeletal/muscular)

Maturation—the modification within the individual's neurophysiological system

Development—the modification of the bodily processes in order to perform spontaneous behaviors and adapt to the environment

Developmental process—the manner, rate and sequence of acquiring behavior

Environment—everything with which an individual interacts including the self, other persons, objects, the earth, space and the relationship within space

Spatiotemporal adaptation process

a. Assimilation—the sensory process of taking in or receiving information that is external to and/or within the self system

b. Accommodation—the response or the motor process of adjusting the body to react to the incoming stimulation

c. Association—The organized process of relating the sensory information with the motor act and of relating present and past experiences with each other

d. Differentiation–the process of discriminating those external elements of a specific behavior that are pertinent to a given situation, distinguishing those that are not and thereby modifying or altering the behavior in some manner

Sensorimotor sensory—involves the sensory input (assimilation), sensory output (accommodation) and sensory feedback (association and differentiation)

Perception—the individual's sensory judgment and feeling evolving through repeated experiences in the environment

Postural strategies—controlled movement

Movement strategies—promote and sequence changes in patterns of the body or body parts to give rise to purposeful action

Purposeful activities—are directed toward goals outside the body or to events and activities within the environment and thus become environment centered

Purposeful behavior—self-starting actions which are body-centered and concerned with innate goals, e.g., to sit, to stand

Skill—appropriate use of posture and movement in relation to the effort (speed, timing, exertion, space, control) for performance of an activity

Efficiency of performance—relationship between the amount of work that is accomplished and the force or energy expended to accomplish the action

Accuracy of performance—is the perception or judgment of direction, distance, control and time of actions

Reflexes and reactions—describe specific responses or series of responses to particular sensory input or combination of sensory input. Reactions are distinguished from reflexes by their greater complexity and inconsistency of the response

Mobility—actions produce "move ability"

Stability—actions produce "stay ability"

Primitive phase—infant adapts fetal movements to develop undifferentiated movement strategies, facilitating mobility by means of primitive reflexes

Transitional phase—undifferentiated movement and holding strategies that are adapted to movement synergies and weight-bearing patterns by means of chain reactions

Mature strategies—differentiating mobility and stability functions and developing automatic balance reactions to distribute mobility and stability muscle tone appropriately

Postural and perceptual sets—not well defined, has to do with the grouping or organizing of strategies which are consistently selected to achieve specific outcomes

Self. system—reflects the person's uniqueness which evolves from the developmental process

Preparation—both the preliminary and ongoing process of enhancing the neural and muscular functions for their readiness and use as posture and movement strategies

Facilitation—continued successive application of the necessary stimulus to elicit an adaptive response

Adaptation—is an organized process of modification in which a child assimilates everything that is happening, accommodates to these experiences and associates, differentiates and integrates the new experiences to those previously acquired

Spatiotemporal stress—the challenge of the environment exceeds the functional capacity to adapt, and lower level SMS behaviors are used to adapt to the environmental demands

Dysfunction—the inability to perform effectively and interact with the environment

Developmental disability—the result of any condition, trauma, deprivation, or disease which interrupts or delays the sequence and rate of normal growth, development and motivation

Primitive dysfunction—characterized by the influence of primitive, lower level behaviors being utilized repeatedly to the environment

Pathological dysfunction—may include primitive patterns but is accompanied by abnormal muscle tone and abnormal reflexive behavior

Not Defined

Autonomy
Competence
Level of competence
Sense of mastery

EXPECTED RESULTS

1. Prevention—occurs when the child engages in activity that is designed to keep distress from occurring or to hinder secondary complications from the initial identified problem
2. Modification—occurs when the child facilitates change within the self system which is brought about by his own participation with actions/activities
3. Remediation—the process of engaging a child with activity that is designed to correct, remedy or improve his skill level
4. Compensation—occurs in therapy when the activity promotes another aspect of performance or substitutes a different form of action
5. Maintenance—activity that helps the child keep in condition and retain the acquired appropriate functions

ASSESSMENT INSTRUMENTS

Assessment areas
  Developmental history of the child's occupational performance
  History of the child
Process/procedures
1. Collect and review past data, interview child and family and other persons involved with the child
2. Clinical observations—analysis and synthesis of findings, recording and reporting

INTERVENTION STRATEGIES

1. Media—purposeful activity, toys and games
2. Methods

a. Use activities that provide a successful experience for the child-feedback.
b. Use a variety of activities which permit repetition of action.
c. Preparation activities—normalizing postural tone, increasing range of motion, strength-promoting subcortical attention, securing a balance of inhibitory-facilitory state
d. Facilitation—stimuli may include position, activity, child or therapist.
e. Use of self-directed activities
3. Equipment—not stated specifically
4. Prerequisite skills
None required—model starts at level of child's performance and development

SUMMARY

The spatiotemporal adaptation model is based on the process of adjusting posture and movement sequences to the gravitational demand of space and temporal demands of timing movement. The development of spatiotemporal adaptation is viewed as a spiraling process which includes the integration of sensory input or assimilation, motor output or accommodation and sensory feedback which includes association and differentiation (Fig. 10.8). During spatiotemporal adaptation primitive postures and movements are modified and integrated into purposeful behaviors. Purposeful behaviors are the foundations for the development of complex strategies which are adapted to perform purposeful activities and develop skills. The ability to perform with skill, efficiency and accuracy facilitates the attainment of a unique self system and the quest for autonomy and competence.

The concept of spatiotemporal adaptation has been applied by Gilfoyle and Grady to the development of purposeful behaviors including creeping, sitting, rolling, standing and walking, as well as to purposeful activities and skills. To illustrate the effects of adaptation and development each behavior or activity is divided into three stages of acquisition. The primitive stage includes the initial postures or movements, the transitional stage includes the intermediate behaviors and the mature phase includes the final level of performance and skill. Figure 10.9 is an example of phases involved in learning the creep. The same stages are applied to sitting, rolling, standing and walking and personality development.

Spatiotemporal stress occurs when the child is unable temporarily to meet the demands of the situation with the strategies or behaviors available. Normal stress occurs in response to gravity, complexity of movement or requirements of the activity. Gravitational stress occurs when a more secure posture or a higher level posture is needed. Stress produced by complexity of movement occurs whenever a situation interrupts the automatic monitoring and blending of muscle functions. Stress due to requirements of the activity or skills occurs when there is an interruption in the automatic use of recently established perceptual sets.

Spatiotemporal distress occurs when the amount of stress is out of

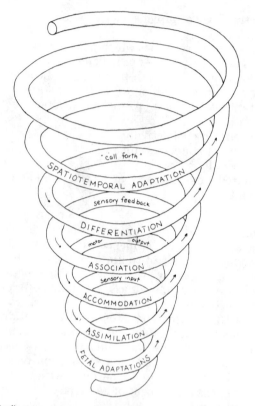

Figure 10.8. Spiraling continuum of spatiotemporal adaptation. (Reproduced from E. M. Gilfoyle *et al.* (19), with permission from Charles B. Slack.)

control or cannot be managed. Abnormal stress conditions may result from abnormal assimilation such as sensory deprivation, abnormal accommodation such as abnormal tone, or abnormal association and differentiation, such as faulty sensorimotor sensory integration.

Analysis and Critique of the Spatiotemporal Adaptation Model
FRAME OF REFERENCE

The frame of reference is consistent with the views of occupational therapy as far as it goes. However, there appears to be a lack of reference for the final outcome of spatiotemporal adaptation. Certainly, the spiraling continuum must reach a point beyond rolling, sitting, walking and self-identity before death. A review of the model offered in the text provides no clues. Within the text, the words competence, autonomy, independence and mastery are mentioned but never tied into the models. The lack of end point will be discussed further in concepts.

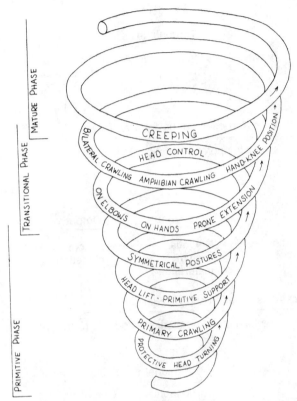

Figure 10.9. Key behaviors of creeping. (Reproduced from E. M. Gilfoyle *et al.* (19), with permission from Charles B. Slack.)

CLARITY

Spatiotemporal adaptation is a complex model and as such has numerous assumptions and concepts. Only the major assumptions and concepts were included in the review. Those assumptions which were summarized from existing literature and the concepts used within the primitive transitional and mature stages were not included because they do not affect the overall effectiveness of the model in explaining how spatial and temporal elements relate to movement and adaptation.

The assumptions which were identified present an interesting array of models. Within the first three pages of text six different conceptual models were identified by the authors. These are illustrated in Figures 10.10 to 10.16. Although the subject matter of the models is legitimate, the differences between two models dealing with the same subject seem confusing. For example, there are two models of spatiotemporal adaptation (Figs. 10.10 and 10.11) and two on goals (Figs. 10.12 and 10.13). One

MODELS OF PRACTICE

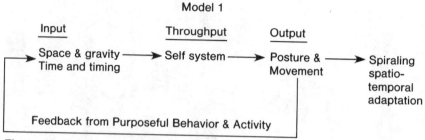

Figure 10.10. Spatiotemporal adaptation: Model 1. (Data from E. M. Gilfoyle *et al.* (19, p 3).)

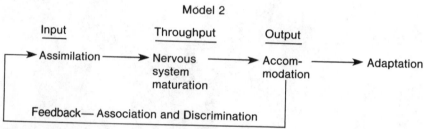

Figure 10.11. Spatiotemporal adaptation: Model 2. (Data from E. M. Gilfoyle *et al.* (19, p 48).)

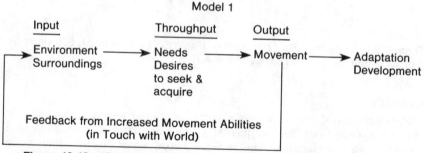

Figure 10.12. Goal: Model 1. (Data from E. M. Gilfoyle *et al.* (19, p 1).)

of the goal models states that the ultimate goal is adaptation and development. The other states that competence, autonomy and independence are the ultimate outcomes. This confusion is continued into the chapter on the model for therapy which adds the goal of mastery to the list. Within the lists of concepts only adaptation and development are defined. Thus the concepts are not much help in determining which or how many of the goal statements are valid. The models of spiraling adaptation are likewise of no assistance, since none of them include a

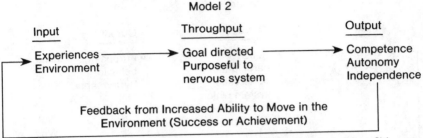

Figure 10.13. Goal: Model 2. (Data from E. M. Gilfoyle *et al.* (19, p 2).)

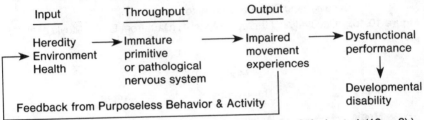

Figure 10.14. Model of dysfunction. (Data from E. M. Gilfoyle *et al.* (19, p 2).)

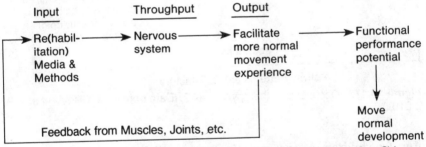

Figure 10.15. Therapy model. (Data from E. M. Gilfoyle *et al.* (19, p 3).)

final goal but simply trail off into space. Basically, the reader is left with a series of models which form a good foundation for the use of developmental and adaptive concepts but do not provide a logical ending.

Another example of duplicate models are those used to explain the process of occupational therapy (Figs. 10.16 and 10.17). Again, there are several goals from which to select. However, perhaps more confusing is the fact that the purposeful activity appears as the input for the first occupational therapy model, while in the second model purposeful activity is stated as an output. Actually, both uses are correct and logical. The term purposeful activity can be used to describe the media which stimulate interest or attract attention. For example, toys are purposeful activ-

Model 1

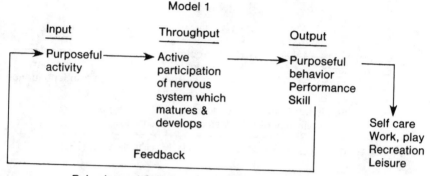

Behavior and Skill are Satisfactory

Figure 10.16. Occupational therapy: Model 1. (Data from E. M. Gilfoyle *et al.* (19, p 3).)

Model 2

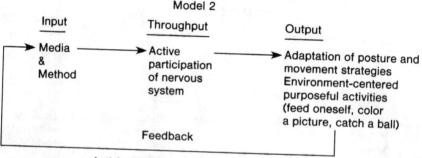

Activity Patterns are Satisfactory

Figure 10.17. Occupational therapy: Model 2. (Data from E. M. Gilfoyle *et al.* (19, p 210).)

ities for children. At the same time, purposeful activity can mean to be active or to act more in a purposeful manner. For example, catching a ball is a purposeful activity in which the person moves the body and segments which permit the ball to land and stop in the hands. Because of the double meaning of purposeful activity, occupational therapists must be careful to describe what is meant when the term is being used. Furthermore, if both definitions are being used, care must be taken so that the audience knows which meaning is being applied in each reference.

Finally, Figures 10.17 and 10.18 are designed to show the differences between occupational therapy and physical therapy. Physical therapy is viewed as body-centered, while occupational therapy is viewed as environment centered. Such a view needs further clarification for adequate analysis.

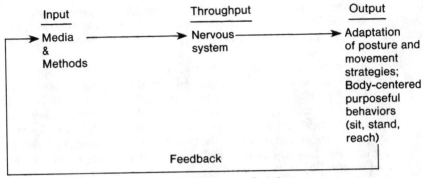

Body—Centered Behaviors are Satisfactory

Figure 10.18.   Physical therapy model. (Adapted from E. M. Gilfoyle *et al.* (19).)

UNIQUENESS

The uniqueness of the spatiotemporal model is the attempt to systematically analyze a number of basic developmental milestones into specific posture and movement strategies which progress from primitive to transitional to mature behaviors. Unfortunately, the analysis is limited primarily to motor behavior. Only one sensory modality, vision, and one psychological aspect, self-identity, are discussed. The effects of space, time and motion on social activities such as group interactions and role performance are not included.

RESEARCH GUIDE

The concept of spatiotemporal adaptation should be very useful to occupational therapists in developing research proposals. Numerous possibilities for research topics exist. These include:

1. What is the spatiotemporal process of hearing development?
2. How does spatiotemporal adaptation affect social interaction development and role performance?
3. Do different spatial environments affect the quality of spatiotemporal adaptation?
4. Do competence, achievement and mastery develop out of a spatiotemporal spiraling process?
5. Can independence and autonomy be described by the spatiotemporal process?
6. Could problem solving and decision making be learned using the spatiotemporal process as a model?
7. How does the increasing ability to discriminate space and time affect spatiotemporal learning in the cognitive domain?

ELABORATION AND REFINEMENT

Elaboration would be useful to expand the spatiotemporal adaptation model into the psychological and sociocultural areas. Many examples have been discussed already in the critique. The spatiotemporal adaptation process could be even more useful if the development of competence, autonomy, social interaction, and role performance were shown to follow a similar spiraling progression.

Refinement is needed to clarify the goal of spatiotemporal adaptation and the relationship of therapy skills to spatiotemporal distress. As Figures 10.12 and 10.13 show, the goals are unclear. Figures 10.16 and 10.17 illustrate the need to clarify the function of occupational therapy, a refinement of how knowledge of space and time is affected by the spatiotemporal process. In other words, how does the cognitive knowledge of time and space help the person influence or change the environment instead of responding to it.

SPECIALIZATION

The model of spatiotemporal adaptation has been built within the pediatric area of specialization. The model builders attempted to describe how the practice of occupational therapy can be maintained within the specialty area. However, the model of spatiotemporal adaptation itself does not integrate the practice of occupational therapy into the total framework. It would be helpful for pediatric specialists to see an expanded model of spatiotemporal adaptation which includes spatiotemporal distress and dysfunction and then leads to the practice of occupational therapy. The author has attempted to interpret the model builders' descriptions into a series of possible conceptual models (Figs. 10.12 to 10.17). These models, though, may not illustrate completely the concepts envisioned by Gilfolye and Grady.

EXPLANATORY USEFULNESS

The concept of spatiotemporal adaptation is useful primarily in explaining the development of familiar milestones, such as sitting and walking. The concepts of stress and distress are useful in suggesting the continuum between normal and abnormal progression. In particular, the model illustrates that each skill is the result of prior performances which began at a primitive level and progressed through a transitional phase to a mature or recognized skill level.

The spatiotemporal model attempts to show how occupational therapy and other therapy interact with a child who shows spatiotemporal distress. However, the goals of spatiotemporal adaptation are unclear, and the process of therapy is not completely clear which limits the model's usefulness as an explanatory tool.

COMMONALITY

The commonality with other professions is primarily through the concept of development and partially through the emphasis on posture and movement. Nearly all the professions and consumer groups are interested in development and the problems of delayed development. The spatiotemporal model provides considerable information on the development of milestones. Professions which are concerned with the development of posture and movement, such as physical therapy, recreation and physical education, also can learn from the model of spatiotemporal adaptation. Furthermore, some attempt has been made to clarify the therapeutic role of occupational and physical therapy. Further, differentiation of the recreational therapist and adapted physical educator could be useful by indicating their role in relation to posture and movement skills.

PRACTICE MODELS

Practice models and theories based on the spatiotemporal model will need to identify more clearly the methods which promote adaptation and reduce the impact of distress. While some methods have been identified by the model builders, there remains a need to further clarify and verify intervention strategies.

There may be a need to develop better assessment instruments as well. Specifically, the model stresses that behaviors and skills involve a process, a progression and a sequence of behaviors which transform into a mature skill. Many assessment instruments test primarily for primitive behaviors or for mature skills. Few provide a continuum of phase development related to a given skill. Assessments which stress the evaluation of the primitive and transitional phases as well as mature skill development could serve to improve the assessment capacity of therapists and developmental specialists. A summary of the spatiotemporal adaptation model is provided in Table 10.5.

ACTION AND DOING MODELS
Actions and Achievement Model—Meyer

FRAME OF REFERENCE

The material for this model of action and achievement predates the model of occupational therapy discussed under the section on time and space. Action and achievement is contained in a paper given by Meyer to a graduating class of student nurses in 1916 at the Sheppard and Enoch Pratt Hospital where Dr. Dunton worked (22). The paper was not

Table 10.5
Spatiotemporal Adaptation Model Criteria Summary

Evaluation Criteria	Very Good 1	Moderately Good 2	3	4	Very Poor 5
Frame of reference	x				
Clarity			x		
Uniqueness		x			
Research guide	x				
Specialization		x			
Elaboration/refinement				x	
Explanation		x			
Commonality		x			
Practice model		x			

published, however, until 1952. The assumptions and concepts are consistent with those of the model of occupational therapy but do not include specific reference to time binding. Meyer does not provide clues as to the source of his thinking, but the rationale is consistent with his other writings. The model is very incomplete. Only assumptions are given. However, the rationale for the use of activity or occupation seems important from a historical perspective.

ASSUMPTIONS ABOUT MAN AND ACTION

1. Man's mind shows its metal most clearly in what man does, and what man says and thinks and feels is but a help toward action.
2. Action is both the foundation and the climax of mental life.
3. Talk and feeling and thinking are but a way to action and depend for their wholesomeness on action.
4. Our emotions find their best solutions and corrections in the quiet achievement of no matter how small a task.

ASSUMPTIONS ABOUT OCCUPATIONS

1. A lack of the wholesome effects of some manual work or concrete performance with the natural rewards of satisfaction is apt to drive the human being into a hypertrophy.
2. A lack of performance may dry up those gifts of nature which are meant to be guides to actions and which if cultivated by themselves alone may lead to troubling fermentation of thought and fancy.

ASSUMPTIONS ABOUT HEALTH AND ACTION

1. The bulk of nervous and mental diseases have long figured as disorders of feeling, and these present to a large extent difficulties in the outlets of activity.
2. Our general health may be helped wonderfully by being made to turn to a system of formal exercises, and to turn exercise into terms of natural occupation.
3. Action has its effect on the attitude of the body, and the attitude of the body is, in the end, the condition and starting point for any activity and achievement.

ASSUMPTIONS ABOUT OCCUPATIONAL THERAPY

1. Action and achievement are the healthiest forms of suggestion and persuasion.
2. Therapy should lead to healthy care along the road of simple activity.

CONCEPTS

Activity—manual work or concrete performance with the natural rewards of satisfaction.

Action—the foundation and the climax of mental life

Achievement—getting some work or things done

SUMMARY

The model of action and achievement was stated for the benefit of nurses who had been trained in the rise of occupational therapy prior to formal courses in occupational therapy alone. The major assumption is that action and activity provide the reality orientation, satisfaction and sense of achievement that mental activity alone cannot give. Furthermore, action shows a person's true being, whereas talk, feeling and thinking are only a first step which by implication may go astray and are at best only a help toward action. The model of action and achievement is one of the earliest to provide a rationale for the use of activity or occupation as a therapeutic medium. Figure 10.19 illustrates the model of action and achievement.

Doing and Purposeful Action Model—Fidler and Fidler

FRAME OF REFERENCE

The model of doing and purposeful action by Fidler and Fidler (23) is based on the studies of play by Jerome Bruner, Jean Piaget and Mary Reilly. The sense of mastery and competence is drawn from Eric Erickson and Robert White. The relatedness to nonhuman objects is described by Harold Searles and the development of the sense of "I" is drawn from John Dewey.

Central to the model of doing and purposeful action is the role of performance and skill development in the process of human adaptation. Without doing and action the individual is prone toward psychopathology or dysfunction.

ASSUMPTIONS ABOUT ACTION

1. Action is essential to human existence.
2. Action is both the *product* of a mental image that sets the objective and the *creator* of a mental image.
3. It is through action with feedback from both nonhuman and human objects that an individual comes to know the potential and limitations of self and the environment so as to achieve a sense of competence and intrinsic work.
4. The drive to action transformed into the ability to "do" is fundamental to ego development and adaptation.
5. Humans are dependent upon their social and cultural environments

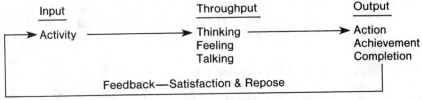

Figure 10.19. Model of action and achievement.

for learning and developing the action patterns necessary for both survival and satisfaction.

ASSUMPTIONS ABOUT DOING

1. Doing is a means for communicating feelings and ideas, expressing and clarifying individuality and achieving gratification.
2. Doing enables the development and integration of the sensory, motor, cognitive and psychological systems, serves as a socializing agent and verifies one's efficiency as a competent contributing member of one's society.
3. Doing can mediate between one's inner and outer world, nurture the capacity to invest, teach realistic responses to success and failure, provide concrete evidence of one's capacities and limitations, test the reality base of fantasy and perceptions, and validate the ability to achieve and influence one's environment.
4. Both the quality and variety of doing is critical for ego development and adaptation.
5. Activity or doing must match the individual's sensory, motor, cognitive, psychologic and social maturation as well as their developmental needs and skill readiness.
6. Different periods in the life cycle demand different configurations of skills.
7. The balance among performance skill clusters in terms of proportion of time, attention and energy allocated to each is critical in achieving and maintaining a way of life that is satisfying to self and others and is health-sustaining.
8. The level and kind of skills and the balance among them at any one point are determined by age, developmental level, unique biology and culture.
9. Activity or doing must be recognized by the sociocultural group as relevant to their values and needs.
10. The meaning and worth of one's doing or mastery is appreciably determined by the views and values of significant others.

ASSUMPTIONS ABOUT HEALTH AND DYSFUNCTION

1. A reduction in doing generates pathology.
2. When action does not follow thought, perception is distorted and the critical learning that comes from confronting the consequences of an act is precluded.
3. When the motivation or ability to act on mental images or ideation is blocked or inhibited by forces in the environment or by sensori-motor deficits, coping behavior and adaptive skills are not learned.

CONCEPTS

Doing—is purposeful action directed toward the intrapersonal, interpersonal or nonhuman environment through the process of investigating, trying out, and gaining evidence of one's capacities

Humanization—the process whereby the individual becomes a person whose actions are gradually transformed into behavior that concomitantly satisfies individual needs as well as contributes to societal development

Performance—the ability to care for and maintain the self in an independent manner, satisfy one's personal needs for intrinsic gratification, and contribute to the needs and welfare of others

Action, acting—the produce of a mental image that sets the objective and the creator of a mental image

Gratification, intrinsic—requires no social reward or ratification from others (White)

Not Defined

Purposeful action
Action patterns
Adapt, adaptation
Cope, coping
Personal integrity
Self actualization
Acculturation
Sense of mastery, mastering
Achieve, achievement
Sense of competence, efficiency
Exploratory learning
Random activity
Adaptive skills
Sense of value
Social role identity
Balance

EXPECTED RESULTS

   a. Facilitate learning and change
   b. Help maintain a state of health

ASSESSMENT

   Procedures—determine nature and level of individual's
   a. Intact skills
   b. Skill limitations
   c. Balance among performance skill clusters.
   Identify those components or subsystems of performance that inhibit or prevent skill development, including:
   a. Sensory, motor, psychologic and social deficits
   b. Human and nonhuman factors in the environment that impact on being able *to do.*

INTERVENTION

   1. Media—not mentioned
   2. Methods
      a. Match activity experiences to the individual's defects, learning readiness, intact functions and values.
      b. Provide action learning experiences necessary for the develop-

ment of the critical components of performance and for skill acquisition.

3. Equipment—none given.
4. Prerequisite skills—not stated.

SUMMARY

Doing and purposeful action is a model based on the constructs drawn from social and individual psychology that discuss human action and the role of doing and purposeful action in in development, adaptation and human existence. The major assumption is that doing and purposeful action enable the individual to learn those performance skills which are necessary to create a balance of skill clusters which in turn will maintain the self, satisfy individual needs and contribute to the society at large (Fig. 10.20). Conversely, the model suggests that psychopathology and dysfunction are the result of deficient opportunities for doing and purposeful action (Fig. 10.21). Thus, the role of occupational therapy is to determine the problems in doing and purposeful action by assessing the nature level and balance of performance skills. Implementation involves matching the activities to individual deficits, learning readiness, intact facts and values.

Graded Occupation Model—Hall
FRAME OF REFERENCE

Hall's model (24) of graded occupation was a reaction to the accepted rest cure treatment of a now rare disorder called neurasthenia which is

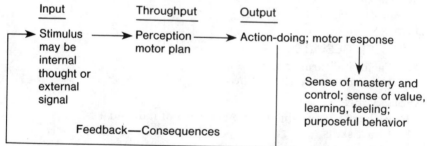

Figure 10.20.   Action and doing model.

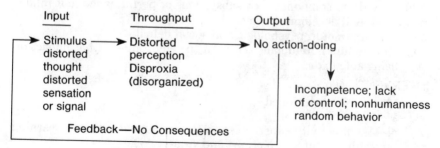

Figure 10.21.   No action or doing model.

characterized by feelings of weakness and lowering of body and mental tone. The prevailing theory of etiology was that neurasthenic patients were suffering from overwork which had piled up poisonous waste products in the system. Rest would permit the wastes to be deposed and health would return.

Hall (25) felt that faulty living patterns such as wrong occupation or poor habits were involved, as well as a tendency to worry about small problems. Treatment should therefore be aimed at correcting the faulty living patterns by changing interests, occupations and habits. In 1906, Hall (26) was granted $1000 from the Proctor Fund of Harvard University "to assist in the study of the treatment of neurasthenia by progressive and graded manual occupation" at the Devereau Mansion in Marblehead, Massachusetts.

ASSUMPTIONS ABOUT MAN AND OCCUPATION

1. It is normal and right for a man to be busy (24).
2. There is in mankind an inborn love of making things, of creating complex beautiful objects (24).
3. Manual work is wholesome and developmental (26).
4. Rational occupation of some kind is an essential of sound and successful living (27).

ASSUMPTIONS ABOUT HEALTH AND DISEASE

1. Faulty living may be an important etiological factor in neurasthenia (neurosis) (24).
2. Idleness, long continued, is a menace not only to the proper functioning of the body but also the morale and spirits of the individual (31).
3. The unoccupied hand and mind always court confusion and degeneration (25).
4. Life without aim or ambition is a sick life (29).
5. Occupation without results is actually depressing (25).

ASSUMPTIONS ABOUT THE USE OF OCCUPATION AS THERAPY

1. Occupation of the body and mind are indispensable in the treatment of the functional nervous diseases (30).
2. The ideal life for the neurasthenic should be one of occupation (25).
3. There is a great need to lift the neurasthenic out of his symptoms by bringing about through a gradual process the conditions of a normal life, a life of pleasant and progressive occupation (24).
4. A suitable occupation of hand and mind is a very potent factor in the maintenance of physical, mental and moral health in the individual and in the community (26).
5. A suitable occupation may be a valuable remedy when (26)
   a. An unsuitable occupation has been the rule
   b. A suitable occupation has been misused or
   c. Idleness has been the habit.
6. Manual work is best for it is objective and wholesome and trains to accuracy and precision of movement (24).

7. Manual work used as a remedy aims to introduce a new and objective interest, gradually forcing its adoption and increasing its prominence until the mental and physical habits of the patient are grounded about this wholesome center (27).
8. The more useful the work, the better its therapeutic effects (31).
9. Patients should be taught self-sufficiency by closely following thought with the actual doing of work (30).

ASSUMPTIONS RELATED TO OCCUPATIONAL THERAPY

1. Occupational therapy at first amuses then actively interests the patient (33).
2. The effort should interest the patient and lend itself to a graded arrangement (32).
3. The rest and play should be measured until all need for caution and reserve is past (32).
4. We cannot mold our patients all alike after one pattern; each will give a different interpretation and value to his work and each must preserve his individuality (24).
5. The best way to restore lost or impaired function is by use (32).

CONCEPTS

Economic strength (*conservation of energy*)—to do deliberately and without undue excitement what simple manual work may be deemed advisable, *i.e.*, to grasp the saw without a crushing grip (26)

Graded effort—starts with light work, simple process work which shows and guides pleasant results and short work periods (32)

Principle of indirection—arousing interest and ambition in a new and unsuspected way (33)

System of parallels or equivalents—using new paths to attention, patience and sustained effort when old paths to reach an objective are blocked (33)

Leisure—well earned repose (34)

Idleness—forced upon us (34)

Principle of substitution—put something new and better such as interest or belief in self in place of old sense of inadequacy and old worries (34)

Industrial system of treatment or work cure—a division of the 24 hours into changeable periods of work, rest and recreation, plenty of air, wholesome food, wise suggestions and such medical treatment as may be indicated (26)

EXPECTED RESULTS

1. We are dealing with matters of everyday living and are concerned with two things—the attitude of the patient toward his environment and also with that environment (25).
2. We should sidetrack the vicious trains of thought and habits of living and substitute a less harmful, saner and more rational life (24).

3. We should substitute a simple but positive efficiency which will reorganize the life of the individual on better lines (24).
4. The work cure takes the patient as he is and seeks first to improve the mental and moral condition by substituting for the well known confusion and faulty habits of life a simpler and saner order of living (27).
5. The one great end to be obtained is self-forgetfulness and a pride and satisfaction in work and in life.

ASSESSMENT INSTRUMENTS
None mentioned.

INTERVENTION STRATEGIES
1. Media
   a. Pottery making and glazing
   b. Hand weaving, rug making and fabrics
   c. Spinning
   d. Fabric dying
   e. Basket making, discarded, not profitable
   f. Wood carving, discarded, not profitable
   g. Metal work, discarded, not profitable
   h. Leather, discarded, not profitable
2. Methods
   a. Treatment begins with bed rest, but gradually patient is asked to do more.
   b. Hours of rest gradually shorten and hours of work made longer until a day is full.
3. Equipment
   a. Kiln
   b. Patterns wheel
   c. Looms
   d. Spinning wheels
   e. Bobbin winders
   f. Vats for color dye
4. Precautions
   No specific precautions given.

SUMMARY
Graded occupation was built on an idea that faulty living, not overwork, was the basis for neurasthenia. Hall organized his treatment regime into a 24 hour per day program which included changeable periods of work, rest and recreation, fresh air, wholesome food, wise suggestions and medical treatment when necessary. He started his patients on small doses of work which he gradually increased. The work was usually manual in nature such as pottery or weaving.

Hall developed five concepts which are useful to occupational therapy today. One is graded effort which is the process of starting out with light, simple work for short periods of time and gradually increasing the complexity and time. A second is economic strength or conservation of energy which involves using only the strength and energy needed to get the job done. The third is the concept of indirection in which interest or ambition is aroused through the use of something novel or new to the person. The fourth concept of substitution follows the third. Substitution involves replacing an old undesirable feeling, belief or interest with a new and better one. The fifth concept of parallels or equivalents follows the fourth. Equivalents involve the use of alternate pathways to getting and maintaining attention when the old ones are blocked.

Hall used all five concepts in his treatment program. He graded the effort expected of his patients in terms of complexity and time. He observed and corrected faculty uses of energy conservation. He used occupations and activities which were novel to his patients and thus not associated with old faulty habits (indirection). He organized the treatment program so that patients learned to substitute the new attitudes and habits of living for the old faulty ones. Finally, he felt that work and leisure occupations could be viewed as equivalents in terms of performance requirements. If the patient refused to work, Hall used a leisure activity to gain the same level of performance from the person.

Activities Model—Cynkin
FRAME OF REFERENCE

The activities model by Cynkin (35) is drawn from a variety of sources, including psychologists, psychiatrists, anthropologists, neurologists and occupational therapists. The model is an eclectic approach to the use of activity in a therapeutic process.

ASSUMPTIONS ABOUT MAN AND OCCUPATIONS

1. Activities of many kinds are characteristic of and essential to define a human existence.
2. Activities are carried out as part of the procedures of man's day to day living.
3. Activities involve a process of "doing."
4. Activities can be learned.
5. Activities are socioculturally regulated by a system of values and beliefs and thus are defined by and in turn define acceptable norms of behavior.
6. Activity patterns can be equated with function.
7. Activities delineate and differentiate an idiosyncratic style for each individual.

ASSUMPTIONS ABOUT HEALTH

1. An individual leads a most satisfying way of life if able to carry out a set of activities approved by the group but also fulfilling personal needs and wants.
2. Change in activities-related behavior can move in a direction from dysfunctional (unacceptable) to functional (acceptable).
3. Activities themselves, systematically selected and combined in patterns tailored to each individual, are means for the development or restoration of function.

4. Change in activities-related behavior from dysfunctional toward functional takes place through motor, cognitive, and social learning.

ASSUMPTIONS ABOUT OCCUPATIONS

1. Activities have properties which can be classified, including attributes, sets, rhythms and frequencies, patterns of sequence, time dimensions and interpersonal field.
2. Activities can be grouped into categories under such headings as work-related, leisure time, social, recreational and self-care.
3. Activities occur in a field of action which encompasses
   a. The environment in which the specific activity takes place
   b. The roles that govern the conduct of the activity both implicit and explicit.
4. Activities have time dimensions based on a socioculturally determined view of how much time is good and proper to spend on specific kinds of activities.
5. Activities change with the stages of development which
   a. Recognize milestones that signal the progress attainment of critical developmental steps toward physical, mental, social and emotional maturity
   b. Become associated with specific age groups in terms of physical, mental or emotional readiness for performance.

ASSUMPTIONS ABOUT LEARNING ACTIVITIES

1. Activity needs a sustained sequence, a habitual routine, so that attention can be held by shutting off irrelevant impressions.
2. To achieve the sense of accomplishment, or competence, requires a task that has some beginning and some terminus.
3. An activity must have some meaningful structure to it if it requires skill that is a little beyond that now possessed by the person.
4. The "teacher" must be a day to day working model with whom to interact and not a model to imitate.
5. Activities encourage a give and take situation or reciprocity that requires a person to fit one's efforts into an enterprise.

ASSUMPTION ABOUT OCCUPATIONAL THERAPY

Occupational therapy assumes that in the doing comes the reward, either in the process itself or in the attainment of a successful end result.

CONCEPTS

Health and function—manifested in the ability of the individual to participate in socioculturally delineated and prescribed activities with satisfaction and comfort

Ill health or dysfunction—inability of the individual to carry out the activities of every day living in those patterns designed and approved by the community

Will to learn—the intrinsic motives for learning, including curiosity

Meaning of activities—includes being familiar to the individual, arousing positive associations and tending to elicit approval from others

Relevance of activities—the relationship of activities to the real world to which the individual has to return and belong

EXPECTED RESULTS

None stated.

ASSESSMENT INSTRUMENTS

1. Types
   a. Activities history—the story of the individual's activities life
   b. Activities inventory—produces a chronological listing of specific activities that have helped to form the pattern of the individual's everyday life
   c. Object history—uncovers feelings and associations about the significant objects, human and nonhuman, that have been connected with activities
2. Procedures—directed at answering the following questions:
   a. Who is this individual who has come for help?
   b. What is this individual's activities configuration in terms of past and present experience and future wishes?
   c. What is the sociocultural activities configuration of the group to which this individual belongs?
   d. What are the physical, intellectual, emotional and interpersonal skills required to perform these activities in ways that are individually satisfying and socioculturally acceptable?
   e. Which of these skills does the individual have?
   f. Which of these skills have never been developed?
   g. Which of these skills has the individual lost, temporarily or permanently?
   h. How long have the skills been lost or unavailable?
   i. What are the possibilities for the following?
      1. Regaining lost skills
      2. Compensating or substituting for lost skills
      3. Achieving new skills
   j. What are the probabilities, given realistic constraints, of acquiring these skills?

INTERVENTION STRATEGIES

1. Media—analysis
   a. Appropriate activities should be meaningful and relevant to the patient/client and to the setting.
   b. Practical activities should be administered quickly and easily, completed within time frames imposed and fit within budgetary restrictions.
   c. Versatile activities should lend themselves by virtue of their properties and characteristics to a variety of processes, end products and situations.
   d. Adaptable activities should be adaptable to individuals and thus to different patient needs.

2. Methods
   a. Selection—activities are selected on the basis of patient/client needs based on criteria stated under media.
   b. Structuring—the breakdown of each activity in ways that make it therapeutic.
   c. Scheduling—integrating activities into the patient/client's daily schedule.
   d. Interaction—the therapist serves as a competence model, facilitator, advocate and a counselor.
   e. Environments—consists of arranging physical settings, people and objects to facilitate activity.
   f. Theory—use of procedures consistent with a particular theoretical rationale.
   g. Process—the stages of an occupational therapy program including initial assessment, planning, implementation and termination.
   h. Equipment—specialized to be applied or attached to:
      1. The patient/client, *e.g.*, splints, slings, prostheses, weighted cuffs-functional devices
      2. Objects in the environment, *e.g.*, bath rails, jar opener, armrests
      3. Activities apparatus, padded grips, easels, pulley and weights.
3. Equipment—not stated.
4. Prerequisite skills—none stated.

SUMMARY

The activities model focuses on what is the nature of activities, what makes activities therapeutic, how activities can be used to promote function and reduce dysfunction and how therapy occurs. Cynkin discusses the rationale and beliefs about activities in terms of human existence, socioculture values, health promotion and functional performance. She explores how activities can be categorized, classified and configurated. Categories include work-related, leisure time, social, recreational and self-care. Classifications include environmental requirements, interpersonal transactions, rules, tools, etc. Configurations are the patterns of use in a time period, such as a day.

Cynkin suggests that activities promote function through learning that is meaningful and relevant to the person. When activities are used for reducing dysfunction, the therapist must understand the nature of dysfunction, the rationale for various management techniques, the constraints of limitations of activities, the methods which can be employed, the tools and environments required and specific techniques in terms of therapeutic potential. Finally, Cynkin discusses the process or stages of therapy, including initial assessment, planning, implementation and termination. The process illustrates how activities are incorporated into actual therapy situations.

Analysis and Critique of Action and Doing Models

FRAME OF REFERENCE

Models of action and doing follow the same basic division according to meta model philosophy. Occupational therapy from its formal beginning in 1910 to 1920 has struggled to maintain a dual existence and explain the rationale for action and doing within its media. The models presented in this section convey the organismic and humanistic models of action and doing in relation to activity. Actually, these models have had less influence than the one outlined in Figure 10.22. The medical model of action and activity produced rationale and activity analysis based on diagnostic categories and emphasizes the potential role of the activity in reducing the affects of undesirable behavior while increasing the desired behavior. The locus of control is with the institutional staff, while the individual is a pawn.

In contrast, the models presented in this section illustrate the use of action and activity to increase the individual's abilities and skills in dealing effectively with the internal and external environment. The locus of control is maintained within the individual who is viewed as the primary actor or originator of behavior.

CLARITY

Probably no other area of occupational therapy has been discussed more and understood less than the effect of action on health and role of activity in gaining, regaining and maintaining health. When action is discussed by Meyer and the Fidlers, it is clearly a process which begins within the person as a mental mechanism and ends in an activity or occupation. The activity or occupation becomes a confirmation of the mental process which the individual can assess in terms of what the mental process initiates vs. what actually was done. The feedback is the result of the action on the activity which is either a success or a failure in comparison to the action plan. Repetition of action and activity

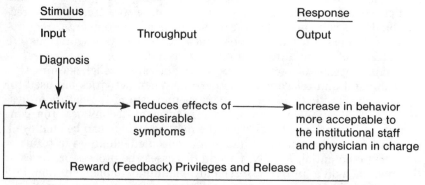

Figure 10.22.   Medical model of action and activity.

normally leads to ego development, adaptation, achievement, mastery or competence according to Meyer and the Fidlers (Fig. 10.23). In contrast, the medical model of action and activity views action as a response and activity as the stimulus to produce that action response. Activity is used to control action, not as an inherent part of the action.

It is important to provide some working definitions of terms which do not seem to appear in occupational therapy literature with any degree of regularity. Action is the doing of something. Specifically, the word is used in occupational therapy to convey the idea that a person is acting or moving as a whole being. When the word action is used in a more limited sense, such as the action of a muscle, the point should be clarified.

Definitions of activities should, likewise, be clarified. An activity is what is being acted upon through the individual's action. The activities of occupational therapy therefore are usually external to the individual. This use of the word "activity" is thus different from the action or activity of an internal organ such as the heart's pumping activity and different also from a mental activity such as thinking. Probably the word "function" should be used in relation to the heart's action and the word "process" should be used to clarify the action of thinking.

The next word problem concerns purposeful action or activity. There are three major actions and two major outcome criteria related to purpose. Purpose may be applied to an individual, to the therapist or to society. Purpose may have a wide variety of intended action and values. When the phrase "purposeful activity" is used, how has the concept of purpose been determined? Probably, the ultimate purposeful activity is one which the individual, the therapist and society all agree has the same intended action and value.

Cynkin, in her model, has addressed the issue of purpose by talking about meaning and relevance. Meaning is used to refer to individual beliefs and feelings about an activity, while relevance is used to convey

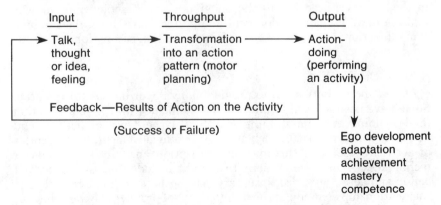

Figure 10.23. Humanistic model of action and activity.

the social view of activity. She does not mention the third variable, that of the therapist's personal bias and professional assessment of the individual and social attitudes toward a specific activity. Occupational therapists must continue the task of clarifying and refining the concept of purposeful activity because it is central to theories of the profession.

A fourth concept which needs to be clarified is that of classifying activity media. Nowhere in literature is there a sanctioned list of which activities occupational therapy uses. None of the model builders described in this section was willing to take on the problem either. Small wonder occupational therapists are accused of using other professions' media and moralities. Occupational therapists are not certain as to what is "mine" and thus are confused about what is "yours."

The fifth concept which needs attention is that of defining and describing the methods, techniques or approaches which action and activity make possible. Again, the profession has no recognized list. Hall presents the only model which describes some real attempts to identify the therapeutic potential of activities in terms of recognizable methods or techniques.

These comments about a lack of recognized methods and techniques do not overlook the many attempts to classify the media according to one or more characteristics of the medium. Classifications are useful, but the real value is in developing identifiable methods based on the techniques.

UNIQUENESS

Occupational therapy has over the years viewed itself as unique because of the use of activity to promote health. Unfortunately, many others also make the same claim. However, most of these professions use only one category or classification of activity, such as sports, dance, poetry, music or art, whereas occupational therapy traditionally has used all of those plus others. Perhaps the uniqueness of occupational therapy does not lie in the activities used but in the understanding of action and doing in relation to all human development and performance. If so, the explanation of action must be more pervasive in the occupational therapy literature.

RESEARCH GUIDE

Action and activity seem to provide many opportunities for research. Some have been alluded to already. These include (a) the role of action in developing and maintaining health, (b) the types of actions and activities which are useful such as gross or fine movement, (c) categories of activities useful in therapy, (d) description and use of methods or techniques. Other research activities might include the effectiveness of action and activity vs. drugs, surgery, psychotherapy or incarceration or the relationship of action to the development of problem solving behavior, a sense of mastery or competence, and adaptive or coping behavior.

SPECIALIZATION

To date, specialization in relation to action and activity has been in terms of selecting to use or selecting not to use certain activity as media. For example, some therapists apparently have decided to use only the media associated with sensory integration, while others have decided not to use anything that is considered to be a craft activity. Such apparent specialization may be more detrimental than helpful in promoting occupational therapy as a service-oriented profession. If craft activities can promote the development and maintenance of useful actions which facilitate individual function then crafts should not be banned from use because the therapist does not believe that crafts are worthy of being a professional medium.

ELABORATION AND REFINEMENT

There appears to be plenty of room for both elaboration and refinement of action and activity. Elaboration is needed to determine the sequences of actions which provide the skills for adaptive behavior. The role of exploration, curiosity, manipulation and play all need to be explored.

Refinement is needed to pinpoint outcome criteria. How can mastery of action be measured? What is a person who is competent in an activity able to do? How many actions are needed to adapt and cope to a given environment? How do the actions or activities involved in adapting to an institution differ from those involved in successful community living. Is there a sequence of action development? How can actions once developed be maintained? Is the process of redeveloping actions the same as the ones that develop actions? Can the same or similar activities be used?

EXPLANATORY USEFULNESS

The role of action and activity in human development and behavior would be assumed to be a very useful explanatory tool. In reality, occupational therapists have only scratched the surface of the potential for using action and activity as therapy. Techniques have been used but not described or not verified as instruments of change. For example, graded activity has been known at least since 1906. Where is literature to support the use of graded activity and how is a person assessed to determine what grades of activity are needed? In other words, the potential value of action and activity as a means of explaining something about occupational therapy is great, but the current knowledge is far too limited.

COMMONALITY

The use of activity is very common in therapeutic programs. The growing number of single modality professions makes the point of commonality obvious. In terms of action and activity, the occupational therapists may have to explain the difference between, rather than the commonality among, various disciplines. Perhaps the real point is that occupational therapy used action and activity as the means to develop, redevelop or maintain functional skills and promote adaptive behavior for successful and satisfying living. The concept is deceptively simple. Medicine is used to much more complicated concepts. Society has come to expect that complicated concepts and processes are the rule and normative standard. Occupational therapists must convince medical personnel and society that a simple sounding concept still has a significant impact on the health and function of a human being.

PRACTICE MODEL

Developing a good practice model based on action and activity should be easy to do. There certainly are enough basic models from which to choose. Figure 10.24 is an overview of models discussed in this section. Table 10.6 is a summary of the criteria used to evaluate the models.

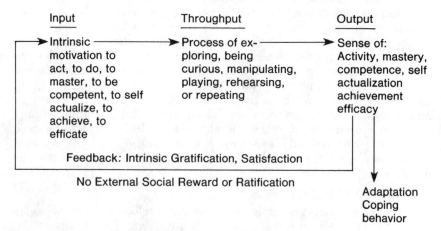

Figure 10.24.   Overview of action models.

Table 10.6
Action and Doing Models Criteria Summary

Evaluation Criteria	Very Good 1	Moderately Good 2	3	4	Very Poor 5
Frame of reference	x				
Clarity			x		
Uniqueness		x			
Research guide	x				
Specialization			x		
Elaboration/refinement		x			
Explanation		x			
Commonality		x			
Practice model		x			

PATTERN AND SEQUENCE MODEL
Developmental Model—Llorens
FRAME OF REFERENCE

The model of development proposed by Llorens (36, 37) is an attempt to integrate or combine several theories which use the concept of development and growth (pattern and sequence) as the central theme of the theory. The developmental theories include the neurophysiological development as contributed by Ayres, the physical, social language, sociocultural and daily living skill development as outlined by Gesell, the eight psychosocial stages described by Erickson, the dynamics and organization of personality described by Freud and the development of intellect as provided by Piaget.

Another major concept related to development is that of adaptive behavior and skills. Havighurst, Mosey, Pearce and Newton have been used as references for the development of coping in and mastery of the environment.

Both development and adaptive behavior have in common the assumption that finality or outcome is the result of a sequence or pattern cycle and order. Each step in the sequence is viewed as dependent upon the successful resolution of the developmental "crisis" which occurs in the previous step. Any event or experience which interrupts or stops the sequential relationship from one step to the next causes dysfunction in the organism.

ASSUMPTIONS ABOUT MAN

1. The human organism develops horizontally (simultaneously) in the areas of neurophysiological, physical, psychosocial and psychodynamic growth and in the development of social language, daily living and sociocultural skills at specific periods of time.
2. The human organism develops longitudinally (chronologically) in each of these areas in a continuous process as he ages.
3. Mastery of particular skills, abilities and relationships in each area of neurophysiological, physical, psychological and psychodynamic development, social language, daily living and sociocultural skills, both horizontally and longitudinally, is necessary to the successful achievement of satisfactory coping behavior and adaptive relationships.
4. Mastery is usually achieved naturally in the course of development.
5. The fundamental endowment of the individual and the stimulation of experience received within the environment of the family come together to interact in such a way as to promote positive early growth and development in both the horizontal and longitudinal planes.
6. Later the influences of extended family, community, social and civic groups assist in the growth process.
7. Physical or psychological trauma related to disease injury, environ-

mental insufficiencies or intrapersonal vulnerability can interrupt the growth and development process.

8. Growth interruption will cause a gap in the development cycle resulting in a disparity between expected coping behavior and adaptive facility and the necessary skills and abilities to achieve same.

ASSUMPTIONS ABOUT OCCUPATIONS AND PERFORMANCE

1. The areas of occupational performance are work, education, play, self-care and leisure.
2. Performance involves complex behaviors that require efficient physical skills and well organized intellectual, social, and psychological abilities.
3. The skills and abilities that are supportive to adequate occupational performance may require development and integration during the course of remediation.
4. Supportive skills and behaviors necessary for successful occupational performance include, (a) adequate sensory perception and cognitive integration, (b) motor coordination, (c) interpersonal-social skills, (d) the ability to relate to human and nonhuman objects and (e) the ability to respond to and effectively interact with the environment as required by the culture.
5. Dysfunction or potential dysfunction in any one of the occupational performance areas may render the individual nonfunctional.

ASSUMPTIONS ABOUT OCCUPATIONAL THERAPY

1. Occupational therapy is an applied health field.
2. The scientific base for intervention is rooted in the biological, behavioral and social sciences and in the knowledge of the inherent properties of activities and relationships.
3. The art of the practice of occupational therapy is learning to combine appropriate information from the basic science fields with the knowledge of sensorimotor developmental, symbolic and daily life activities and interpersonal relationships to help individuals solve problems in their ability to function.
4. Occupational therapy is concerned with facilitating or promoting optimal growth and development in all ages of man.
5. Evaluation of behavior and performance is necessary to determine the need for occupational therapy. Occupational therapy treats problems and potential problems in occupational performance.
6. Occupational therapy through the skilled application of activities and relationships can provide growth and development links to assist in closing the gap between expectations and ability by increasing skills, abilities and relationships in the neurophysiological, physical, psychosocial, psychodynamic, social language, daily living and sociocultural spheres of development as indicated both horizontally and longitudinally.

* 7. Occupational therapy can provide growth experiences to prevent the development of potential maladaptation related to insufficient nurturance in neurophysiological, physical, psychosocial, psychodynamic, social language, daily living and sociocultural spheres of development both horizontally and longitudinally.

CONCEPTS

Occupational therapy—is a problem-solving process involved with the treatment and training of the ill and disabled for restoration of function, and intervention into the lives of the well and able for prevention of disability and maintenance of health

Neurophysiological—refers to those aspects of development that are related to nervous system control of bodily functions and vital processes

Physical or physical motor—refers to observable coordinated physical behavior

Psychosocial—refers to those aspects of behavior that integrate psychodynamic and social factors

Psychodynamic—refers to interactive psychological factors within the organism

Social language—refers to the development of verbal and nonverbal communication skills

Sociocultural—refers to those factors dedicated by and learned within the culture for social interaction

Activities of daily living—refer to routine tasks of everyday life

Developmental tasks and ego adaptive skills—refer to behaviors required of the organism for adaptive functioning

Adaptive functioning—is the result of the satisfactory integration and assimilation of all functional areas of growth and development

Occupational performance—includes work, education, play, self-care and leisure areas which are carried out consistent with cultural requirements of the human organism at given ages and stages of development

Developmental analysis—the process by which occupational therapy determines the extent or lack of disruption and the appropriate evaluation and intervention to be undertaken

Sensorimotor integration—refers to the ability to perceive accurately and integrate sensory stimuli and indicate an appropriate adaptive response through motor behavior

Affective development—ability to comprehend and express emotion, feeling, feelings, and mood factors in behavior and to initiate and respond appropriately to contact with others

Object relationships—ability to establish and adaptively use relationships with human and nonhuman objects to satisfy human needs

Sensory activities—activities that primarily stimulate the senses through the influence of human objects, both self and others

Developmental activities—activities that involve the use of nonhuman objects in play, learning and skill achievement

Symbolic activities—activities that utilize human and nonhuman objects specifically to elicit affective responses and involve the individual in satisfying needs and learning to cope with emotions

Daily life tasks/activities of daily living—those tasks that are required routinely in day to day living

Mastery (described, but not defined)—generally the skill or ability to do activities and engage in interpersonal relationships

Not Defined

Adaptation
Adaptive behavior and skills
Coping behavior
Developmental mastery
Supportive behavior and skills
Work
Education
Play
Self-care
Leisure
Prevention
Remediation
Maintenance

EXPECTED RESULTS

1. Mastery of the developmental tasks and adaptive skills.
2. Achievement of developmental mastery for successful adaptation.
3. Prevention of maladaptation.
4. Maintenance of health.
5. Assisting the person to develop or regain the capacity to function adaptively in the areas of occupational performance is the major focus for prevention, remediation and maintenance in occupational therapy practice.
6. Development of supportive skills and behaviors.
7. Attainment of adaptive functional ability in occupational performance.

ASSESSMENT INSTRUMENTS

1. Techniques
   a. Personal interview—oral or written
   b. Observation of behavior—anecdotal or noted
   c. Review of medical history and other records—written or oral
   d. Testing procedures—informal, formal, standardized and unstandardized
2. Areas to be assessed
   a. Neurophysiological—observation and sensorimotor testing
   b. Physical—observation and sensorimotor testing
   c. Psychosocial—observation and projective testing

d. Psychodynamic—observation and projective testing
e. Social language—observation and developmental testing
f. Daily living—observation and developmental testing
g. Sociocultural—observation and developmental testing
h. Intellectual development—observation, developmental testing and specific intellectual assessment
i. Age, life roles, sex

INTERVENTION STRATEGIES

1. Media and modalities
   a. Sensory Activities
      1. 0–2—touching, being touched, cuddling, hugging, moving, exploring, looking
      2. hearing, tasting, smelling, identifying sounds and objects, physical exercise, balancing, motor planning
      3. 3–6—listening, learning, practicing, skilled tasks and games
      4. 6–11—reading, writing and numbers
      5. 12+—work and leisure activities
   b. Developmental play—see equipment
   c. Symbolic activities
      1. 0–2—biting, chewing, eating, blowing, cuddling in "mothering" relationship, throwing, dropping, messing, collecting, destroying
      2. 3–6—destroying and exhibiting
      3. 6–11—control and mastery
   d. Interpersonal
      1. 0–2—"mothering" relationship, parallel play
      2. 3–6—parallel play in small groups
      3. 6–11—individual interaction, groups, teams and clubs
      4. 12+—individual interaction group and teams
   e. Daily living—not given
2. Methods, techniques and approaches
   Analysis and application of sensory, physical, psychodynamic, social, practical, attention and skill aspects.
3. Equipment for developmental activities
   a. 0–2—blankets, dolls, animals, sand, water, books, blocks, food, trips, gross movement toys, pull toys, play ground equipment, clay, crayons and chalk
   b. 3–6—being read to, coloring, drawing, and painting
   c. 6–11—scooters, wagons, collections, puppets and building tasks
   d. 12+—craft equipment for weaving, carving and modeling, machinery
4. Prerequisite skills—previous developmental stage

SUMMARY

The model by Llorens is made up of three sections. The first section includes a number of developmental theories which illustrate the expectations, behaviors and needs of the developmental-human organisms (Fig. 10.25). In the second section, Llorens outlines the activity areas

MODELS OF PRACTICE

SECTION I
DEVELOPMENTAL EXPECTATIONS. BEHAVIORS & NEEDS
(Selected for illustrative purposes)

NEUROPHYSIOLOGICAL-SENSORI-MOTOR Ayres	PHYSICAL-MOTOR Gesell	PSYCHOSOCIAL Erikson	PSYCHODYNAMIC Hall Grant/Freud	SOCIO-CULTURAL Gesell	SOCIAL-LANGUAGE Gesell
0-2 Sensorimotor Tactile functions Vestib. functions Visual, Auditory. Olfactory, Gusta-tory	0-2 Head sags Fisting Gross motion Walking Climbing	Basic Trust vs. Mistrust/Oral Sensory Ease of feeding Depth of sleep Relax. of bowels	0-4 Oral Dependency Init. aggress. Oral erotic activity	Individual mothering person most important Immediate family group important	Small sounds Coos Vocalizes Listens Speaks
6 mo.-4 Integration of Body Sides Gross motor plan. Form & space perc. Equil. resp. Post. and bilat. int. Body sch. dev.	2-3 Runs Balances Hand pref. established coordination	Autonomy vs. Shame & Doubt/Muscular-Anal Conflict between holding on & letting go	0-4 Anal Independence Resistiveness Self-assertive-ness Narcissism Ambivalence	Parallel play Often alone Recognizes extended family	Identifies objects verb. Asks "why?" Short sentences
3-7 Discrimination Refined tactile Kinesth.., Visual, Auditory, Olfact.. Gustatory funct.	3-6 Coordination more graceful Muscles devel. Skills develop	Initiative vs. Guilt/Locomotor-Genital Aggressiveness Manipulation Coercion	3-6 Genital-Oedipal Genital interest Poss. of opp. parent Antag. to same parent Castration fears	Seeks companionship Makes decisions Plays with other children Takes turns	Comb. talking and eating Complete sent. Imaginative Dramatic
3 - Abstract Thinking Conceptualization Complex relat. Read, write, numbers	6-11 Energy development Skill practice to attain proficiency	Industry vs. Inferiority/Latency Wins recognition thru productivity Learns skills & tools	6-11 Latency Prim. struggles quiescent Init. in mastery of skills Strong defenses	Group play & team activities Independence of adults Gang interests	Language major form of communication
Continue develop. Conceptualization Complex relat. Read, write, numbers	11-13 Rapid growth Poor posture Awkwardness	Identity vs. Role Confusion/Puberty & Adolescence Identification Social roles	11 - Adolescence Emancip. from parents Occup. decisions Role experiment Re-exam. values	Team games Org. important Interest in opposite sex	Verbal language predominates
Development presumably maintained	Growth established and maintained	Intimacy vs. Isolation/Young Adulthood Commitments Body & Ego mastery	Outgrow need for parent validation Identify with others	Group affil. Family, Social, Civic, Interest	Non-verbal behavior also used to communicate
Alterations begin to occur in sensory functions conceptualization and memory	Alterations begin to occur in motor behavior, strength, and endurance	Generativity vs. Stagnation/Adulthood Guiding next generation Creat.. productive	Emotional responsibilities may lessen Phys. and econ. independ. accepted Shift from survival to enjoyment		
Alterations in sensory functions, conceptualization, and memory	Alterations in motor behavior, strength, and endurance	Ego Integrity vs. Despair/Maturity Acceptance of own life cycle	Continued growth after middle age Inner trend toward survival		

Figure 10.25. Schematic representation of facilitating growth and development. (Reproduced with permission from L. A. Llorens (37).)

ACTIVITY OF DAILY LIVING Gesell		SECTION II FACILITATING ACTIVITIES & RELATIONSHIPS (Selected)					SECTION III BEHAVIOR EXPECTATIONS & ADAPTIVE SKILLS		
		SENSORI-MOTOR ACT.	DEV. ACT.	SYMBOLIC ACT.	DAILY LIFE TASKS	INTER-PERS. RELAT.	DEVELOPMENTAL TASKS Havighurst	EGO-ADAPTIVE SKILLS Mosey, Pearce & Newton	INTELL. DEVELOP. Piaget
Recognizes bottle Holds spoon Holds glass Controls bowel		Tact. stim. Visual, Aud., Olfact., Gust. stim.	Dolls Animals Sand Water Excursions	Biting Chewing Eating Blowing Cuddling	Recog. food Hold feed. equip. Use feed. equip.	Individual Interaction	Learning to Walk Talk Take solids Elimination	Ability to respond to mothering Mastering of gross motor responses	Motor skills Integrated
Feeds self Helps undress Recog. simple tunes No longer wets at night	E	Phys. exer. Balancing Motor planning	Pull toys Play grnd. Clay Crayons Chalk	Throwing Dropping Messing Collecting Destroying	Feeding Dressing Toileting	Individual Interaction Parallel play	Sex difference To form concepts of soc. & phys. reality To relate emotionally to others Right Wrong To devel. a conscience	Ability to respond to routines of daily living Mastery of 3 dimen. space Sense of body image	Investigative Imitative Egocentric
Laces shoes Cuts with scissors Toilets indep. Helps set table	V A L	Listening Learning Skilled tasks & games	Being read to Coloring Drawing Painting	Destroying Exhibiting	Feeding Dressing Toileting Simple Chores	Individual Interaction Play small groups		Ability to Follow directions Tol. frustrations Sit still Del. gratification	Egocentricism reduced social. incr. Lang. rep. motor
Enjoys dressing up Learns value of money Responsible for grooming	U A	Reading Writing Numbers	Scooters Wagons Collections Puppets Bldg.	Controlling Mastery	Feeding Dressing Grooming Spending	Individual Interaction Groups Teams Clubs	Learn phys. skills Getting along Reading, writing Values Soc. attitudes	Ability to perceive, sort, org. & utilize stimuli Work in groups Mas. of inanimate obj.	Orders exper. Relates parts to wholes Deduct.
Interest in earning money	T I	All of the above available to be recycled	Weaving Machinery tasks Carving Modeling	All of the above to be recycled	Feeding Dressing Grooming Pre-voc. skills	Individual Interaction Groups Teams	More mature rel. Social roles Sel. occupation Achieving emot. independence	Ability to accept & discharge resp. Capacity for love	Systemat. approach to prob. Sense of equality
Concern for personal grooming, mate, family	O N			Arts Crafts Sports Club & interest groups Education Work	Feeding Dressing Grooming Life role, skills	Individual Interaction Groups	Selecting a mate Starting family Marriage, home Congenial social group	Ability to function indep. Control drives Plan & execute Purposeful motion	Develop. established and maintained
Accepting and adjusting to changes of middle age							Civic & social responsibility Econ. standard of living Dev. adult leisure act. Adj. to aging parents	Obtain, org. & use knowledge Part. in primary group Part. in variety of relationships Exp. self as accept.	Alterations in other areas may affect
Adjusting to changes after middle age							Adj. to decr. phys. health, retire., death Age group affil. Meeting social obligations	Part. in mutually satis. heterosex. relations	

Figure 10.25.

and some examples which she feels will meet the developmental expectations, behaviors and needs. Finally, in section three, Llorens specifies the behavior expectations and adaptive skills which should result from the interaction of needs and activities. These concepts are rearranged into a systems model in Figure 10.26.

As the first section of the model suggests Llorens views development as a simultaneous process occurring in several areas of function, as well as a chronological process occurring throughout the life-span. Normal function is the result of mastery of particular skills, abilities and interpersonal relationships. Such mastery can be seen in the adaptive and coping behaviors exhibited by the person (Fig. 10.27). Dysfunction caused by overwhelming physical or psychological trauma disrupts the developmental process and results in a gap between the skills and abilities available and the adaptive or coping behavior which is expected (Fig. 10.28). Therapy provides the opportunity to develop or regain the skills and abilities through the application of selected activities and relationships (Fig. 10.29). When the skill and abilities are combined, the person is able to master the level of occupational performance required in work education, play, self-care and leisure.

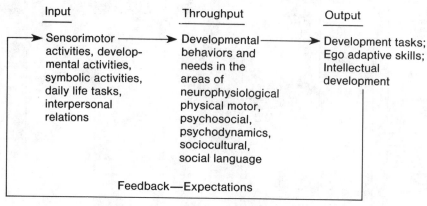

Figure 10.26.   Occupational therapy process.

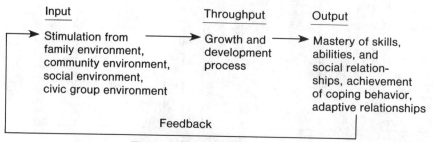

Figure 10.27.   Model of function.

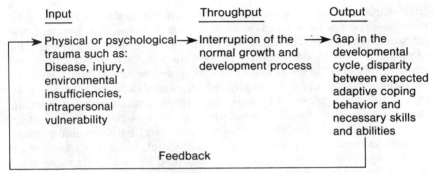

Input	Throughput	Output
Physical or psychological trauma such as: Disease, injury, environmental insufficiencies, intrapersonal vulnerability	Interruption of the normal growth and development process	Gap in the developmental cycle, disparity between expected adaptive coping behavior and necessary skills and abilities

Feedback

Figure 10.28. Model of dysfunction.

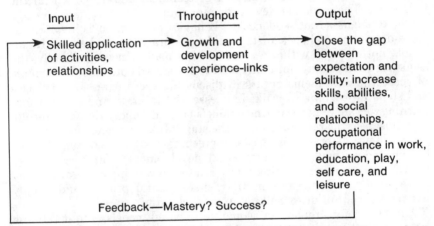

Input	Throughput	Output
Skilled application of activities, relationships	Growth and development experience-links	Close the gap between expectation and ability; increase skills, abilities, and social relationships, occupational performance in work, education, play, self care, and leisure

Feedback—Mastery? Success?

Figure 10.29. Model of the occupational therapy process.

Analysis and Critique of the Developmental Model

FRAME OF REFERENCE

Llorens' model of development is based on theories of development which have stressed the sequential nature of growth development as an orderly process. All of the theories are consistent with the organismic metamodel as Llorens uses them. Although age as a reference for sequence is common, other sequential procedures can be used, such as a series of steps or operations in a task, a progression from simple to complex or other hierarchical arrangement.

CLARITY

The major assumptions regarding sequence concern whether the order is fixed and invariant, and whether the order is correct or the best order given current information. Most model builders and theorists select the invariant hierarchical approach. Stages, levels and phrases are viewed as a fixed sequence through which each individual progresses or fails to progress. Llorens does not state *per se* that she views development as a fixed sequence, but the theorists upon which the model is based tend to view progression as a fixed sequence; thus Llorens has assumed the invariant concept by default if not by design. The advantage of a fixed sequence is that model building is simplified in both construction and explanation. Human development is viewed as lawful and logical with no deviations which must be explained in terms of normal, typical or functional progression. All deviation can be explained as abnormal, atypical or dysfunctional. The solution becomes obvious. Treatment or intervention should be directed toward changing the abnormal atypical or dysfunctional development in the direction of normal, typical or functional development within the established sequence of progression. Difficulties in obtaining change can be explained as inadequate therapist learning, faulty assessment, or lack of technical knowledge within the profession. The model, however, remains intact.

The problem is that sequences of behavior may not be as invariant as some developmental specialists would have practitioners believe. In addition, not all steps within a stage or level may be needed. Finally, the sequence of steps may not really lead to the stated outcome. An example of these three problems occurs in discussing the progression of stages and steps in learning to walk. Is it essential to crawl and creep before learning to walk or can scooting on one's bottom achieve the same results and thus meet the requirements of the stage? Likewise, must homolateral precede heterolateral (cross-pattern) creeping on all fours or can one step be omitted without damage to total development? Furthermore, are crawling, creeping or scooting really related to walking at all or do they serve some other purpose in the developmental process and simply happen to occur prior to walking in most children?

Another major problem in sequentially based models is to determine whether all the steps have been identified so that a complete profile is obtained. The lack of identification of a step in normal development may not be of any consequence. In abnormal development, a missing step could provide the link toward more normal growth and development. The dramatic examples of incomplete sequences have occurred in microbiology where identification of a missing enzyme or amino acid have provided the answer to a serious health problem. Complete knowledge of sequence is no less important in occupational therapy and could be just as dramatic if the facts were known. The problems of the tactilely or touch-defensive child could be such an example if therapists could outline a sequence of steps or sequences of steps to normalize every tactilely or touch-defensive child. Other areas of incomplete sequence appear in the adult and aging years.

A third problem in sequence is illustrated by Llorens' model. When a model builder borrows other developmental sequences, the borrower must determine whether each sequence is needed and is in correct order. Otherwise, the problems of the first model will appear in the second. Furthermore, if the first model builder or theorist changes the initial model or theory, the second model builder has to change the second model or defend the original position.

All three of the problems in sequentially oriented assumptions illustrate the complexity of model building. A model is only as good as the material on which it is built. A model is only useful if others believe it to be useful. If there is doubt regarding the building materials or the usefulness in application, the model may be attractive but unused.

If assumptions can be problematic, concepts can be also. First of all, concepts without working definitions which explain how the concept or construct is used in the model seriously reduce the communication value and potential use of the model. This point has been stressed in Chapter 2. The Llorens model is another example of missing definitions. In particular, some of her outcome words are not defined. What exactly is meant by adaptation, mastery, coping behavior and adaptive behavior and skills? How can the practicing therapist hope to determine whether the outcome has been achieved if the outcome is not defined so that criteria can be deduced from it?

Related to lack of outcome definitions is the problem of definitions of the sequential progression. If one concept must come first the definition should include that point. If the concept is the third in a series, the definition should state the number three position. Llorens has sidestepped the issue of sequential progressive concepts. They are implied in the positioning of developmental areas in the model and again in the listing of assessment areas. However, nowhere does she state that neurophysiological development is the first or most central area of development. A simple model of interlocking rings could have illustrated the relationship of developmental areas throughout the life-span (Fig. 10.30). Such a model provides the rationale for the concepts and for order of assessment procedures and analysis. The model also points out inconsistencies. In the definitions of the concepts social language appears before sociocultural development, but thereafter in the text the two are reversed (37). Which way was intended?

UNIQUENESS

The trend in sequenced based models within occupational therapy has been to stress the combination and interaction of developmental sequences rather than working with only one or two sequences. Such an integrated approach could provide occupational therapy with a unique base. The base is accomplished by identifying the interacting and integrating areas of development and by showing how the integration processes facilitates or triggers further growth and development. The key concepts become maturation vs. learning as the facilitation or trigger mechanism. Llorens does not address the mechanism by which growth and development is facilitated or triggered. Ultimately, occupational therapists must know the degree to which their efforts to provide an optimal environment can be expected to produce results. Maturation traditionally has been considered to be fairly immune to efforts to hasten the process, although environmental opportunity may maximize the effects. On the other hand, learning has been considered to be less affected by the passage of time and more receptive to efforts which may

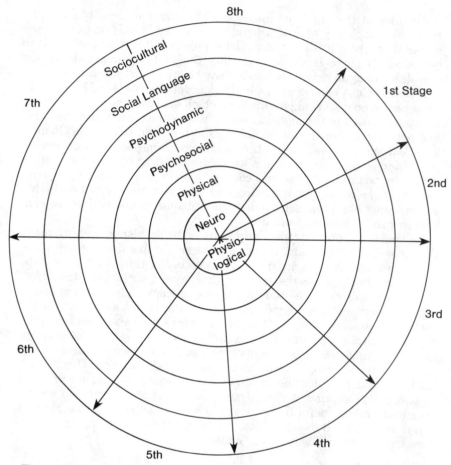

Figure 10.30. The relationship of developmental areas throughout the life-span.

increase the amount of learning by manipulating the environment. Thus those areas of development which respond to learning interactions offer more opportunity for therapy intervention techniques than do maturational areas.

RESEARCH GUIDE

Sequential tasks always need research to verify the order of the items as well as the authenticity of the items themselves. Developmental sequences usually need, in addition, expansion of items in later years. Llorens' model is no exception. Except for Erickson's theory, the other theorists do not have much to say about development or decline in the adult and aging years. Research in life-span development in the years after adolescence could expand greatly the knowledge of human performance in all the areas Llorens uses in her models.

Another area of research is the development of better assessment instruments. Again, the real need appears to be assessment of adults and aging in all developmental areas.

SPECIALIZATION

Developmental and sequential processes provide many opportunities for specialization. A person can specialize in one area of development or in one type of sequential process. Another option is to specialize in one age or stage of development or in one step within a process. Making a decision probably is the most difficult part of determining an area of specialization within development or sequential process.

ELABORATION AND REFINEMENT

As mentioned under Research Guide, a major need for elaboration is in the areas of development concerned with adulthood and aging. In particular, the roles and tasks of the aging individual need elaboration.

Refinement would be useful in describing the role of adaptation, coping and mastery in development. Outcome criteria in terms of adaptive skills and behaviors need to be specified as mentioned under concepts.

EXPLANATORY USEFULNESS

Development is an easy method to use in explaining the changes in human behavior and ability. It has been popular since Arnold Gesell started his extensive studies in 1911. Llorens' model probably explains the process of occupational therapy better than it explains occupational therapy. Section I of the schemetic representations of facilitating growth and development (Fig. 10.25) suggests the areas in which occupational therapy is interested and assesses. Section II lists some of the media and modalities used by occupational therapy in promoting development. Finally, section III outlines some of behaviors and skills toward which occupational therapy intervention might be directed.

COMMONALITY

Development and developmental sequence have been used as a frame of reference for the study of children for many years. Psychology, nursing and education have had courses in development within the curricula for some time. In recent years, life-span development courses have become popular also. Therefore, development as a concept is understood by a number of professions. The problem is to identify in what ways occupational therapy's approach to development is different from others, as mentioned under the section of Uniqueness. Other professions assess developmental sequence in various areas and plan programs based on the information. Occupational therapists must show that they are able to assess problems in the sequence of development and plan programs to correct or minimize the sequential problems.

PRACTICE MODEL

The opportunity to develop practice models based on development and sequential process is as wide as the areas of potential specialization. The

Table 10.7
Developmental Model Criteria Summary

Evaluation Criteria	Very Good 1	Moderately Good 2	3	4	Very Poor 5
Frame of reference	x				
Clarity			x		
Uniqueness		x			
Research guide		x			
Specialization	x				
Elaboration/refinement			x		
Explanation			x		
Commonality	x				
Practice model	x				

focus of models should be better assessment techniques and better intervention strategies which address the needs of facilitating development throughout the life-span. A summary of the criteria used to assess the developmental model are provided in Table 10.7.

References

1. Meyer A: Remarks on habit disorganizations in the essential deteriorations, and the relation of deterioration to the psychasthenic, neurasthenic, hysterical and other constitutions. In Winters C: *The Collected Papers of Adolph Meyer*, Vol. II, Baltimore, Johns Hopkins Press, 1951.
2. Meyer A: The philosophy of occupation therapy. *Arch Occup Ther* 1:1–10, 1922.
3. Meyer A: *Psychobiology*. Springfield, Ill, Charles C Thomas, 1957.
4. James W: *Principles of Psychology*, New York, Holt, Rinehart & Winston, 1890, vol 1, p 114.
5. Slagle EC: *A Syllabus for Training of Nurses in Occupational Therapy*, 2nd ed. Utica, NY, State Hospitals Press, 1933.
6. Slagle EC: Occupational therapy in relation to mental and nervous disease. *Bull Presbyterian Hosp* 49:5–8, 1922.
7. Slagle EC: Training aids for mental patients. *Arch Occup Ther* 1:11–17, 1922.
8. Slagle, EC: A years development of occupational therapy in New York State Hospitals. *State Hosp Q* 8:590–603, 1923.
9. Slagle, EC: The department of occupational therapy. *Institutional Q* 10:29–32, 1919.
10. Kielhofner G: Temporal adaptation: a conceptual framework for occupational therapy. *Am J Occup Ther* 31:235–242, 1977.
11. Neville A: Temporal adaptation: application with short-term psychiatric patients. 34:328–331, 1980.
12. Laken A: *How to Get Control of Your Time and Your Life*. New York, Wyden, 1973.
13. Barsch RH: The concept of temporal tolerance in the brain-damaged child. *Am J Occup Ther* 17:101–105, 1963.
14. Green HB: Temporal stages in the development of the self. In *Study of Time*. New York, Springer, 1975, vol 2, p 1–19.
15. Knapp RH: Attitudes toward time and aesthetic choice. *J Soc Psychol* 56:79–87, 1962.
16. Braley LS, Freed NH: Modes of temporal orientation and psychopathology. *J Consult Clin Psychol* 36:33–39, 1971.
17. Liben LS: Spatial representation and behavior: multiple perspectives. In Liben LS, Patterson AH, Newcombe N: *Spatial Representation and Behavior Across the Life Span*. New York, Academic Press, 1981.
18. Pick HL, Lockman JJ: Frame of reference to spatial representation. In Liben LS,

Patterson AH, Newcombe N: *Spatial Representation and Behavior Across the Life Span.* New York, Academic Press, 1981.
19. Gilfoyle EM, Grady AP, Moore JC: *Children Adapt.* Thorofare, NJ, Slack, 1981.
20. Gordon IJ: *Human Development from Birth Through Adolescence.* New York, Harper & Row, 1969.
21. Gilfoyle EM, Grady AP: Posture and Movement. In Hopkins H, Smith H: *Willard and Spackmans' Occupational Therapy.* Philadelphia, Lippincott, 1978.
22. Meyer A: What is the safest psychology for a nurse? In Winters E: *The Collected Papers of Adolph Meyer.* Baltimore, Johns Hopkins, 1952, vol 4.
23. Fidler GS, Fidler JW: Doing and becoming: purposeful action and self-actualization. *Am J Occup Ther* 32:305–310, 1978.
24. Hall HJ: The systematic use of work as a remedy in neurasthenia and allied conditions. *Boston Med Surg J* 152:29–32, 1905.
25. Hall HJ: Neurasthenia. A study of etiology. Treatment by occupation. *Boston Med Surg J* 153:47–49, 1905.
26. Hall HJ: Work-cure. *J Am Med Assoc* 54:12–14, 1910.
27. Hall HJ: Manual work in the treatment of functional nervous diseases. *J Am Med Assoc* 55:295–297, 1910.
28. Hall HJ: Out-patient workshops—a new hospital department. *Mod Hosp* 1:101–103, 1913.
29. Hall HJ: Orthopedics and the sanatorium. *Boston Med Surg J* 169:678–680, 1913.
30. Hall HJ: Occupation therapy in organic disease. *Boston Med Surg J* 171:228–229, 1914.
31. Hall HJ: Remunerative occupations for the handicapped. *Mod Hosp* 8:383–386, 1917.
32. Hall HJ: Graded effort in convalescence. *Boston Med Surg J* 185:625–627, 1921.
33. Hall HJ: Forward steps in occupational therapy during 1920. *Mod Hosp* 16:245–247, 1921.
34. Hall HJ: *Occupational Therapy: A New Profession.* Concord, Mass, Rumford Press, 1923.
35. Cynkin S: *Occupational Therapy Toward Health Through Activities.* Boston, Little, Brown, 1979.
36. Llorens LA, Schuster JA: Occupational therapy sequential client care recording system: a comparative study. *Am J Occup Ther* 31:367–371, 1977.
37. Llorens LA: *Application of a Developmental Theory for Health and Rehabilitation.* Rockville, Md, American Occupational Therapy Association, 1976.

CHAPTER 11

Descriptive Models: Occupational Areas

OCCUPATION MODELS

Activities of Daily Living

HISTORY

Although daily living activities have been a concern of the occupational therapist for many years the systematic evaluation of such activities did not begin until 1935. In that year, Sheldon (1), a teacher of orthopedic physical education, published a list of daily living activities for children. In 1945, Deaver and Brown (2) published a rating scale of 37 items based in part on Sheldon's work. Deaver is credited with coining the term activities of daily living. The first scale printed in the occupational therapy literature appeared in the first edition of Willard and Spackman (3) which is based on the scale developed by Deaver and Brown. The first scale developed and published by an occupational therapist appears in the *American Journal of Occupational Therapy* in 1950 (4). Livingston developed a form to assess cerebral palsy patients in their skills and record their achievements. Since that time, seven additional scales have been published which credit an occupational therapist as a major or contributing author (5–11).

ASSUMPTIONS

The author has been unable to locate a systematic list of assumptions for ADLs. The major assumptions which underpin the use of ADLs in occupational therapy seem to be as follows:

1. ADLs are a measure of functional skills which a person performs in daily living.
2. ADLs are necessary prerequisites to entering the employment market.
3. ADLs represent a collection of socially acceptable and sanctioned behaviors.
4. ADLs are a set of performance standards which measure or outline the parameters of acceptable deviation from the norms of behavior.
5. ADLs directly affect the role behaviors which a person can perform.
6. ADLs may affect a person's self concept and sense of self worth.
7. ADLs may be influenced by the interactive influence of physical, psychological, social, economic and cultural factors.
8. ADLs performance is an integration of skills in the motor, sensory, cognitive, intra- and interpersonal performance areas.

CONCEPTS

Physical demands of daily life—includes acts inherent in ordinary daily living, such as, locomotion and traveling activities, self-care activities and hand activities (2) (Early description of ADLs)

Functional training—involves the physical reconditioning of the person through a carefully devised exercise and activity program in order to make the person able to handle the body in the most efficient way, so that the person will be as independent as possible (1)

Activities of daily living—the performance of the activities necessary during the course of an ordinary day for independence (1)

Architectual barriers—physical restraints to a person's movement about the environment

ASSESSMENT INSTRUMENTS

1. Goals of ADL evaluation and implementation
   a. Assess the present level of independent and dependent functioning.
   b. Determine in which activities the person needs further learning and practice opportunities.
   c. Determine in which activities assistive devices may be needed.
   d. Assess changes in level of function by repeated evaluation.
   e. Provide data to assist in the decision to discharge to home or to another care facility.
   f. Determine the speed, frequency and efficiency with which a person performs one or more ADLs.
2. Evaluation procedures
   The most common evaluation procedure is a form on which a person's capabilities are recorded. Forms are used for three main purposes. The first purpose is to record and assess the present level of independence and dependence in an institutional setting. Based on the record an intervention program can be developed and revised to include learning or relearning experiences supplying aids and equipment or providing assistance where independence is not possible or incomplete. The second purpose is to evaluate the level of performance in the person's home environment. Based on the performance level, recommendations for changes and adaptations can be made to simplify and to make safer a number of activities. The third purpose is to identify persons who need special care but are not currently receiving such attention. Based on the number of tasks which the person is unable to perform, a decision can be made as to whether the person needs a protective environment or whether other persons and community resources can substitute and fulfill the functions which the person is unable to do. It is important to keep in mind that independence involves motor, sensory, cognitive, emotional and social skills; thus activities of daily living should be

assessed in persons with problems in mental health as well as those with physical disabilities. ADLs also should be assessed whenever a change is made in the use of any special aids or adapted equipment to determine impact on independent functioning.

3. Areas of assessment

The use of ADL evaluation forms tends to vary according to the types of disorder (acute and chronic, pediatric or elderly), the type of disease or the type of request (intake, discharge, homebound). Thus, the variety of forms is endless. The more common items are:

a. Physical self maintenance
   1. Dressing and undressing
   2. Feeding or eating
   3. Personal hygiene—teeth, hair, face, nails
   4. Toileting
   5. Transfers (bed to chair)
   6. Ambulation or mobility

b. Instrumental self maintenance
   1. Write name or write a letter
   2. Shop for food
   3. Plan, prepare and serve meals
   4. Clean house or apartment
   5. Use telephone
   6. Use public transportation
   7. Count money
   8. Carry on basic conversation

c. Other items include: posture; use of wheelchair; time management; use of needle and thread; use of splints, braces or prosthesis; turn lights, television or water faucet on and off; open and close door, window or drawer; use scissors; plug in electric cord; hang up garments; understand signs for safety or direction.

4. Scoring

The early ADL evaluation forms stressed speed of performance (1), but occupational therapists adopted a recording system which stressed the ability to perform as well as the time required. This performance-based approach may have been related to the fact that the ADL forms were used to assess the children with cerebral palsy. For example, Connell (5) recorded the time and grade based on a five point rating scale as follows:

N (normal)—no apparent involvement

G (good)—able to perform activity with speed and accuracy in spite of involvement

F (fair)—able to perform activity, but with slowness and inaccuracy of movement

P (poor)—partial performance

0—unable to perform activity

In the 1960s some forms such as Dinnerstein (6) continued to use scoring systems which included quality of performance and amount of time, but others, such as Schoening (7), dropped the timing requirement for speed and accuracy. Schoening used a five point scale which is coded as "zero for completely dependent, one for patient requiring extensive assistance, two for moderate assistance, three for minimal assistance and/or supervision, and four for independence." By the time the test was published in 1973, the scoring system was simplified to zero for totally dependent, one, for almost but not quite dependent, two for all other possibilities, three for almost, but not quite independent, and four for totally independent.

In 1972, Potvin (9) devised a test which scored by the time only, while in 1976, Casanova and Ferber (10) evaluated performance only. Thus the 1970s did not see a consistent scoring criterion for ADL evaluation forms. This lack of criterion measurements continues to be symptomatic of the state of the art in ADL evaluation.

INTERVENTION STRATEGIES

1. Media
   a. Form boards—practice boards for buttoning, zipping, snapping, door fasteners, etc.
   b. ADL dolls—same concept as a form board
   c. Practice clothes—clothes used to practice ADL skills which may be oversized, reinforced or have a variety of button hole sizes, snaps, hooks, etc.
   d. Adapted devices or equipment—built up handles, elongated handles, nonskid surfaces, Velcro fasteners
   e. Normal clothes, devices and equipment
2. Methods, techniques
   a. Forward chaining—teach first step, then second step to the end of the task sequence
   b. Backward or reverse chaining—teach last step first, then second to last backwards to first step
   c. Selected task—teach hardest to learn task first, then integrate into normal sequence
   d. Clinic or classroom practice—practice skills in isolation from normal setting and out of time sequence
   e. Normal environment and time—actual performance at the normal time of occurrence
   f. Dry run—actual performance but not in the normal time sequence or visa versa
   g. Simplification—remove or combine certain tasks in the sequence
3. Equipment
   Form boards—toys or garments, adaptive devices and equipment
4. Prerequisites and precautions

a. Observe for "gadget tolerance." Some people have a limited capacity to relate to and use new objects in their environment.
b. Observe safety rules during check-out and use of adaptive devices and equipment

SUMMARY

Activities of daily living consists of determining the tasks a person needs to perform in everyday life and facilitating the performance of those tasks. Most commonly, the tasks are centered around self maintenance activities, such as feeding, dressing and grooming. However, community-based skills may be included also, such as time management, catching a bus, cashing a check or shopping for groceries.

When a person has difficulty performing ADLs because of physical limitations, certain adaptations to equipment or alterations of the environment may be made to facilitate performance. Many adapted devices are available for feeding, dressing, grooming and preparation of foods. Some alterations to the environment might include building a ramp, removing thresholds, widening a door, rearranging the furniture or removing slippery rugs.

Assessment of ADL skills usually is accomplished by using a check sheet to record performance. Several types of record keeping forms are available. The limitation of forms is what and how items are measured. Intervention strategies include a choice of media and techniques. A variety of form or practice boards, toys and equipment are available. Techniques include a number of basic teaching methods, such as forward or backward chaining and the use of adapted devices within the teaching sequence.

Analysis and Critique of the ADL Model

FRAME OF REFERENCE

Assessment and intervention of activities of daily living grew out of a concern to know what daily activities a person could perform. Sheldon (1) gives three reasons for recording such activities; (a) to know if the physical education work was actually useful to the child in daily life; (b) to have an accurate standard of judging improvement in the child's activity; and (c) to work out given standards of activities for various types of handicaps. In actual use, Sheldon reported that the recording helped to disclose problems that might otherwise be overlooked, provided additional information to muscle testing for program planning and established a standard or goal for the intervention program.

Deaver and Brown (2) stress that daily life, as well as daily work, imposes many physical demands on a person which are taken for granted by the average person. For the disabled person, the demands of daily life and daily work may be beyond the available coping mechanisms and threaten independence. Brown (2) states the aim of a daily living program is to promote self-reliance. Clearly these ideas are consistent with those of occupational therapy.

CLARITY

The assumptions about ADLs appear fairly clear, but the problem of concepts is far from clear. The major problem is deciding what activities should be considered ADLs. A summary of eight instruments developed totally or in part by occupational therapists illustrates the problem (Table 11.1). There are 32 items listed which could be reduced or expanded, depending on a person's choice or perspective. Some attempt at uniformity and clarity would seem to be desirable if only among occupational therapists.

Lawton and Brody (13) suggest that ADLs can be divided into two major categories, physical self maintenance and instrumental self maintenance. Physical self maintenance includes toileting, dressing, eating, grooming, ambulation and bathing. Instrumental self maintenance includes use of the telephone, shopping, food preparation, housekeeping, laundry, use of private and public transportation, finances and medication. Thus, physical self maintenance is concerned with those activities which directly affect the maintenance of the body and the self which must be done for basic survival in most cultures, whereas instrumental self maintenance is concerned with those activities which directly affect the maintenance of the body and the self in our culture.

Various concepts are used to describe clusters of behaviors which seem to be related. *Eating or feeding* are the terms more frequently used to refer to the concept of chewing, biting, drinking, using utensils, cups, glasses or plates, and using adapted equipment or devices. *Hygiene or personal hygiene* are the terms used to describe brushing hair and teeth, shaving, nail care, washing the face and body and putting on makeup. *Communication* commonly includes writing, speaking, typing, reading and telephoning. *Dressing and undressing* includes putting on or taking off items of clothing. Dressing may include fastening devices, or the category may be separate. Fastenings include buttons, zippers, snaps, hooks and sometimes shoe lacing and tying. *Transfers* is the concept of moving from one place to another, such as from bed to chair. Other transfers may include the toilet, tub, shower, wheelchair, or car. *Ambulation and mobility* both refer to the ability to move about and include walking independently, use of crutches or cane, or use of a wheelchair. *Toileting* includes all activities related to normal functions, as well as the use of catheters, suppositories and sanitary napkins or tampons. *Cooking or meal preparation* includes all planning of a meal, opening cans, packages or jars, mixing ingredients, turning on the oven and stove and setting the table. A *miscellaneous* category may include a number of other common activities, such as turning on or off light switches, television sets, radio or record players, opening or closing drawers, windows or doors plus many other items.

UNIQUENESS

If occupational therapists are going to claim ADLs as a unique area of assessment and management, they are going to have to hustle. Of the 31

Table 11.1
Summary of Categories Found on ADL Forms

	Gersten	Benjamin	Livingston	Schoening	Potvin	Dinnerstein	Connell	Casanova
Toileting		X	X			X		X
Teeth care	X	X			X			X
Bathing	X	X	X					X
Hair Care		X	X	X		X	X	X
Dressing/undressing	X	X	X	X	X	X	X	X
Make up						X		X
Sharing		X				X		X
Posture			X					X
Nail care			X				X	X
Housekeeping								X
Meal planning								X
Telephone					X		X	X
Bus								X
Shopping								X
Meal preparation		X						X
Meal serving								X
Eating/drinking	X	X	X	X	X	X	X	X
Clean up								X
Writing letter			X					X
Utilities			X			X	X	X
Locomotion/travel		X		X			X	
Transfers	X	X		X		X		
Wheelchair						X		
Ambulation	X					X		
Interpersonal relations						X		
Bed				X				
Bowel and bladder		X		X				
Games			X					
Preparation of tea		X						
Use of taps/faucets		X						
Stairs		X						
Sit up	X							

published instruments viewed by the author for this section, only four were authored by occupational therapists. Another four listed an occupational therapist as a contributing author. Of the 23 remaining instruments, 11 listed a physician as a primary author, five listed a physical therapist, four listed a doctor of philosophy and one each listed a social worker, nurse and teacher. ADL instruments and programs are everywhere.

It would appear that occupational therapists have a problem of image and authority. What occupational therapists say they do and what literature reveals is quite disparent. Of the eight scales in which occupational therapists are credited as authors, only the four which appear in the occupational therapy journals list the occupational therapist as the senior author. None of these four include any normative data, or provide any information on validity or reliability. An evaluation tool which does not provide information on these three areas cannot be considered a serious evaluation instrument. If occupational therapists are going to be recognized as authorities in the problems of daily living, then occupational therapists must become more visible in the area of assessment which includes evaluation tools that meet the criteria of test construction currently in existence. Furthermore, these evaluation tools must be available in a variety of formats which relate to the problems of people in different environments. The problem of suitability or construct validity is another major concern of ADL evaluation and implementation.

Some authors admit that ADL forms are developed frequently on the basis of intuition or face validity rather than on construct validity (10, 11). In other words, the author selects items that seem logical to include based on the author's judgment and observation. Little attempt is made to determine if in fact the items are the ones which most significantly affect a person's performance in that person's actual living environment. Thus, it is possible for a person to achieve top marks on the ADL evaluation tool but not be able to function independently in the actual living environment, because the significant items for that person were not assessed during the ADL evaluations. Thus, the problem of determining what should be evaluated is essential to the construction of an ADL evaluation form, and such determinations cannot be made solely on the basis of what "looks good" to the test developer. Modifications and adjustments must be made as the instrument is used in actual practice during the research development phase.

Hoberman et al. (14) have suggested that the criteria for the development and use of any given ADL test should be based on two objectives: first, the test should reveal useful information, and second it should be administratively practical. These objectives are not unique to ADL evaluations, but the subobjectives are. Regarding the objective of producing useful information, Hoberman suggests five subobjectives. (a) The instrument should show a person's ability or lack of ability to perform a variety of activities which are representative of those encountered in daily living. (b) The data which the instrument provides should include a measure of the person's proficiency in performing activities in terms of the time required, the assistance needed to perform the tasks safely and the endurance or tolerance level which the person has for each activity. (c) The instrument should assist in ascertaining the reasons for failures, such as lack of muscle power, poor balance, inadequate training, fatigability or apprehension. (d) The instrument should provide data on which to base a conclusion about the person's current level of function and predictions to the amount of future progress that may be expected. (e) The instrument should provide information on which to form an opinion as to the person's present and probable future status, as to whether the person will require a protected learning environment or become capable of independent living and as to whether assistive devices or adapted equipment will be needed to perform some or many activities.

The second objective that the test be administratively practical has seven subobjectives. One, the test should be applicable to persons who (a) are in bed, in a wheelchair or able to walk, (b) require or do not require assistive devices and adapted equipment and (c) have varying degrees of motor ability. Two, the instrument should permit repeated reevaluations of persons as the intervention procedures progress. Three, the instrument should be constructed so that repeated administrations can be recorded on one form to facilitate comparison of data and the interpretation of progress. Four, the instrument should provide separate indices of function independence for different classifications of persons such as those who are confined to bed or wheelchair or those who are ambulatory. Five, the scoring system should be devised so that it reflects not only the number of activities performed but the facility or ease with which the activities were performed. Six, the instrument should be as concise and brief as possible by eliminating any duplication of activities and avoiding the testing of persons on certain skills which are clearly above the functional level, such as young children or severely disabled persons, or clearly below the functional level, such as an adult or an ambulatory person. Seven, the instrument should be as simple as possible to administer, score and interpret. These ideal requirements are difficult to meet, but do provide a framework for test construction and assessment of current instruments. Most tests which appear in the literature appear to have severe limitations as to purpose and data provided.

RESEARCH

Research using ADL forms has been widespread. One major problem in the use of ADL forms for research purposes in occupational therapy is to determine the best measurement systems and scoring criteria.

ADLs can be divided easily into the categories of total independence and total dependence, but the stages in between are more difficult to measure. For the most part, ADLs must be measured using a rank order system. Thus, an activity can be evaluated by adding such rating criteria as semiindependent and semidependent or uses adapted equipment and requires human assistance. The problem with all rank order measurements is that equal distance between any two ranks is not possible. One cannot determine if the same amount of performance is required for a person to move up a rating scale from dependent to semidependent as from semiindependent to independent. Thus, the steps between the rating criteria may not be equal. Therefore, when numbers are added to the rating scale to facilitate scoring, a problem arises, because numbers do have equal distance between each other. As a result, it becomes easy to superimpose an ordinal system of measurement in which the distance between any two adjacent ratings is equal onto a rank order system of measurement in which the distance between any two adjacent ratings may be unequal. The real impact of such measure and scoring difficulties is observed when the results of ADL evaluations is interpreted. For example, suppose that a person is completely dependent on all ADL functions on the first evaluation. In 2 weeks the person is reevaluated and is rated as semiindependent. Two weeks later, however, no measurable change has occurred. Possible interpretations are the patient is uncooperative, poorly motivated or reached the maximum level of performance which could be expected. Any of these interpretations could lead to discharge. However, there is another interpretation based on the scoring criteria. This interpretation suggests that more effort may be required to move up the rating scale from semidependent to semiindependent than from totally dependent to semidependent.

It could be hypothesized that the normal progression takes 2 weeks to move from totally dependent to semidependent but that 4 weeks is required to move from a rating of semidependent to semiindependent. If so, the person described above may be making satisfactory progress at the time of the second reevaluation and may be cooperating fully with the rehabilitation program.

A second problem concerns the comparison of two or more persons' experience in an intervention program such as rehabilitation. If the scores such as 0, 1, 2, or 3 are used, the real impact of the rehabilitation program may be misinterpreted. Assuming that one of the stated purposes of the program is to increase the level of function of persons in the area of ADLs a researcher could determine how many persons increased their level of function as indicated by changing scores on the ADL evaluation within 2 weeks after being admitted. If the researcher is unaware that normal progression is actually 2 weeks between scores 0 and 1, 4 weeks between 1 and 2 and 6 weeks between scores 2 and 3, the researcher may conclude that the program is ineffective because few persons receiving initial scores of 1 or above make any significant, *i.e.*, measureable change. The researcher has fallen into the trap of the ordinal scale and assumed that the numbers mean equal performance levels, time requirements or both and therefore is unaware that ADL evaluations actually are based on rank-ordered measurements.

A third problem is the use of ADL evaluations in outcome criteria.

Numerous efficacy studies of rehabilitation have used ADL scales as a criterion measurement of the outcome of a rehabilitation program. The hypothesis is that good rehabilitation programs will have "graduates" which maintain or improve their ADL scores a year or more after leaving the program.

Unfortunately, ADL intervention programs do not work like a good vaccine. That is, ADL programs do not prevent loss of function. The program only increases the potential for function but cannot guarantee that the functions will be used or maintained. Changes in life-style, living environment and health states influence the level of ADL functioning. Failure to consider these variables may result in an inaccurate assessment of a rehabilitation program.

Once all the problems of item selection, measurement criteria and scoring procedures are solved, there appears to be some good hypotheses which could be posed by a researcher concerning the role of ADLs in rehabilitation outcome and social independence. These hypotheses could be stated as follows:

1. Performance of ADLs is central and basic to the goal of achieving independent functioning.
2. The more independent a person is in ADL performance, the more likely the person is to be able to maintain independent living.
3. There is a core of ADLs which a person must be able to perform alone in order to live independently.
4. The performance of ADLs is a functional measure of the success of a rehabilitation program.
5. ADLs are subject to a valuing scale which determines one's social scale of dependence-independence.

SPECIALIZATION

Many occupational therapists probably feel that they specialize in ADL assessment and management. Such an emphasis on daily living tasks would seem to be a logical concern for occupational therapists. Moreover, ADLs assessment and management could provide a specialization in assessment development and standardization, and a specialization in the efficacy of occupational therapy programs by using ADL instruments as outcome criteria.

Some of the advantages therapists have in specializing in ADLs is the combined knowledge of sensory motor skills, social values and expectations, and work efficiency. When total independence is not a feasible goal, therapists can assist in helping a person decide which ADLs should be done alone and which can be best accomplished with assistance. Such decisions suggest a hierarchy of ADLs in which society does or does not provide alternative forms. For example, society permits and sanctions having one's hair groomed and cleaned by others. However, there are no social options for toileting skills. When another person helps with toileting, a person's independent status is lost. On the other hand, some ADLs appear to have a partial option. For example, a person can have one's teeth cleaned by a dental assistant without fearing loss of status but perhaps not every day.

The occupational therapist does appear to have a unique view of ADLs which would serve the purpose of specialization. However, occupational therapists must develop the viewpoint into tangible results for others to see.

ELABORATION AND REFINEMENT

Elaboration of ADLs is needed to determine more accurately the role of ADLs in social interaction and approval. Specifically, society appears to have a system of values attached to ADLs which has not been well explored. Knowledge of such values could be very useful in planning and implementing programs. The relevant aspects appear to be skill and performance and age up to a certain point. If a person performs or functions at an above minimal level of performance, society accepts the individual as independent. Performance below the minimum level is viewed by society as too dependent and the value is negative (Fig. 11.1).

Refinement, on the other hand, is needed to determine exactly what ADL skills are needed for function in various environments. Perhaps, also the skills should be subdivided, as Lawton and Brody (13) suggest, into physical and instrumental self maintenance for clarity and ease of assessment. In addition, as mentioned under Uniqueness and Research, the problems of measurement and scoring need attention.

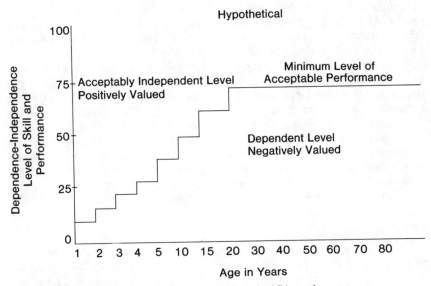

Figure 11.1. Scale of independence in ADL performance.

EXPLANATORY USEFULNESS

ADL performance should be easy to explain to others at a basis level. Almost everyone does daily living tasks and either wants to maintain the current level of performance or increase performance. Thus, most people can identify quickly the purpose and role of ADLs in everyday living. What is more difficult to explain is that ADLs are not as simple or basic as may appear at first glance. ADLs are the result of integrating a number of subskills into patterns of routine performance. As long as the subskills and patterns remain intact, the performance is fairly routine. However, disturbances in the subskills or patterns caused by illness, injury, or normal aging may result in far ranging changes which seem to the nontrained eye to be unrelated. For example, why does pain in the shoulder affect writing with the hand? Most people are unaware of the role the shoulder muscles and joints have in facilitating the use of fingers to hold a pen and write.

Thus, the concept of ADLs as important is easy to describe, but the learning or relearning of task performance is more difficult to explain. However, the role of the occupational therapist is tied to both the concept and the performance. Occupational therapists need to provide better explanations of ADL performance.

COMMONALITY

ADLs are a common subject matter with several other health disciplines and with educators. Nurses and physical therapists in particular are concerned with ADL assessment and performance. Unfortunately, the concern tends to hinder rather than help occupational therapists in attempts to interact with nurses and physical therapists regarding the use of ADLs in program planning. Everyone tends to want to do the ADLs totally or not at all. Somewhere in between usually is most helpful to persons who need the help.

The area of ADLs would seem large enough for everyone to get a "piece of the action." Perhaps more attention should be paid to developing a professional interrelated pattern of dealing with ADLs which stress a connectedness rather than a pattern which stresses separateness. With educators, the problem is more concerned for providing technical assistance. Educators know the teaching-learning methods. What they lack is information from anatomy, physiology, kinesiology and neurobiology which provides the functional and dysfunctional aspects of performance. Educators and occupational therapists can work together well in helping people to learn or relearn ADLs if the talents of each are combined for a common purpose.

PRACTICE MODELS

Good practice models depend upon good assessment instruments. The primary problem in practice model development is the failure to create and test effective assessment tools for evaluating ADL skills. Therefore, development of better assessment instruments should be the primary step in practice model construction. A summary of the criteria used to critique the ADL models is given in Table 11.2.

PRODUCTIVITY
Prevocational Model

FRAME OF REFERENCE

Prevocational evaluation and training has been known to occupational therapists since the early leaders started writing about it (15–17). As a legitimate area of rehabilitation, however, the date 1936 is mentioned most frequently (18). In that year, the Institute for Crippled and Disabled in New York City began a prevocational unit to measure the capacities of disabled persons along the lines of those techniques being used to assess able bodied people for prospective employees. Nevertheless, little expansion of activity occurred until after World War II. In 1954, the Vocational Rehabilitation Amendment Act provided educational funds for medical specialists, and the Medical Facilities Survey and Construction Act provided funds for prevocational units to be included in rehabilitation centers. Occupational therapists became one of the major sources of prevocational evaluators because of their knowledge of disability and activity. In the 1970s, however, occupational therapy involvement diminished as other personnel, especially vocational counselors, became more involved and started enforcing standards which occupational therapy did not meet. Also, the interest among occupational therapists seemed to diminish.

Prevocational evaluation and training is a term used in vocational rehabilitation in the 1950s. The term today is "work adjustment." However, most of the literature in occupational therapy uses the term prevocational, so both terms will be used interchangeably. Prevocational or work adjustment activities seem to have three basic parts which make up a working definition. These are the processes of (a) learning the meaning, value, and demands of work; (b) modifying or developing attitudes, personal characteristics and work behavior and (c) developing

Table 11.2
ADL Models Criteria Summary

Evaluation Criteria	Very Good 1	Moderately Good 2	3	4	Very Poor 5
Frame of reference	X				
Clarity			X		
Uniqueness			X		
Research guide		X			
Specialization	X				
Elaboration/refinement		X			
Explanatory usefulness		X			
Commonality	X				
Practice model		X			

the functional capacities required to obtain the optimum level of vocational development. Each prevocational or work adjustment program emphasizes various aspects or combinations of the three processes. Thus, the variations of programs is endless.

ASSUMPTIONS

The following assumptions are a synthesis of the literature:
1. Productive skills are developed in a sequential developmental pattern (19).
2. The rate of productive skill development is variable.
3. Productivity fulfills extrinsic and intrinsic needs.
4. Some people have inadequately developed productive skills which lead to dysfunction in productive performance.
5. Dysfunction in productive performance reduces the opportunity to fulfill extrinsic and intrinsic needs through productivity.
6. Dysfunction in productive performance may negatively affect performance in self maintenance and leisure.
7. Prevocational assessment and training (work adjustment) can facilitate the development of productive skills.
8. Improved productive performance may increase the probability of productivity fulfilling extrinsic and intrinsic needs.
9. Improved performance in productive skills may influence positively the performance of self maintenance and leisure activities.
10. Improved performance in productive skills may facilitate individual placement in a specific work setting at a selected job or vocation.

CONCEPTS

Prevocational evaluation—an assessment, prior to work training, of the client's potential as a worker, giving special attention to his ability to learn and to retain job skills, social amenities, work tolerances, good work attitudes and habits and personal responsibility (20)

Prevocational training—a program which introduces the client to the meaning of work in society, the characteristics of successful employees, the expected characteristics of an employer and the responsibilities of wage earners, and which prepares him to participate in, and profit from, additional structured vocational instruction (20)

Work—refers to all types of productive activity paid or unpaid, regardless of locale, whether in workshops, institutions, industry, business or the home (21)

Work aptitude—one's natural ability or general suitability to work; sometimes refers to a measure of that ability (20)

Manual dexterity—ability to coordinate one's hands to accomplish basic, specific tasks, *i.e.*, inserting, collating, dialing a telephone, etc (20)

Worker trait—characteristic required to perform a function of an occupation (20)

Work environment—surroundings and the conditions under which an individual performs the occupational duties, including light, equipment, cleanliness and type of supervision (6)

Work or job analysis—involves the systematic study of an occupation in terms of: what the worker does in relation to data, people, and things; the methodology and techniques employed; the machines, tools, equipment, and work aids used; the materials, products, subject matter, or services which result; and the traits required of the worker (22)

Work adjustment program—An individualized, structured and planned, closely supervised, remedial work experience, designed to promote the acquisition of good work habits, to increase physical and emotional tolerance for work activity and interpersonal relationships, and to modify attitudes and behavior which inhibit the satisfactory performance of work (22)

Work sector—the field in which productive activity or work takes place (21)

Work roles—the norms and standards of behavior which are assigned by society to each productive activity (21)

Work adjustment—characterized by the relationship of the work personality to the range of typical work roles in the work culture (21)

Work potential—measured capability of the individual to perform in a competitive job (20)

Work personality—the individual's traits, habits and attitudes related to the concept of employment and the reaction to that concept (20)

EXPECTED RESULTS (23, 24)

1. Assist in determining the aptitudes, interests and abilities through systematic and supervised sampling in the major occupational areas of clerical work, skills and semiskilled occupations, service and subprofessional occupations.
2. Provide a specified period for the evaluation of the patient's performance in actual work situations.
3. Assist the patient in developing work confidence.
4. Assist the patient in developing acceptable work habits.
5. Determine work tolerance in actual or simulated work situations.
6. Provide opportunities for experimentation in the adaptation to vocational equipment to meet the requirements of a work situation.
7. Assist individuals who lack knowledge or contact with a work setting to gain experience in work roles.
8. Assist individuals who lack the functional capacities to perform in a work setting to learn or relearn specific work skills.
9. Assist individuals who lack a sense of direction, identity or purpose in the productive market to gain or regain a work personality.
10. Assist individuals who lack socially learned skills to develop one to one and group interaction skills.

ASSESSMENT INSTRUMENTS

1. Areas
   a. Sensory motor skills—range of motion, muscle strength, endurance, tolerance, coordination, dexterity, perception, sensation
   b. Cognition—skill, attention span, follow directions, judgment, organization, analysis, categorization, resourcefulness, initiative, memory synthesis
   c. Intrapersonal skills—work habits, work attitudes, work values, work interests, emotional adjustment
   d. Interpersonal skills—relationships to peers, relationship to authority, group interaction skills
   e. ADL skills
   f. Productive work skills
2. Examples
   a. Sensory motor tests (25)
      1. Minnesota Rate of Manipulation Test
      2. Pennsylvania Bimanual Work Sample
      3. Crawford Small Parts Dexterity Text
      4. Minnesota Spatial Relations Test
   b. Intelligence tests (25)
      1. Wechsler Adult Intelligence Scale
      2. Wechsler Intelligence Scale for Children—Revised
      3. Stanford Binet Intelligence Scale
      4. Peabody Picture Vocabulary Test (therapist could administer)
   c. Aptitude and achievement tests (25)
      1. Adult Basic Learning Examination
      2. Peabody Individual Achievement Test
      3. SRA Reading and Arithmetic Indexes
      4. Tests of General Educational Development
      5. Wide Range Achievement Test
      6. Differential Aptitude Tests
      7. General Aptitude Test Battery
   d. Vocational inventories, interests and values (25)
      1. Strong Vocational Interest Blank
      2. Kuder Preference Record
      3. Minnesota Vocational Interest Inventory
      4. Allport-Vernon-Lindsey Study of Values
      5. Super's Work Values Inventory
   e. Work samples (25)
      1. Tower System
      2. Philadelphia Jewish Employment and Vocation System
      3. Singer Vocational Evaluation System
      4. Valpar Component Work Sample Series
      5. McCarron-Dial Work Evaluation System
      6. Talent Assessment Program
      7. Wide Range Employment Sample Test

3. Assessment forms developed by occupational therapy
    1. Prevocational Motor Skills Inventory—Brown and Van der Bogert (26)
    2. Evaluation of Work Behavior—Ayres (27)
    3. Work Evaluation Progress Report—Ireland (28)
    4. Physical Capacities Evaluation—Reuss *et al.* (29)
    5. Testing Performance Summary—Cromwell (30)
    6. Performance Evaluation Report—Sattely (31)
    7. Prevocational Unit Forms—Swenson (32)
    8. Work Adjustment Program Evaluation Report—Llorens (33)
    9. Pre-vocation Evaluation of Rehabilitation Potential—Ethridge (34)
    10. Work Assessment—Bailey (35)
    11. Physical Capacities Evaluation—Smith (36)
    12. Workshop Trainee Evaluation—Trombly and Scott (37)
    13. Prevocational Evaluation Patient Progress Form—Pedretti (38)

INTERVENTION STRATEGIES

1. Media
    a. Tools and equipment used in jobs
    b. Arts and crafts
    c. Books on occupational careers and requirements
    d. Job wanted notices
    e. Interview forms
2. Methods and techniques
    a. Behavior modification—changing an individual's behavior in the direction which is desirable in terms of functioning in society.
    b. Job exploration—process of exposing a handicapped individual to vocation information that will increase knowledge of the world of work.
    c. Job task—actual, single work activity taken specifically from a particular occupation.
    d. On the job evaluation—utilization of an actual job setting to give the client the opportunity to experience the specific requirements necessary to do the job and gauge the client's ability to fulfill the specific requirements of the job.
    e. On the job training—a planned experience in an actual work situation through which the client, under supervision, learns to perform all job operations of an occupation.
    f. Work personality development—increasing or modifying the individual's traits, habits and attitudes related to work productivity and employment.
    g. Work readiness—preparing the person's physical, mental and emotional resources for entry into productivity and employment.

h. Work sample—an evaluation of an actual work task; operation of component of an occupational area.

i. Workshop—place where the individual learns and practices productive work tasks for experience. Pay may be received.

j. Work tolerance—increasing the person's ability to endure the requirements of the job duties without performing in an unsatisfactory manner, such as stopping work activity.

k. Work training—organized form of instruction which provides information and skills that are important to the performance of tasks involved in an occupation.

l. Simulation of role play—technique of creating an environment as similar to an actual work situation as possible to permit try out and review of tasks or situations involved in job performance.

m. Task analysis—breakdown of a particular job into its component parts.

n. Work adjustment training—program designed to help the individual form a work personality that will enable the individual to increase productivity and handle the daily demands of employment. Includes development of self-confidence, self-control, work tolerance, ability to handle interpersonal relationships and understand the nature and process of work.

o. Work evaluation—comprehensive process designed to assess the individual in terms of occasional development by systematically utilizing work as the focal point for assessment and vocational exploration.

p. Work habit development—increasing the personal traits essential for getting and holding a job, such as maintaining regular work hours, following directions, etc.

q. Job seeking skills training—increasing or modifying those skills which will enable a person to seek out job vacancies and apply for them, such as filling out applications and handling a job interview.

r. Work therapy—usually designed to use work experience to change the work personality so the person can function in a normal work situation.

SUMMARY

In 1916, Herbert Hall (39), later president of the American Occupational Therapy Association, said "prevocational training is defined as any mental or physical activity undertaken for the purpose of determining the general aptitudes and vocational tendencies of an individual, or for the purpose of overcoming educational or physical deficiency preparatory to full vocational training. When prevocational training is medically prescribed, it is occupational therapy." It is clear that Hall felt that occupational therapy had a definite role in prevocational training and that the role the preparatory stages in learning or relearning a productive occupation.

The intervening years between 1916 and 1954 saw occupational therapists struggling to find exactly what the role of occupational therapy was in relationship to prevocational activities. In 1954, the newly amended Vocational Rehabilitation Act seemed to point the way. Money was available to support prevocational units in medical facilities. Occupational therapists became active in programs designed to assist clients to learn or relearn how to work and be productive. Practice models were evident from several areas. There were personal and work adjustment programs designed to prepare a person for work, such as Cromwell (30), Ireland (28), and Llorens (33). There were work skills and ability programs designed to determine what specific talents a person had, such as Combs (18). Finally, there were physical capacities and tolerance programs which determined the person's performance assets and limitations in work situations, such as Reuss (29). These and other examples of similar practice models abounded until the late 1960s. Thereafter, a sharp drop in interest occurred.

Several problems seem to have combined to cause a loss of interest. The cost of medically oriented prevocational programs became too expensive to operate, the vocational rehabilitation counselors gained some of the skills which occupational therapists had been providing, occupational therapists became interested in sensory motor problems and occupational therapists had not advanced a theory or model to explain their role in productivity.

Some occupational therapists have begun the process of building theories and models of occupation, work and productivity (see chapter 9). Other therapists will have to expand upon the work already done to establish a permanent role for occupational therapy in prevocational evaluation and work adjustment.

Analysis and Critique of the Prevocational Model

FRAME OF REFERENCE

One of the major problems in the area of productivity appears to be a lack of identified philosophy among occupational therapists regarding the role of work. As a profession, occupational therapy has little theoretical explanation as to why people work, what is personally obtained from working and how people learn to work as a developmental task. Fidler and Fidler (40), Maurer (41), and Reilly (42) have made initial attempts to define and describe the role of work in a framework of occupational therapy, but all requires further elaboration and refinement. The Fidlers have stressed the value of doing as a reality-orienting agent. Hart (43) had made the same point by stating that work involves a continuous adaptation to reality. Work involves such tasks as observing, measuring, perceiving and copying which in turn require attention and thinking applied to present situations. Certainly occupational therapy has the media to provide opportunities for doing and performing. The problem is what kinds of doing and performing are most helpful in building work-related skills.

Maurer has stated that vocational development is a developmental or sequentially learned process. Therefore, stages of work development should be identifiable. Four areas are suggested by Maurer which could be analyzed into stages and substages. These areas are identification with the worker, acquiring basic habits of industry, elaborating the self concept and learning to handle and adjust to authority. Again, these areas seem feasible to attain within the known media and methods of occupational therapy. The problem is one of organization and synthesis.

Reilly has emphasized the need to develop competence, mastery and achievement in the work-play continuum. Performing an activity or task provides the opportunity to gain a sense of competence and mastery. Occupational therapists add the dimension of structuring the task in the environment so the person has a maximum chance of success which may never have been experienced prior to therapy.

The problem of learning or relearning to work seems to be especially severe among the chronically disabled. Long-term problems in mental health, severe developmental delay and multiple handicapping conditions are difficult for vocational and rehabilitation counselors to handle. Perhaps, occupational therapists should direct efforts toward increasing work skills within these three groups using the concepts based on doing, development, competence and achievement. The models in Figures 11.2 and 11.3 summarize a possible approach to work and productivity based on the three frameworks provided by Fidler, Maurer and Reilly integrated with problems suggested by Gellman (10).

Another related problem is that of cost. Running a prevocational unit in a medical setting is expensive. When federal funds were available, the financial considerations were not as critical. However, when finances are determined by state appropriations, insurance or direct client payment, the cost becomes important. According to Wegg (44), little study of cost effectiveness was considered. No information was available as to the cost of work adjustment of prevocational evaluation in relation to vocational placement or between a prevocational center in a medical setting as

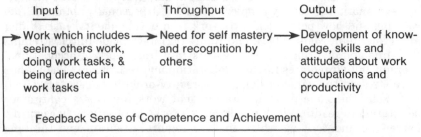

Figure 11.2. Model of work and productivity development.

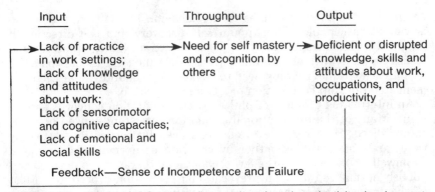

Figure 11.3.   Model of deficient or disrupted work and productivity development.

opposed to a nonmedical setting. Work as an outcome may not be suitable in acute settings. Evaluation may be possible, but the learning or training probably is best accomplished in a community setting. Furthermore, learning work as a major goal without considering ADLs and leisure skills is not consistent with the concept of balance and a total activity schedule. Community or outpatient settings permit more opportunities to view work as part of a total living pattern.

CLARITY

Most of the definitions of concepts have come from literature other than occupational therapy. However, the assumptions are based on a synthesis of occupational therapy literature on work and prevocation evaluation and training.

The occupational therapist needs to be aware that many of the existing models and theories of vocational education are based on the mechanistic and reductionistic philosophies. Nadolsky (45) has summarized the existing vocational theories into three major orientations, the individual trait, the environmental setting and the individual environmental relationship. The individual trait orientation is based on the assumption that the organism is essentially the sum of its parts which can be isolated and measured. Another assumption is that the person is incapable of self-discovery or self-direction. Both are characteristic of mechanistic philosophy.

The Environment Setting Orientation is based on the assumption that jobs can be duplicated and controlled so that a person's performance can be measured for fitness to the job. Self-discovery and self-direction are unnecessary since vocational placement is largely a matter "of matching job requirements to individual performance skills." These assumptions also are more consistent with mechanistic rationale.

The Individual Environmental Relationship Orientation is the only one of the three consistent with the organismic philosophy. Evaluation is based on the assumption that the relationship of the individual to the environment is important in assessing behavior. In addition, the person is viewed as capable of maximum self-discovery and self-direction if provided with the opportunity to choose between events, situations and tasks related to work and productivity. Models and theories of productivity for occupational therapy need to be based on the Individual Environment Relationship Orientation or a similar approach.

An interrelated problem of philosophical orientation concerns assessment. Many of the prevocational evaluations are standardized or semistandardized. However, the evaluations used by occupational therapy were rarely standardized either by criterion or normative techniques. Cromwell (30) was one of the few occupational therapists to develop and publish normalized data on prevocational evaluation procedures. Most of the forms used in occupational therapy were nothing more than checklists which required little skill to use or interpret but did not indicate a definite relationship between prevocational performance and latter job performance. The lack of skill or use of skill to develop better evaluations consistent with a frame of reference seems to be related to the decreased use of the occupational therapists in prevocational units. Occupational therapists working in programs to improve productivity must be prepared to develop and administer assessment procedures consistent with the organismic philosophy.

UNIQUENESS

Although the prevocational and work adjustment area has been taken over by the work evaluators, there may be other areas which occupational therapists can pursue. Perhaps, the uniqueness of productivity for occupational therapists lies in the understanding of the relationship of a person to work. The understanding involves the belief that through work a person changes materials into something else and is changed in the process. The change produced by the work becomes a part of a person's identity and becomes a means of centering and discovering the self (46). Work and productivity are a part of the fabric of life and contribute to the whole functioning of an individual.

RESEARCH

Research is needed in many areas. For example:

1. What developmental tasks are most related to productivity, work adjustment and adaptive behavior in the worker role?
2. What is the sequence and integration of the developmental tasks?
3. How does dysfunction in productivity occur and what are the performance deficits?
4. Does play behavior provide an index to later productive potential?
5. How do interests and values relate to productive skills development?
6. What productive roles are available to chronically handicapped persons and retired persons?
7. What is the relationship between leisure and productive skill development?

8. What services and program formats can occupational therapy provide to facilitate the development, integration and implementation of productive skills and role fulfillment in productivity?

SPECIALIZATION

Productivity and prevocational programming seem to be logical areas of specialization for occupational therapists. The major hurdle is to develop programs consistent with the philosophy of occupational therapy, that is, the programs must be based on concepts of self-discovery and competence followed by achievement and self-identity. Perhaps, also the concept of recognition should be stressed in terms of contribution to any part of society such as a living unit and that payment in money is not the only form of social recognition. Such values as "sharing the load" and "doing one's part" are just as valid a recognition of achievement as money and may be more feasible with chronically disabled persons.

ELABORATION AND REFINEMENT

The frame of reference for productivity and prevocational programming needs elaboration to encompass the concepts of occupational therapy as a humanistic, wholistic and developmentally oriented professional. Productivity should be viewed as contributing to a sense of self which interacts with rather than reacts to the environment.

Refinement is needed in assessment to learn more about the person's interests and values in productivity in addition to evaluating skills. Programs of intervention need to be directed at involving the person in productivity that is manageable whether or not the job pays in real money.

EXPLANATORY USEFULNESS

At present, prevocation and work adjustment provide a very limited explanation for the role of occupational therapy in productivity. Further, development and expansion are needed to explain the scope of how occupational therapists view work, occupation and productivity. The most useful part of prevocation and work adjustment is the focus on assessment. The assessments may point the way for model building which will explain the role of development in skill building competence and achievement.

COMMONALITY

Prevocational evaluation, training and work adjustment obviously are a common ground with vocational rehabilitation specialists and counselors. One major problem for occupational therapists has been to identify their role or type of expertise as different from vocational evaluators and work adjustment specialists. Teachers are another group with whom occupational therapists may find commonality or overlap. Teachers have become specialists in career development. As occupational therapists examine stages of productive work development, they may find that teachers have proposed similar models.

PRACTICE MODELS

Further, development of new practice models or refinement of the existing models discussed in summary section will depend in part on building better theoretical models. Most of the existing models have become better developed by vocational specialists than by occupational therapists. Sources for better practice models seem to be available in the works of Fidler and Fidler (40), Maurer (41) and Reilly (42) as discussed in the frame of reference section of the critique. A summary of the evaluation criteria is provided in Table 11.3.

Play Model—Reilly

FRAME OF REFERENCE

Reilly has used a variety of the systems and theories as the background for her analysis of play. These include general systems, organizational theory, appreciative system, field of imagination, symbolization theory, information theory, universal grammar theory, exploratory drive theory, competence theory and achievement theory.

General systems as developed by Bertalanffy and Boulding are used as to provide concepts relating to macro and micro level concerns and adaptive behavior. Organizational theory provides the concepts of hierarchy. The appreciative theory of Vickers is used to explain the value of play in relation to external and internal reality. Symbolization, universal grammaticality and learning theory are used as a basis for the concept of rules as a third means of information processing. Finally, the exploratory drive of curiosity as described by the competence theory of White and McClelland's achievement theory are used to develop a hierarchical system of play behavior.

ASSUMPTIONS ABOUT MAN AND PLAY (47)

1. Play is a spontaneous activity (p. 123).
2. Play develops in a hierarchical process (p. 124).
3. Play is learned, adaptive behavior (p. 126).

Table 11.3
Prevocation Models Criteria Summary

Evaluation Criteria	Very Good 1	Moderately Good 2	Moderately Good 3	Moderately Good 4	Very Poor 5
Frame of reference		X			
Clarity			X		
Uniqueness		X			
Research guide	X				
Specialization	X				
Elaboration/refinement		X			
Explanatory usefulness			X		
Commonality	X				
Practice model		X			

4. Play is related to the energy system of value (p. 126).
5. Play emerges through and is motivated by (energy force), a system of values or an appreciative system as opposed to instincts or needs (p. 127).
6. Play is derived from imagination which is drawn from three action systems—central nervous system, symbolization process and language (p. 132).
7. Play is based on a rule symbolization language process which asks "What is this?" and operates through conflict and curiosity (p. 140).
8. Play is a subsystem of information and language which provides for the rules for action regarding sensorimotor activity, objects and people and thinking (p. 144).
9. Play behavior occurs in the three hierarchical stages of curiosity—exploratory, competency and achievement (p. 145).
10. Play behavior involves sensory experience, practice, repetition, imitation, competition, mastery and risk taking (p. 146).
11. Play in a chronological or longitudinal sense is the antecedent preparation area for work (48).

ASSUMPTIONS ABOUT HEALTH AND PLAY, OCCUPATIONS AND PLAY AND OCCUPATIONAL THERAPY AND PLAY

Not stated.

CONCEPTS (47)

Play—a biosocial phenomenon (p. 122)

Spontaneous activity—an internal behavior which will act without dependence upon external stimulation (p. 123)

Hierarchical process—involves change which occurs quantitatively from small to large and from simple to complex and qualitatively from lower to higher forms of behavior (p. 124)

Behavior energy (motivation, drive)—described as occurring in three evolutionary stages—instinct, need and values (p. 126)

Adaptive behavior—described as occurring in three time-spans—evolution, development and learning. Learning involves the fastest change (p. 126)

Appreciative system—a system for making judgments based on the quality of relevant mental faculties, stored and retrievable material at the individual's disposal and the state of readiness to see or value things in one way or another (p. 129)

Learning—described as a product of the interaction of external facts of reality with internal values (p. 131)

Imagination—described as involving the use of symbols and actions . . . and as a device for processing information (pp. 131–132)

Rule symbolization process—one of three language systems. It is based on nervous system's sensorium which responds to curiosity and conflict encounter in exploratory behavior and responds by asking "What is this?" (p. 140)

Symbols—translate sensation into meaning (p. 136)

Exploratory behavior—behavior that is engaged in for its own sake and is the product of an autonomous capacity to be interested in the environment (p. 146)

Competency behavior—characterized by a drive to deal with the environment, to influence it actively, and to be influenced by it through feedback mechanisms (p. 146)

Fragmentation—process of repetition with various forms such as interruption of an activity sequence before reaching the normal goal behavior, the enacting of fractional sequences, the repetition of fractional sequences and the reordering of sequences (p. 147)

Achievement behavior—competition with a standard of excellence which focuses on performance (p. 147)

Achievement motivation—the striving to increase, or keep as high as possible, one's own capability in all activities to which a standard of excellence may apply and where the execution of activities may succeed or fail (p. 148)

Adaptation—described as a change process (p. 126)

Interests—described as based on the principle that man notices only those aspects of reality that interest the person (p. 130)

Instincts—described as an energy force which occurs first in the evolutionary process (p. 126)

Needs—described as an energy force which occurs second in the evolutionary process (p. 126)

Values—described as an energy force which is newest in the evolutionary process (p. 126)

EXPECTED RESULTS

Since there is no discussion of dysfunction, there are no specific outcomes or goals of intervention.

ASSESSMENTS INSTRUMENTS

Table 11.4 outlines the names of instruments, content areas and yield of the published assessment developed within the model of play.

INTERVENTION STRATEGIES

Some of the articles on assessment instruments suggest media and methods which could be used in intervention programs, but there is no consensus on which media or methods belong to the model of play.

SUMMARY

Reilly's model of play is based on the assumption that play is a multidimensional phenomena which attempts to explain how man acquires play behavior and for what purposes such behavior is used. Play is viewed as a biosocial phenomenon because it is a living behavior which increases in complexity over time and is acquired from interaction with the environment.

Play is a function of the learned mechanism of adaption which is the latest and has the shortest time-span in molding the human species. Learned adaption is acquired through the energy or behavior force of valuing or appreciation. Thus, play is related to the valuing appreciation force. The valuing appreciation force has three types of regulators: self-regulation, coherence and action. Play seems to involve the third regulator type. The action regulator operates by (a) noticing that which is of interest and matches an internal schema, (b) weighing or comparing the information and, (c) advocating the optimal or balanced condition which then is formed into new schemata to be added to the learned.

The acquisition of all human behavior is outlined in Figure 11.4 with emphasis on learned adaptation. Figure 11.5 outlines the acquisition of play behavior. Play is derived from the mental process of imagination which functions through the central nervous system, symbolization and language. The central nervous system contributes through sensation and the sensorium the initial question of "What is this?" Symbolization contributes words, dreams, and most significant, rules, which involve sensorimotor activity, objects and people, and thinking processes. Finally, language, through the information process, contributes myths, composed of word symbols, dreams composed of visual imagery and play composed of rules of action. Myths and words become the basis for thinking and logic. Dreams and visual imagery are the basis of feeling and relationships. Play and rules of actions form the basis of a reality about the environment and its technology (Fig. 11.6).

In the final analysis, play contributes to the development of rule-constructed language whereby the individual knows inner and outer reality. The key motivation or energy source is the exploratory drive of curiosity which provides the information to formulate the rules of action (Fig. 11.7).

Curiosity can be subdivided into three stages which roughly parallel the developmental stages used by Piaget. The three stages are explanatory, competency and achievement. Exploratory motivation leads to exploratory behavior which is done for pure enjoyment. Competency motivation leads to competency behavior in which tasks are practiced and mastered. Achievement motivation leads to achievement behavior in which performance is measured against a standard of excellence. These substages of curiosity are illustrated in Figure 11.8.

Ultimately, play, according to Reilly, contributes to and is preparation for work behavior. Thus, play is viewed by Reilly as part of the occupational behavior model previously discussed. However, play is a subject area with many potentials and thus is considered here as a separate area which could be developed in a number of ways.

Table 11.4
Instruments Content Areas and Yield of Published Assessments for the Model of Play[a]

Content Area	Name[b]	Clinical Yield
History, development	Play history (49, 50)	Interpretation of past play experience with materials, actions, people and settings. Age Range: Birth–16 yr
Intrinsic motivation	Guide to observation of play development (51)	Interpretation of current play with human objects and nonhuman objects Age range: Birth–11 yr
Rules/skills	Guide to play observation (52)	Interpretation of current play in dimensions of generation of rules, achievement of objective, skilled act with objects, people and flexibility of skills Age range: Not specified
Symbol formation, creativity	Growth gradient (53, 54)	Interpretation of current symbolic creative art expressions in dimensions of a maturity profile, creative profile, human schema/symbols, space symbols, color and design schema Age range: 2–18 yr
Cognition, games	Guide to assessment of cognition (55)	Interpretation of current level of cognition in dimensions of concrete operations and formal operations Age range: 7–12 yr
Exploratory play	Play scale (56)	Interpretation of current play in space management, material management, limitation, participation Age range: Birth–6 yr
Development	Play skills inventory (57, 58)	Interpretation of current play in dimensions of sensation, motor ability, perception, intellect Age range: 8–12 yr
Imitation	Guide to status of limitation (59)	Interpretation of current status of imitation process in dimensions of child, role models, family organization and physical environment Age range: Not specified

[a] Reprinted with permission from L. L. Florey: *American Journal of Occupational Therapy* 35:520, 1981.
[b] The numbers following the name of the pilot instruments or guides indicate references to the published material.

Table 11.4—Continued

Content Area	Name[b]	Clinical Yield
Play	Specification for a play milieu (60)	Examination of balance of human, nonhuman, qualitative, quantitative elements in milieu
		Age range: Not specified
Art/games	A play agenda (61)	Specification for environment, experiences, activities that promote risk-taking and decision making
		Age range: Birth–12 yr

Analysis and Critique of the Model of Play

FRAME OF REFERENCE

Reilly's model of play is based on a very comprehensive frame of reference which permits the development of a comprehensive rationale. All of the major references are consistent with the organismic and systems models. Perhaps, the major problem is to establish a source for imagination. Is imagination an evolutionary product which is present at birth along with the primitive reflexes or does it develop concurrently with sensorimotor exploration?

CLARITY

The model of play is primarily an outline of the rationale for viewing play as a significant aspect of human behavior. The assumptions do not state what role play provides in developing or maintaining health and what goes wrong in ill health or dysfunction. Likewise, no real attention is given to assumptions regarding play as an occupational role or the use of occupational therapy as a means of dealing with dysfunction. Although some assumptions are provided in the model of occupational behavior, the lack of statements in the extensive writing on play reduces the effectiveness of the model on play as a tool for developing practice models in occupational therapy. Some assistance is provided by the many graduate student theses dealing with play, but the formulation of assumptions remains incomplete.

The formulation of concepts is somewhat more complete. Descriptions are available, and although working definitions are not always present, the major problem is to understand how the concepts interrelate. One or more visual models would have been extremely helpful. The sheer volume of complex concepts seems to decrease the comprehension rate when text alone is present.

UNIQUENESS

The model of play appears to be a unique formulation of an important aspect of human behavior and activity. Play, behavior and skills appear to have a real impact on the performance level of adults. Lack of normal

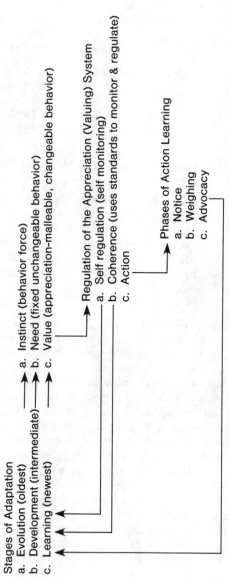

Figure 11.4.   Acquisition of human species behavior.

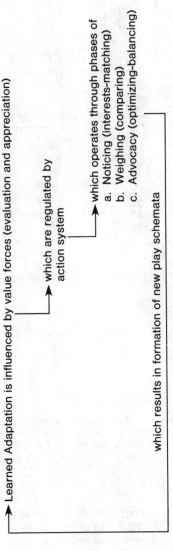

Learned Adaptation is influenced by value forces (evaluation and appreciation)

which are regulated by action system

which operates through phases of
a. Noticing (interests-matching)
b. Weighing (comparing)
c. Advocacy (optimizing-balancing)

which results in formation of new play schemata

Figure 11.5. Acquisition of play behavior.

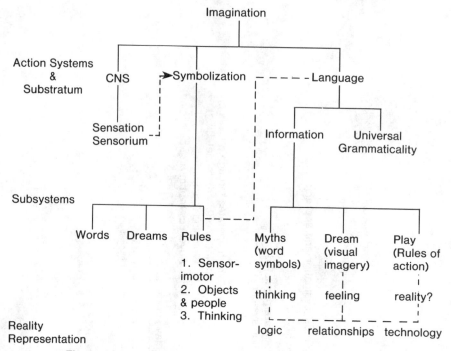

Figure 11.6. Model of the development of play behavior.

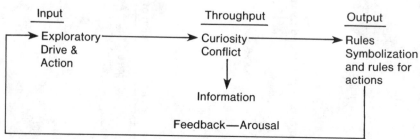

Figure 11.7. Model of the development of a rule construct process.

or usual play behavior and skills could account for some performance deficits seen in adolescents and adults. Likewise, the loss of performance capacity could be regained by use of the progressive stages in play behavior development. The problem is to complete the model's assumptions and firm up the relationship of concepts.

RESEARCH GUIDE

The model of play along with the occupational behavior model has provided a rich source of information for graduate student thesis material. Those students who studied play have developed a number of clinical

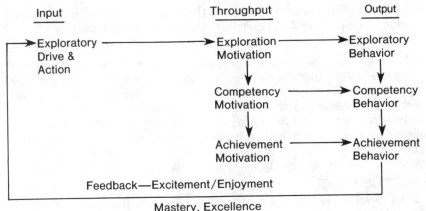

Figure 11.8.   Substages of curiosity.

assessment instruments. These instruments expand the knowledge of how play occurs but do not complete the assumptions regarding play and health, occupation and therapy. A number of questions remain which include:

1. What are the major play skills which a child usually acquires?
2. Can a taxonomy of play skills be developed?
3. What work skills are derived from play skills, and what is the sequence, if any?
4. Are play skills related to or the same as leisure or recreation skills?
5. What techniques can therapists use to promote better play skills?

SPECIALIZATION

The model of play could lead to a number of opportunities for specialization. Age of persons served is the most obvious. However, as the model of play yields more information about dysfunction, there may be several subtypes of dysfunction which require special intervention programs. For example, sensory integration problems might become known as a specific subtype of play dysfunction.

ELABORATION AND REFINEMENT

Elaboration is needed to complete the assumptions regarding play and health, play and occupation, and play and occupational therapy. Elaboration also is needed to identify techniques and methods. Refinement is needed to better define the concepts and to organize the assessment instruments into a systematic assessment profile.

EXPLANATORY USEFULNESS

The model of play may provide a useful explanation of the role of play in normal development. With further expansion, the model may provide an explanation of how the lack of certain play behaviors can affect negatively the development of certain skills such as social or work skills in adult life. The potential for use is there, but the model in its present form is incomplete and difficult to explain in a succinct manner.

COMMONALITY

There are some points of commonality between the model of play and other professions models, such as systems approach, organizational theory and the concept of competence. However, other frames of reference such as imagination, symbolization and information theories are less well known to other health personnel educators and consumers. The model of play in its present form is not easily understood by other disciplines. Further clarification will be needed if the model of play is to serve as a means of communicating the concepts of occupational therapy to others.

PRACTICE MODEL

The development of practice models based on the model of play is limited because there are no assumptions about health, occupation and occupational therapy. The only source of guidance within the model of play itself is a hierarchical or development approach in which a player at the exploratory level is encouraged to move on to competence and achievement, and tasks or activities are graded from simple to complex. Another possibility would be to combine the model of play and the occupational behavior model which would provide more complete assumptions and concepts. A summary of the criteria used to evaluate the model of play are provided in Table 11.5.

Leisure Model

FRAME OF REFERENCE

The author has been unable to find any model specifically related to the development and integration of leisure activity in the occupational therapy literature. Leisure is considered separately from play because play is viewed as preparation for both productivity and leisure. A model on leisure, therefore, should address the skills needed to organize and implement a program of leisure activities. Such a model could include a preparation phase which is based on play.

Table 11.5
Model of Play Criteria Summary

Evaluation Criteria	Very Good 1	Moderately Good			Very Poor 5
		2	3	4	
Frame of reference	x				
Clarity			x		
Uniqueness	x				
Research guide	x				
Specialization	x				
Elaboration/refinement		x			
Explanatory usefulness		x			
Commonality			x		
Practice model			x		

Another consideration is to develop a model which responds to the beliefs and values consistent with occupational therapy. Models of leisure exist currently in the leisure counseling and recreation literature (62). Generally, the models consist of four purposes. The first purpose is to provide an opportunity for disabled persons to have the most therapeutic recreative experience possible (recreation participation). The second purpose involves the provisions of recreation services and opportunities to provide treatment or therapy such as health restoration, remediation, habilitation or rehabilitation which will change or ameliorate the effects of illness and disability (therapy). A third purpose is to assist individuals in establishing and expressing an independent leisure life-stype by eliminating leisure barriers, developing leisure skills and attitudes, and optimizing leisure functioning (leisure education). Finally, the fourth purpose is to provide leisure resource information to well persons or communities who seek or need assistance to engage in desired interests (leisure counseling).

Occupational therapy models can be unique in the approach to leisure by stressing the need for balance between the occupational activities of self maintenance, productivity and leisure and by stressing the integration of all activity into a whole configuration. Also, occupational therapy has the focus of viewing occupational activities as substitute or equivalent approaches to a goal. As Herbert Hall (63) stated, one activity may be used as a substitute for another when performance of the first activity is blocked or no longer can meet a need. Equivalent occupations relate to the use of one kind of occupation for another. Hall felt that leisure activities were effective in building or rebuilding productive skills when actual work activity might be too strenuous, not available or not adaptable to the client's situation. Through transfer of training, Hall felt that skills such as endurance and workmanship gained through leisure activity could be applied to work situations later.

ASSUMPTIONS ABOUT MAN AND LEISURE

1. Man must perceive a motivation, freedom and opportunity to engage in the leisure experience (64).
2. Man will seek leisure as a form of aesthetic participation, a value-laden perception for his well-being (64).
3. Man has a need and a responsibility to "order" or structure the waking hours around personal well-being (64).
4. Man seeks to understand the meaning of various life experiences, including leisure and work (64).
5. Man's perception of the concepts of job, work and leisure are learned (64).

ASSUMPTIONS ABOUT HEALTH AND LEISURE

1. Leisure assists in the development of inner resources (capacity for effort and relation) and the ability to adapt and cope with environmental influences (64).
2. Satisfying leisure behavior contributes to good mental health and positive human behavior (64).

3. A significant relationship exists between personal adjustment and performance in the leisure role (64).
4. There is a positive relationship between leisure time activities and satisfactions in childhood and good psychological adjustment as an adult (64).
5. Leisure contributes to the potential for self actualization (64).
6. Inability to deal with free time leisure is a sign of maladaptive behavior (64).
7. Lack of a positive adaptation to leisure results in maladaption and poor adjustment (64).

ASSUMPTIONS ABOUT LEISURE OCCUPATIONS

1. Leisure occupations are those which a person chooses (is free to choose) to do as opposed to those which must be done (productive) (65).
2. Leisure occupations are those which are carried out within the concept of perceived freedom and without perceived constraint or compulsion (65).
3. Leisure occupation may be engaged in for the activity itself (intrinsic motivation), for a reward or payoff (extrinsic motivation) or both (65).
4. Leisure occupation may be distinguished between an instrumental (interim) or final (end) goal (65).
5. Leisure occupations which are performed are pure leisure and for intrinsic motivation imply that all essential needs have been satisfied (65).
6. Leisure occupations which include leisure and production or self maintenance are both intrinsically and extrinsically motivated, implying that the productive aspect is necessary and has a reward but the individual can quit any time and is aware of the fact (65).
7. Leisure occupations which are performed as leisure- job or leisure self-care and for extrinsic motivation imply that the satisfaction comes not from the activity itself but from its consequences (65).
8. Productivity and self maintenance may be both intrinsically and extrinsically rewarding so that the person enjoys doing the work but also understands the leisure aspect (65).
9. Leisure occupation which is performed as an instrumental goal will be perceived differently by an individual than an occupation which is perceived as a final goal (65).
10. The choice of leisure occupation is bound by social and cultural factors, including economic status, sex and familial experiences (64).
11. The choice of leisure occupation is affected by interests and values (64).
12. The performance of leisure occupations is dependent on performance skills in using environmental resources (64).
13. Leisure time occupations are more meaningful to the extent that they challenge an individual's full potential (66).

ASSUMPTIONS ABOUT OCCUPATIONAL THERAPY AND LEISURE (BY AUTHOR)

1. Occupational therapy can faciliate the development, redevelopment of maintenance of leisure skills.
2. Occupational therapy can provide specific practice opportunities to promote or maintain performance skills in leisure assumptions.
3. Occupational therapy can help organize leisure occupations into a balanced program with self maintenance and productivity occupations.
4. Occupational therapy can facilitate the exploration of attitudes, values and interests in relation to leisure occupations.
5. Occupational therapy can assist in exploring resources for leisure occupation available in the community and determining those most suitable for practical in relation to individual need.

CONCEPTS

Leisure—activity to which the individual turns at will, for either relaxation, diversion or broadening of knowledge (67)

Recreation—consists of activities or experiences carried on within leisure (68)

Dimensions of leisure

a. *Degree of discretion*—leisure may be either freely chosen or determined by work constraints or the pervasive norms of the society (69)
b. *Degree of work relation*—leisure may be independent of work or dependent on the meaning given it by work (69)

Types of discretion

a. *Chosen*—leisure activity which is freely selected and is optional or without penalty (8)
b. *Determined*—leisure activity in which status, role or reward would be diminished or threatened by nonparticipation (69)

Types of work relation

a. *Independent*—leisure activity which is not related to work or the meaning given by work (69)
b. *Dependent*—leisure activity which is related to work, including the economic rewards for tasks performed and the preparation, appearance, community relationship, residence and demeanor required or rewarded by the work position (69)

Categories of leisure

a. *Unconditional leisure*-activity which is freely chosen and independent of the work relation (69)
b. *Coordinated leisure*—activity which is freely chosen but related or dependent on work, such as the businessman who enjoys the country club but is aware that contacts may be made during a friendly golf game (69)

   c. *Complementary or compensatory leisure*—activity which is determined by role expectations or by the need to compensate for work conditions; however, the activity is independent of the work relationship (69)

   d. *Preparation or recuperative leisure*—activity is determined by social expectations and is related to work in that the activity prepares the person for work or helps to recuperate from work (69)

EXPECTED RESULTS (BY AUTHOR)

1. Improve knowledge for performance by the following.
   a. Improvement of problem-solving and decision-making abilities.
   b. Improvement of the valuing or attitude skills of leisure experiences.
   c. Exploration of thoughts and feelings about life-styles, including work and leisure patterns.
2. Focus on performance by the following.
   a. The learning of selected leisure activities.
   b. Implementation of an action plan of leisure activities.
3. Promote self-motivation and goal orientation by setting leisure goals.
4. Facilitate evaluation of leisure activities by reviewing and clarifying the importance of leisure experiences to the individual.

ASSESSMENT AREAS (BY AUTHOR)

1. Reading occupations
   a. Newspapers, magazines
   b. Books, novels, biographies, science fiction
   c. Textbooks
2. Listening occupations
   a. Television, radio
   b. Music, record player, tape recorder
   c. Citizen band, ham radio
   d. Talking books
   e. Telephone
3. Solitary occupations
   a. Lounging, napping
   b. Going for a walk, drive
   c. Shopping or brousing
4. Card playing occupations
   a. Solitary—solitare
   b. Group—bridge, hearts, poker
5. Table game playing occupations
   a. Solitary—quizzes, brain teasers
   b. Group—Monopoly, chess, checkers, billards, table tennis
6. Clubs or organizations occupations
   a. Social clubs—gardens, service
   b. Professional or union

7. Church organization-attending occupations
   Church supper, choir, clubs
8. Cultural activity-attending occupations
   Theater, symphony, exhibits, dance, films, art shows, museums
9. Discussion group occupations
   Book club, social issue club, voter organizations
10. Social activities occupations
    Visiting friends, coffee clutch, dating
11. Volunteering occupations
    a. Women's auxillary, scout leader, YMCA, day camp
    b. Political campaign
12. Performing occupations
    a. Play instrument
    b. Singing
    c. Acting or drama
13. Sports occupations
    a. Passive—attend sporting events, watch on TV, listen on radio
    b. Active—participate in informal or formal leagues
14. Eating and drinking behavior
    a. Eating and/or drinking at home
    b. Eating and/or drinking "on the town"
15. Arts and crafts-making behavior
    a. Drawing, painting, etc.
    b. Ceramics, needlework, woodworking, sewing, cooking, etc.
16. Collecting behavior
    Antiques, stamps, postcards, etc.
17. Gardening behavior—raising plants, flowers
    a. Indoors
    b. Outdoors
18. Attending entertainment behavior
    a. Movies
    b. Nightclubs
19. Raising and training, observing, showing pets behavior
    Cats, dogs, birds, fish, rodents, reptiles
20. Picture taking, developing occupations
    a. Stills—photographs, slides
    b. Movies
21. Building and repair occupations
    a. Furniture
    b. Automobiles
    c. Appliances
    d. Structures
22. Writing occupations
    a. Letters
    b. Short stories
    c. Books

TECHNIQUES
A. Questions for leisure occupations (by author)
   1. What do you read?
      What printed matter do you read?
   2. Do you listen to the _____?
      Do you enjoy listening to (the) _____?
   3. What sort of activities do you do (engage in) when you're alone?
   4. Do you enjoy playing card games?
   5. Do you play any other games?
      What other games do you like?
   6. Do you belong to or attend any clubs or organizations?
      What organizations or clubs do you belong to?
   7. What, if any, church activities do you participate in?
      Do you participate in any church activities?
   8. Are you interested in any culture events?
      Do you attend any concerts or shows?
   9. Do you participate in discussion groups?
      Do you belong to any discussion groups?
   10. What social activities do you enjoy?
       Do you like to go visiting or entertain in your home?
   11. Do you volunteer any of your time to organizations or hospitals?
   12. Are you skilled in any of the performing arts?
       Can you play an instrument, act, dance or sing?
   13. What sports do you like?
       Do you participate or watch?
   14. Where do you enjoy eating or drinking?
       Do you dine out often?
       Do you go out drinking often?
   15. Do you enjoy doing any art or craft work?
       Are you interested in art or craft work?
   16. Do you collect things? What are your hobbies?
       Do you have any hobby collections?
   17. Do you enjoy gardening? Do you raise any plants or flowers in your home?
       Do you have a garden?
   18. Do you go to the movies?
       Do you go to nightclubs?
   19. Do you have a pet?
       Do you raise or keep any animals?
   20. Do you like to take pictures or home movies?
       Do you know how to develop your own film?
   21. Do you enjoy building or repairing things?
       Can you build furniture, repair an electric appliance or car?
   22. Do you enjoy writing?
       What do you write?
B. Interest checklists such as that by Matsatsuya (70)
C. Time logs or activity configurations such as those by Mosey (71)

INTERVENTION STRATEGIES

1. Media—see Taxonomy in Chapter 8 which is based on Overs *et al.* (66)
2. Methods
   A. Use of exercises to clarify values, explore resources, organize time. See Section 1 of Hughes and Mullins (72). The following items from Simon *et al.* (73) appear most useful, but others could be adapted to a leisure focus.

Twenty things I love to do	SN1
Group interview	SN14
Getting started	SN28
Pie of life	SN33
Unfinished sentences	SN37
The free choice game	SN52
Two ideal days	SN57
Self contracts	SN59
Ready for summer	SN71

   B. Practice and performance of leisure occupations to increase skills and develop sense of competence.
3. Equipment
   Variable—depends on choice of leisure occupations
4. Precautions
   Variable—depends on choice of leisure occupations

SUMMARY

The models proposed in this section are designed to suggest a frame of reference and initial theoretical model for examining leisure occupations within the overall framework of occupational therapy. Traditionally, leisure has been viewed as unobligated time and the antithesis of work. Thus, leisure becomes any activity not associated with work for pay which is done in one's free time. These views do not fit into the concept of occupational therapy which holds that occupational areas are interrelated and provide integration and balance.

Figure 11.9 shows an example of the interrelationship of the three occupational areas. There is an aspect of leisure in both productivity and self maintenance. Thus, there are five types of leisure which can be identified. What defines leisure is the degree of choice and degree of relatedness to productivity and self maintenance occupations (Figs. 11.10 and 11.11).

Leisure is also viewed as affected by motivation and goal. Intrinsic motivation is less restrictive on leisure occupations, but extrinsic motivation is involved in some types of leisure. Moreover, both intrinsic and extrinsic motivation may occur simultaneously or in relation to the same event. Goals may be intermediate to accomplish steps in the process which finally achieves an end result.

Pure leisure or unconditional leisure has no strings attached. There is unrestricted choice governed by intrinsic motivation to pursue interests

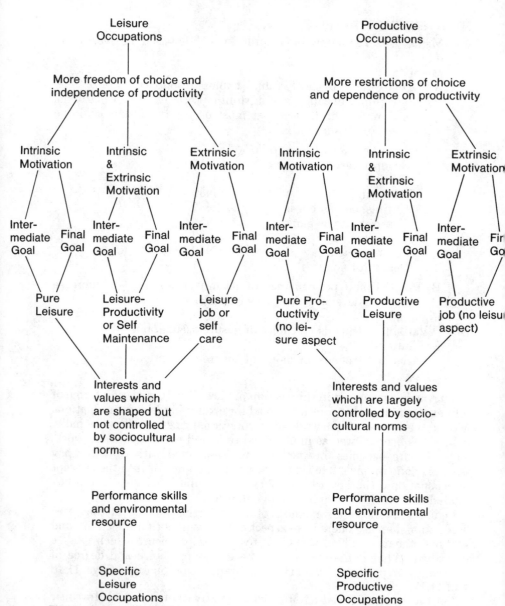

Figure 11.9. Interrelationship of the three occupational areas. (Adapted from J. Neulinger (65).)

and value without regard for their potential contribution to productivity or self maintenance. Limitations are governed only by performance skills and environmental resources. Such leisure occupations are done just for fun. Examples are difficult to give because the conditions, not the activity

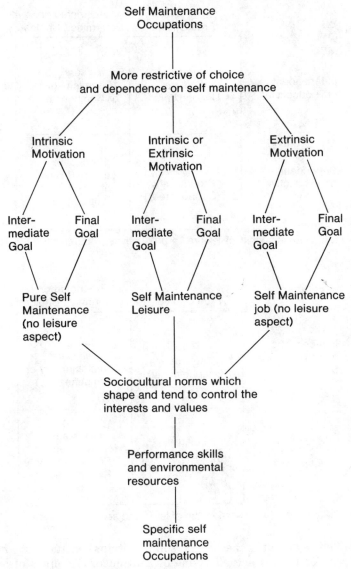

Figure 11.9. *Continued.*

or task, determine the outcome. A person might sew a dress, make a table, go on a trip, play a game, see a movie, and there are many other options.

Leisure productivity or leisure self maintenance is selected by choice but is related to productivity or self maintenance. Intrinsic and extrinsic motivation is involved. Such an occupation usually is of interest to the

	Free Choice	Restricted or Determined Choice
Independent of Productivity	Pure Leisure Unconditional	Leisure job (Complementary or Compensatory
Dependent on Productivity	Leisure Productivity (Coordinated)	Productive Leisure (Preparatory or Recuperative

Figure 11.10. Relationship of leisure to productivity. (Adapted from J. R. Kelly (69).)

	Free Choice	Restricted or Determined Choice
Independent of Self Maintenance	Pure Leisure (Unconditional)	Leisure Self Care (Complementary or Compensatory)
Dependent on Self Maintenance	Leisure Self Maintenance (Coordinated)	Self Maintenance Leisure (Preparatory or Recuperative)

Figure 11.11. Relationship of leisure to self maintenance.

person. The key point is that the person maintains control over whether the activity or task is actually done or continued. Examples of leisure productivity might include repainting a room in the house, helping to build a church, or singing in a group which puts on free programs in the community. Examples of leisure self maintenance might be to bake bread rather than buy it, make a set of dishes from clay, or take a class on financial investments. Since personal control is paramount, any task or activity which obligates the individual is not leisure.

A leisure job or leisure self-care is restricted in choice but is not specifically related to the productive or self maintenance occupations normally done by the individual, although they may be complementary.

The key element is extrinsic reward. Examples of leisure job might include selling the most tickets to a benefit concert to win the ticket selling prize, washing cars to raise money for a social organization or playing on the company-organized bowling team in hopes of winning the conference title. Examples of leisure self-care might include going to a health spa designed to help people lose weight, going to a beauty parlor weekly to have a facial and manicure or wearing expensive jewelery for everyday activities.

Productive leisure is characterized as restrictive in choice, work-dependent and has an extrinsic motivator. However, if the productive occupation is one the person enjoys doing, there may be an intrinsic motivation which is more important than the apparent restrictions. The work becomes satisfying in and of itself so that constraints are not bothersome. The key is the person's perception of and satisfaction with the productive occupation. Examples might include an artist who paints for a living but only when and where the person wants or chooses to work, a salesperson who really enjoys meeting and talking with all kinds of people or a child care worker who really enjoys caring for children and never seems to run out of patience.

Self-care leisure likewise is characterized as restrictive in choice which must be done and has an extrinsic motivator. However, if the self-care occupation is one the person enjoys doing and thus has an intrinsic motivation, that fact is more important than the perception of constraint. The key is the person's internal sense of satisfaction. Examples might include taking a leisurely bubble bath in a sunken tub. Such a bath still meets the social requirement for bathing to remove unpleasant odor. Another example might be dining out at a nice restaurant. Such dining still meets the requirement for regular food intake. A third example might be a person who enjoys dressing for work to show off handmade clothes.

In each leisure situation, the person's perception is as important or more important than the real situation in determining whether leisure exists. A person who is afraid to make choices in unrestricted situations or feels that "having fun" is immoral or socially unacceptable will not have leisure occupations no matter what the situation.

Assessment strategies for leisure occupations involve assessing what the person likes to do and is able to do in terms of skills and resources and in evaluating the values, beliefs and attitudes the person holds about leisure in relation to productivity and self maintenance. Intervention includes clarifying what the person likes best to do, providing structured practice in skill development and use of resources if needed and clarifying values, beliefs or attitudes about leisure. Organizing time for leisure activities may be needed also.

Analysis and Critique of the Leisure Model
FRAME OF REFERENCE

One of the difficulties in developing a model of leisure is a culturally valued concept which changes as the culture changes. In contrast, the concept of work and productivity has continued to have a fairly consistent meaning. Therefore, any model of leisure must be based on a cultural perspective. Since culture is not a uniform entity, a model of leisure will have to provide some flexibility in application.

CLARITY

The term "leisure" is difficult to define because of the variations in cultural values. Kaplan (74) found there were six characteristics or elements to which the term leisure referred. These are: (1) an antithesis to work as an economic function; (2) a pleasant expectation and recollection; (3) a minimum of involuntary social-role obligations; (4) a psychological perception of freedom; (5) a close relation to values of the culture; and (6) often, but not necessarily, an activity characterized by the element of play.

The same issues also affect the statement of assumptions. If leisure is assumed to be unsalaried work then the retired person has all leisure and no work activity. Thus, assumptions about leisure must clarify the real discrimination between productivity and leisure, such as contribution to society vs. contribution primarily to self.

The second issue concerns pleasure and expectation. Leisure usually is considered a pleasant situation or should be undertaken with pleasure in mind, even if the results occasionally are unpleasant. Also, leisure has a past, present and future as do the other occupational areas. The importance of the time reference and expectation is important in relating leisure to older people who may tend to spend leisure time in reflection rather than in expectation of the present and future.

The third issue is to specify the perception of freedom or discretion in relation to leisure. Freedom to engage in leisure pursuits and the discretionary time to devote to leisure activity may be viewed more negatively than positively by people nearing retirement. The development of leisure skills and the use of leisure time are learned behaviors. If such skills are not learned before retirement, the prospect of lots of time and nothing to do may be an unpleasant view.

The fourth issue of values can be illustrated by the same example of a retiree. A culture which values youth and productivity can lead to an interpretation by some retirees that leisure time is the equivalent to being put out to pasture and can lead to a feeling of being "a has been." Such an attitude makes development of a leisure program difficult at best.

A fifth issue is the relationship between leisure, recreation and play and should be addressed. If recreation and play are activities done within leisure, how are recreation and play different? Is the only difference based on age or are there other considerations such as skill development in play or social goals in recreation?

Finally, what is the influence of social roles or leisure? Although leisure activity has been associated with a reduction of social role obligations, leisure activity may still be subject to social review. Interviews for employment or general interest news often include a question about leisure interests. Is leisure activity as free of social obligations as assumed or are there hidden determinants of leisure not readily recognized?

UNIQUENESS

The model presented in the summary contains suggestions for a unique view of leisure through occupational therapy. The approach is designed to look at leisure as one of three major occupational areas which overlap, are interrelated and ultimately integrated in a whole occupational scheme of an individual. As an aspect of the whole, leisure occupation may contribute to dysfunction and lack of balance if leisure skills are not developed or organized into a total profile of occupational tasks.

RESEARCH GUIDE

The lack of models or theories of leisure in occupational therapy has resulted in less research. With the exception of Matsutsuya's study of interests which includes many items for leisure occupation, no real studies of leisure could be located in the published occupational therapy literature.

Some possible research questions are:

1. What is the relationship between play and leisure, *i.e.*, does childhood play facilitate the development of adult leisure values and skills?
2. Do leisure occupations have a possible effect in maintaining or regaining good mental health, *i.e.*, what individual needs can leisure satisfy?
3. Does the performance of leisure occupations improve the role performance of productive and self maintenance occupation, *i.e.*, do people with identifiable leisure occupations perform work and self-care roles better?
4. Do people with identifiable leisure occupations make transitions in life tasks and patterns easier, *i.e.*, with less trauma and problems of adjustment?
5. Do people with identifiable leisure occupations lead more satisfying lives by self-recording and assessment by others?

SPECIALIZATION

Leisure could offer an excellent area of specialization to someone interested in accepting the challenge of developing leisure into a significant topic in the occupational therapy literature. The challenge is to explain the role of leisure as an occupational area, a changing social phenomenon and a means of developing competence and increasing satisfaction for individuals. Based on the information, a more comprehensive model should be possible than presented by the author.

ELABORATION AND REFINEMENT

Elaboration is needed to understand the role of leisure in relation to the other occupational areas. That is to explain what leisure occupations contribute to the total adaptive potential and adaptive pattern at a given time. Leisure needs to have a separate identity which is not just a reflection of productivity but rather a complementary and contributing force in human adaptation.

Refinement is needed to better categorize leisure tasks and to analyze the tasks for better choice selection by individuals. Assessment instruments and intervention strategies need to be developed which increase the involvement of the individual in selecting and learning leisure occupations. The role of leisure as a legitimate goal of intervention needs more recognition.

EXPLANATORY USEFULNESS

The models used in the summary section are designed to show leisure as an entity which is bound into the other two occupational areas. The usefulness of such a model is to illustrate that a functioning, adapting person incorporates all three occupational areas into a total behavior repertoire. Deficiencies in any one occupational area decrease the total adaptive potential of the individual. Thus, leisure is not a spare wheel or a luxury but an integral part of the total system.

COMMONALITY

Leisure is a familiar subject to several other disciplines. Recreational therapists, leisure counselors, corrective therapists, single modality therapists, such as dance, art, poetry, and music and physical education teachers, are all familiar with leisure and recreational activities. The problem is to communicate how occupational therapists view leisure and use leisure activity differently from these other disciplines. Leisure continues to lack a foundation which explores the many aspects that may make up a leisure program. The role of leisure in adaptive behavior is unclear and is seen by many as a luxury role. The possible contribution to performance skills, decision making and problem solving has not been identified so that disciplines can emphasize their contribution.

PRACTICE MODELS

Development of practice models is in part limited by the lack of a basic model. However, some aspects of leisure development and planning have evolved out of other aspects of occupational therapy models. Time organization, development of play skills and practice in general performance skills in sensorimotor, cognitive, intra- and interpersonal areas are examples. General work skills may be useful to leisure occupations also, such as following directions and habits of organization.

Some missing aspects are how to help an individual develop a leisure plan that fits individual needs, how to decide when enough leisure skills have been practice and learned, and how to help people organize life-long leisure plans. Each aspect must be explored in relation to the self maintenance and productive occupational areas and will require unique assessment and intervention approaches or modifications of existing ones.

A summary of the evaluation criteria for the leisure model is presented in Table 11.6.

Table 11.6
Leisure Model Criteria Summary

Evaluation Criteria	Very Good 1	Moderately Good 2	3	4	Very Poor 5
Frame of reference		X			
Clarity			X		
Uniqueness		X			
Research guide				X	
Specialization	X				
Elaboration/refinement			X		
Explanatory usefulness	X				
Commonality			X		
Practice model				X	

References

1. Sheldon MP: A physical achievement record. *J Health Phys Ed* 6:30–31, 60, 1935.
2. Deaver GG, Brown ME: *Physical Demands of Daily Life*. New York, Institute for the Crippled and Disabled, 1945.
3. Willard HS, Spackman CS: *Occupational Therapy*. Philadelphia, Lippincott, 1947, pp 231–233.
4. Livingston DM: Achievement recording for the cerebral palsied. *Am J Occup Ther* 4:66–67, 74, 1950.
5. Connell KA: An occupational therapist's approach to the vocational problems of the cerebral palsied. *Am J Occup Ther* 4:214–233, 238, 1950.
6. Dinnerstein AJ: Evaluation of a rating scale of ability in activity of daily living *Arch Phys Med Rehabil* 46:579–584, 1965.
7. Schoening HA, *et al*: Numerical Scoring of a self-care status of patients. *Arch Phys Med Rehabil* 46:689–697, 1965.
8. Gersten, *et al*: Relation of muscle strength and range of motion to activities of daily living. *Arch Phys Med Rehabil* 51:137–142, 1970.
9. Potvin AR, *et al*: Simulated activities of daily living examination. *Arch Phys Med Rehab* 52:476–486, 498, 1972.
10. Casanova JS, Ferber J: Comprehensive evaluation of basic living skills. *Am J Occup Ther* 30:101–105, 1976.
11. Benjamin J: The Northwick Park A.D.L. index. *Occup Ther (Br)* 39:301–306, 1976.
12. Buchwald E: Functional training. *Phys Ther Rev* 29:491–496, 1949.
13. Lawton MP, Brody EM: Assessment of older people: self maintaining and instrumental activities of daily living. *Gerontologist* 9:179–186, 1969.
14. Hoberman M, Acenia EF, Stephenson GR: Daily activity testing in physical therapy and rehabilitation. *Arch Phys Med* 33:99–108, 1952.
15. Hall HJ, Knox MMC: *Handicrafts for the Handicapped*. New York, Moffat and Yard, 1916, p 126.
16. Slagle EC: Handicrafts used as treatment. *Handicrafter* 1:26–27, 1928.
17. Dunton WR: Occupational Therapy, In Mock H, *et al*: *Principles and Practices of Physical Therapy*, Vol I, Hagerstown, Md, Prior, 1935, vol 1, p 28.
18. Combs MH, *et al*: Vocational exploration. *Am J Occup Ther* 12:64–68, 1958.
19. Maurer PA: Prevocational activities and evaluation for the child and adolescent. *Phys Ther* 48:771–776, 1968.
20. Cawood LT: *Words: Work-Oriented Rehabilitation Dictionary and Synonyms*. Seattle, Northwest Association of Rehabilitation Industries, 1975.
21. Gellman W: The principles of vocational evaluation. *Rehabil Lit* 29:98–102, 1968.
22. Ehrle R, *et al*: Glossary of terms used in vocational evaluation. *Vocational Eval Work Adjustment Bull* 8:85–93, 1975.

23. Redkey H, White: *The PreVocational Unit in a Rehabilitation Center.* Washington, DC, U.S. Department of Health Education and Welfare, Office of Vocational Rehabilitation, 1956.
24. Gellman W: The workshop as a clinical rehabilitation tool. *Rehabil Lit* 26:34–38, 1965.
25. Buros OK: The Eighth Mental Measurement Yearbook. Highland Park, NJ, Gryphon Press, 1978.
26. Brown EM, Van der Bogert M: Prevocational motor skill inventory. *Am J Occup Ther* 7:153–163, 188, 1953.
27. Ayres AJ: A form used to evaluate the work behavior of patients. *Am J Occup Ther* 8:73–74, 1954.
28. Ireland KL: Evaluating work behavior in occupational therapy. *J Rehabil* 23:8–9, 25, 1957.
29. Reuss EE, et al: Development of a physical capacities evaluation. *Am J Occup Ther* 12:1–14, 1958.
30. Cromwell FS: *Occupational Therapists' Manual for Basic Skills Assessment: Primary Prevocational Evaluation.* Four Oaks, Pasadena, Calif, 1960, p 87.
31. Sattely C: Performance evaluation and vocational evaluation In *Work Adjustment as a Function of Occupational Therapy.* Dubuque, Iowa, Brown, 1964.
32. Swenson VW: West Haverstraw Rehabilitation Hospital: Concepts and appraisal of the prevocational program. In *Work Adjustment as a Function of Occupational Therapy.* Dubuque, Iowa, Brown, 1964.
33. Llorens LA: Work adjustment program. *Am J Occup Ther* 18:15–19, 1964.
34. Ethridge DA: Pre-vocational assessment of rehabilitation potential of psychiatric patients. *Am J Occup Ther* 22:161–167, 1968.
35. Bailey D: Ready for work? *Br J Occup Ther* 44:80–83, 1981.
36. Smith SL: Physical capacities evaluation. In Hopkins H, Smith H: *Willard and Spackman's Occupational Therapy*, 5th ed. Philadelphia, Lippincott, 1978, pp 213–218.
37. Trombly CA, Scott AD: *Occupational Therapy for Physical Dysfunction.* Baltimore, Williams & Wilkins, 1977.
38. Pedretti LE: *Occupational therapy: Practice Skills for Physical Dysfunction*, St. Louis, Mosby, 1981.
39. Hall HJ: Occupational therapy in 1921. *Mod Hosp* 18:61, 1922
40. Fidler GS, Fidler JW: Doing and becoming: purposeful action and self-actualization. *Am J Occup Ther* 32:305–310, 1978.
41. Maurer P: Antecedents of work behavior. *Am J Occup Ther* 25:295–297, 1971.
42. Reilly M: The educational process. *Am J Occup Ther* 23:299–307, 1969.
43. Hart HH: Work as integration, *Med Record* 160:735–739, 1947.
44. Wegg LS: The Essentials of work evaluation. *Am J Occup Ther* 31:651–652,1977.
45. Nadolsky JM: Vocational evaluation theory in perspective. *Rehabil Lit* 32:226–231, 1971.
46. Dooling DM: *A Way of Working.* Garden City, NJ, Anchor, 1979, p viii.
47. Reilly M: An explanation of play. In Reilly M: *Play as Exploratory Learning.* Beverly Hills, Calif, Sage Publications, 1974.
48. Reilly M: The educational process. *Am J Occup Ther* 23:299–307, 1969.
49. Takata N: The play history. *Am J Occup Ther* 23:314–318, 1969.
50. Takata N: Play as a prescription. In Reilly M: *Play as Exploratory Learning.* Beverly Hills, Calif, Sage Publications, 1974.
51. Florey L: An approach to play and play development. *Am J Occup Ther* 25:275–280, 1971.
52. Robinson A: Play: the arena for acquisition of rules for competent behavior. *Am J Occup Ther* 31:248–253, 1977.
53. Michelman S: Research in symbol formation and creative growth. In West W: *Occupational Therapy Functions in Interdisciplinary Programs for Children.* Washington, DC, Department of Health, Education and Welfare, 1979.
54. Michelman S: The importance of creative play. *Am J Occup Ther* 25:285–290, 1971.
55. Zorn J: Research in cognitive development. In West W: *Occupational Therapy Functions in Interdisciplinary Programs for Children.* Washington, DC, Department of Health, Education and Welfare, 1970.

56. Knox S: A play scale. In Reilly M: *Play as Exploratory Learning.* Beverly Hills, Calif, Sage Publications, 1974.
57. Hurff J: A play skills inventory. In Reilly M: *Play as Exploratory Learning,* Beverly Hills, Calif, Sage Publications, 1974.
58. Hurff J: A play skills inventory: the competency monitoring tool for the 10-year old. *Am J Occup Ther* 34:651–656, 1980.
59. deRenne-Stephan C: Imitation: a mechanism of play behavior. *Am J Occup Ther* 34:95–102, 1980.
60. Takata N: The play milieu—a preliminary appraisal. *Am J Occup Ther* 25:281–284, 1971.
61. Michelman S: Play and the deficit child. In Reilly M: *Play as Exploratory Learning.* Beverly Hills, Calif, Sage Publications, 1974.
62. Newsletter of the National Therapeutic Recreation Society. Arlington, Va, National Recreation and Park Association, 1982, Concord, Mass, vol 7, pp 5–6.
63. Hall HJ: *Occupational Therapy: A New Profession.* Concord, Mass, Rumford Press, 1923.
64. McDowell CF: *Leisure Counseling: Selected Lifestyle Processes.* Eugene, Oregon, Center of Leisure Studies University of Oregon, 1976.
65. Neulinger J: *The Psychology of Leisure: Research Approaches to the Study of Leisure.* Springfield, Ill, Charles C Thomas, 1974.
66. Overs RP, Taylor S, Adkins C: *Avocational Counseling Manual.* Washington, DC, Hawkins, 1977.
67. Dumazedier J: *Toward a Society of Leisure.* London, Collier-Macmillan, 1962.
68. Kraus R: *Recreation and Leisure in Modern Society.* New York, Appleton-Century-Crofts, 1971.
69. Kelly JR: Work and leisure: a simplified paradigm. *J Leisure Res* 4:50–62, 1972.
70. Matsatsuya JS: The interest check list. *Am J Occup Ther* 23:323–328, 1969.
71. Mosey AC: *Activities Therapy.* New York, Raven Press, 1973.
72. Hughes PL, Mullins L: *Acute Psychiatric Care: An Occupational Therapy Guide to Exercises in Daily Living.* Thorofare, NJ, Slack, 1981.
73. Simon SB, Havve LW, Kirschenbaum H: *Values Clarification.* New York, Hart, 1972.
74. Kaplan M: *Leisure in America: A Social Inquiry.* New York, Wiley, 1960.

CHAPTER 12

Descriptive Models: Sensorimotor and Cognitive Performance Areas

BIOMECHANICAL MODELS

The biomechanical or kinesiological model is based on the mechanical principles of kinetics, the forces which produce, arrest or modify motions of bodies, and kinematics, the geometry of motion without regard to the forces acting to produce motion. The model is based on the assumption that voluntary muscle and control are the result of muscle strength and function, joint integrity and range, and physical endurance or tolerance. Thus it follows that dysfunction of the neuromuscular skeletal system can be corrected or restored through muscle strengthening, improved range of motion, better coordination, and increased endurance.

Reconstruction Model—Baldwin

FRAME OF REFERENCE

Bird T. Baldwin was a psychologist assigned to Walter Reed General Hospital at the end of World War I. In April, 1918, he undertook the task of organizing a department of occupational therapy for soldiers with physical injuries. A knowledge of measurement techniques probably helped Baldwin in his quest to ultimately "isolate, classify, repeat and to a limited degree, standardize and control the type of movements involved in the particular occupational and recreational operation" (1). His goals were the functional restoration and the acquisition of habits of industry for the purpose of helping each patient find himself and function again as a complete man, physically, socially, educationally, and economically.

Baldwin's major contributions to occupational therapy were the (a) use of mechanical appliances to measure and record daily performance for the patient's observation and the therapist's record and (b) understanding the role of intra- and interpersonal factors in overcoming disability through being a member of a social group and making tangible products of economic value.

ASSUMPTIONS

1. The best type of remedial exercise is that which requires a series of specific voluntary movements (1).
2. The voluntary movements should be those involved in the ordinary trades and occupations, physical training, play, or the daily routine activities of life (1).
3. The patient's attention should be repeatedly called to the particular remedial movements involved (1).
4. The movements should be initiated by the patient (1).

5. The movements should be a part of a larger and more complex series of coordinated movements (1).
6. The purposive nature of the movements and the end products of the work offer a direct incentive (motivation?) for sustained effort (1).
7. Periodic measurement of the increase in range and strength of movement helps the patient watch the recovery compare progress with others and overcome plateaus or regressions (1).

CONCEPTS

Palliative—keeping persons cheerful and in good spirits by using work which prevents them from dwelling on their disabilities, decreasing homesickness and fretting over petty annoyances (2).

Remedial—increasing skill and dexterity in the arm and breaking up wrong association, preventing depression and inducing correct habits of thought (2).

Extention—the straightening of a joint (4).

Flexion—the bending of a joint (4).

Abduction—movement away from the body (4).

Adduction—movement toward the body (4).

Rotation—turning or twisting around an axis (4).

Pronation—movement of the forearm in turning the palm of hand down (4).

Supination—movement of the forearm in turning the palm of the hand up (4).

Circumduction—a circular swinging movement (4).

EXPECTED RESULTS (1)

1. Help restore the body to its normal condition as far as is possible.
2. Enable the individual to feel that, despite physical handicap, a person may still be a self-reliant and self-respecting member of the community.
3. Help make the most of mental and physical resources and increase personal efficiency.
4. Provide a means of earning a comfortable livelihood.
5. Aid functional restoration and the acquisition of habits of industry.

ASSESSMENT INSTRUMENTS (4)

1. Range of voluntary movement (range of motion)—a different apparatus was used for each joint.
2. Strength of voluntary movement—a commercial spring balance scale was used.

INTERVENTION STRATEGIES

1. Media (3)
   a. Academic
      1. English, French, Spanish

    2. Arithmetic, geometry, algebra
    3. Trigonometry
    4. Penmanship, left hand writing
    5. Civil service preparation
    6. Physics, chemistry
    7. History
  b. Commercial
    1. Commercial arithmetic and English
    2. Shorthand, stenotyping
    3. Filing and recording
    4. Bookkeeping
    5. Salesmanship
    6. Commercial law
  c. Agriculture
    1. Truck farming out of doors
    2. Vegetable forcing under glass
    3. Growing of flowers
    4. Textbook studies
  d. Printing
    1. Hand composition
    2. Linotype operation
    3. Press work
  e. Mechanical and electrical departments
    1. Oxy-acetylene welding
    2. Wiring for bells, lights and motors
    3. Telegraphy, radio operation
    4. Motion picture machine operation
    5. Machine shop practice
    6. Electrical studies
    7. Mechanical studies
  f. Drafting
    1. Shop drawing, details and assembly
    2. Tracing and blue printing
    3. Architectual drawing
    4. Topographical drawing
    5. Freehand sketching
  g. Woodworking
    1. General carpentry
    2. Framing
    3. Cabinet work
    4. Pattern making
  h. Display painting
    1. Lettering
    2. Sign painting
    3. Poster making
  i. Arts and crafts
    1. Woodcarving
    2. Jewelry making and repairing

      3. Silversmithing
      4. Watch and clock repairing
      5. Engraving
      6. Modeling
   j. Leather work
      Shop repairing
   k. Physical education
      1. Athletic sports
      2. Calisthenics
      3. Gymnastics
      4. Dancing
   l. Rug weaving
      1. Fundamentals of rug weaving
      2. Rug repair
      3. Loom work
      4. Knitting machines
      5. Dyeing
2. Methods
   a. The work selected must involve the movements required by the prescription (1).
   b. Where more than one activity is equally desirable from a curative standpoint, the one with a vocation outlook is assigned unless the person prefers to work along the lines of avocation rather than vocation (1).
   c. Analysis of activities by joint motion should be made for stiff joints. Details are provided in the monograph (4).
   d. Analysis of activities by muscles involved should be made for peripheral nerve palsies. Examples are provided in the monograph (4).
3. Equipment
   A detailed list of equipment and tools is given for the fingers and thumb, wrist and elbow, shoulder, back, knee, ankle, midtarsus and toes (4). The idea of changing the size of the handles is mentioned. Considerations of sizes, shapes, and weights are listed also.
4. Precautions
   The methods were developed for stiff joints and were not considered suitable for peripheral nerve palsies without modification to prevent overstretching. Overstretching-paralyzed muscles was recognized as resulting in irreparable damage.

SUMMARY

Baldwin's contribution to occupational therapy seems to be overlooked in its importance to the development of assessment and implementation for physically disabled persons. His contributions appear to be four. He was the first to measure joint range of motion, to measure muscle strength, to analyze occupations for their use of joints and muscles and to suggest some adaptations to equipment to better achieve desired motions.

In 1918, the practice of occupational therapy in physical dysfunction was far behind the use of occupational therapy in mental health which had origins in the moral treatment of the 1840s. Baldwin appears to have organized some effective media, methods and equipment which continued in use today, although many modifications have occurred. Later developments simplified the measurement of joints when the hand-held goniometer became common, and muscle strength testing is now done with dynamometers or manual measurements. Nevertheless, Baldwin seems to have been the first to establish and use these techniques routinely in an occupational therapy department.

Other aspects of Baldwin's program which have undergone change are the academic and vocational preparation areas. In 1918, many of the soldiers had not had much schooling and education. Many were immigrants or children of immigrants and had not gone to school. Academic education was important to vocational preparation. The year 1918 marked the passage of the Soldiers Rehabilitation Act. Thus, the differentiation between occupational therapy and vocational rehabilitation had not been made.

Orthopedic Model—Taylor

FRAME OF REFERENCE

The orthopedic approach to occupational therapy is based on a knowledge of anatomy and physiology and an understanding of diseases and injuries (pathology). Analysis of joint motion and muscle action also is important (kinesiology).

Marjorie Taylor was an early leader in the practice of occupational therapy in physical disabilities. She was the director of occupational therapy at Robert Breck Brigham Hospital in Boston, Massachusetts, and later director of the Curative Workshop in Milwaukee, Wisconsin, as well as director of the school of occupational therapy at Milwaukee Downer College. In 1954, Taylor retired and was awarded the Award of Merit by the American Occupational Therapy Associaton. Most of her ideas were developed at Brigham Hospital. Since she did not reference her work, the sources are unclear.

ASSUMPTIONS

1. Muscle reeducation should localize the action of certain muscle groups without bringing into play the action of other muscles not needed for the task (5).
2. Paralyzed muscles should be "coaxed" into activity, not forced (5).
3. The exact muscle which has been paralyzed should be developed (5).
4. Contraction of the muscle should be from the point of origin to the point of insertion (5).
5. Flaccidity or weakness should be treated through graded exercise (5).
6. Spasticity or hypertonicity and continued spasm should be treated through relaxation, rhythm and coordination (5).

7. Athetosis or uncoordinated worm-like movements combined with flaccidity should be treated through coordination (5).
8. Contractions or shortening of strong muscles because of lack of balance with weak opponents (5):
   a. Severe cases should be treated with traction.
   b. Less severe cases through strengthening the weak opposing muscles.
9. Exercise should be given in slow rhythm, allowing time for waste products to be carried off to reduce fatigue and irritability of the muscle (5).
10. The joint should go through the whole range of motion to establish the habit of reflex and obtain better coordination in the nerve centers (5).
11. Active voluntary motion is the only agency by which muscles may be strengthened (5).
12. Muscles should not be stretched or strained (5).
13. Occupations involving an entire group of muscles will not strengthen individual weak muscles (5).
14. Exercise increases the strength of muscles and improves circulation (5).

CONCEPTS

Passive exercise—therapist puts the joint through the full arc of motion without the assistance or resistance of the patient (5).

Active exercise—carried on by the patient and made up of assistance-free and resistive exercise (5).

Assistive exercise—performed by patient assisted by the therapist or some mechanical device, such as a pulley or weight (5).

Free exercise—carried on by the patient against the least possible resistance (5).

Resistive exercise—necessitates muscle power which is equal to overcoming the force of gravity (5).

Occupation—any activity in which the patient takes an active part (5).

Muscle reeducation—the localized action of certain groups without bringing into play other muscles whose action is for some reason undesirable (5).

EXPECTED RESULTS (5)

1. Muscle strengthening of individual muscles or muscle groups.
2. Improved circulation.
3. Better coordination in the nerve centers.
4. Establish or reestablish the habit of reflex.
5. Increased areas of motion (range of motion).

ASSESSMENT INSTRUMENTS

No specific assessments are mentioned. Activity analysis of some media is discussed but primarily in terms of intervention.

INTERVENTION STRATEGIES

1. Media (6)
   a. Cord knotting—shoulder, elbow and forearm, wrist and fingers
   b. Braid weaving—shoulder
   c. Mitre sawing—shoulder
   d. Screwing—shoulder, elbow and forearm
   e. Shoulder wheel
   f. Shoulder ladder
   g. Loom weaving—shoulder, elbow and forearm, wrist and fingers
   h. Coping saw—shoulder
   i. Hammering—shoulder
   j. Planing—elbow and forearm
   k. Sawing—elbow and forearm
   l. Sand papering—elbow and forearm
   m. Basketry—elbow and forearm
   n. Leather tooling—wrist and fingers
   o. Woodcarving—wrist and fingers
   p. Game of crokinole (caroms)
2. Methods (6)
   a. Splinting
   b. Use of occupations which require frequent contraction and relaxation
   c. Adjusting the height of the activity for different actions
   d. Adding elastic weights or pulleys to increase resistance-graded exercise
   e. Slings
3. Equipment
   None specifically mentioned.
4. Prerequisites or precautions (6)
   a. Pain lasting several hours.
   b. Fatigue lasting several hours.
   c. Swelling depending on the disorder.
   d. Local heat in the joints.

SUMMARY

The orthopaedic model is based on a thorough knowledge of "mechanical structure of bone and joint formation and the motor structure or muscle group action" (7) plus the knowledge of diseases including symptoms and prognosis. Use of the orthopaedic model in assessment involved examining joint limitations and lack of power in various muscle groups. Treatment was based on analyzing and employing one or more occupations which provided the needed motions to increase strength or range of motion in weak muscle groups without increasing the stronger muscles as well.

Kinetic Model—Licht
FRAME OF REFERENCE

Licht believed that occupational therapy needed to become more scientific and accept the scientific method which stressed cause and effect relations. When the relations were observed in repeated studies, truth could be established.

Sidney Licht, M.D., was a physician and a writer. In 1947, he became the editor of *Occupational Therapy and Rehabilitation* after William R. Dunton, Jr., retired. Licht's interest, however, was in physical dysfunction and not psychiatric disorders. In 1950, Dunton and Licht (8) joined forces to write and edit a textbook of occupational therapy. This book was revised in 1957.

Licht's major contribution to occupational therapy was to develop an outline of objectives for occupational therapy and to establish working definitions of each category. Although the objectives did not encompass the essence of occupational therapy, the definitions have remained useful.

ASSUMPTIONS

1. The scientific method must be applied to occupational therapy if its continued acceptance as therapy is desired (9).
2. Occupational therapy is medically prescribed activity for therapeutic objectives (9).
3. Volitional effort and perserverance are usually necessary to gain the desired end in minimum time (10).
4. Motivation will frequently be related to the pleasure or boredom resulting from exercise (10).
5. Static contraction requires the expenditure of energy and is therefore related to muscle strengthening (10).
6. Muscles which have been immobilized for a longer period will tire more readily from prolonged static contraction than from intermittent contractions (10).
7. Interrupted voluntary rhythmic contractions followed by relaxation even though brief are more desirable (10).
8. Occupational therapy can accomplish more with passive than active motions (10).

CONCEPTS

Kinetic analysis—the identification and classification of active and passive body motions, including muscles, muscle groups and joints required in the execution of a craft, an occupation or activity (10)

Kinetic occupational therapy—related to motion and used to restore or improve muscle strength, joint mobilization and coordination (9)

Metric occupational therapy—related to measurement and used to improve work tolerance and measure progress of tolerance (9)

Tonic occupational therapy—related to tone and use to improve and maintain muscle and mental tone (9)

Cycle of motion—the analysis of the preparatory and effective motion of activity (11)

Type of muscle contraction—the determination as to whether the muscles used are contracted statically, intermittently, slowly or brisky and whether there is passive contraction, extension or stretching (11)

Joint range—the extent of joint motion usually recorded in degrees (11)

Starting position—the stance in which the activity is performed (11)

Realism—analysis should concentrate on the economic use of body mechanics and stress the important motions while reemphasizing incidental or accidental motions (11)

Tool variant—the size and shape of the tool may determine the motions involved (11)

Clinic energy dosage—units of visible work achievement (11)

EXPECTED RESULTS (11)
1. Perseverance of interest and delayed fatigue.
2. Coordination through realistic motions.
3. Strengthening of muscles.
4. Mobilization of joints.
5. Reeducation of unlearned or forgotten motions.
6. Stretching of shortened tissues.
7. Proper alignment of body structures.
8. Prevent contractures.
9. Training in ADLs.
10. Promote physical independence.
11. Prevocational exploration.

ASSESSMENT INSTRUMENT
1. Kinetic analysis outline of crafts and occupation (11).
    a. Cycle of motion including preparatory and effective motion.
    b. Type of muscle contraction
        1. Static or intermittent
        2. Slow or brisk
        3. Passive or active
        4. Flexion or extension
        5. Stretching
    c. Joint range
    d. Accuracy
        a. Joints should not be lumped together.
        b. Both extremeties should be analyzed.
        c. Incidental or accidental motions should be excluded.
    e. Starting position
    f. Realism
    g. Tool variants
2. Assessment of change (11)
    a. Measure rate of movement per unit of time.
    b. Measure number of repetitive motions.
    c. Measure number of inches lost or gained by the medium.
    d. Measure weight loss by the medium such as wood.

INTERVENTION STRATEGIES
1. Media (9)
    a. Agriculture
        1. Animal husbandry
        2. Horticulture

b. Arts
   1. Fine—painting, sculpture, etc.
   2. Graphic—printing, lettering
   3. Dramatic—theatre, radio, cinema
   4. Dance—social, folk, etc.
   5. Literary—bibliotherapy
   6. Music—music therapy
c. Crafts
   1. Hand crafts
   2. Machine crafts
d. Education
e. Industrial and maintenance
   1. Industrial therapy
   2. Hospitals industry
f. Recreational therapy
   1. The arts
   2. Athletics
   3. Social gatherings

2. Methods (12)
   a. Muscle strengthening—increase number, frequency, duration and diurnal periodicity of contractions.
   b. Joint contracton—increase the force applied and duration of the force, decrease the interval between applications of pressure, increase the total duration of each session and number of sessions per day or week.
   c. Factors affecting methods
      1. Effects of gravity can increase or decrease the work component.
      2. Position of the body or body parts also affects the gravitational effect.
      3. Working surface or edge affects the work performance, depending on whether it is sharp or dull.
      4. Various motions may interfere with desired effects and need to be prevented.
      5. The weight or shape of a tool handle may interfere with performance if not selected for the disability.
      6. Energy is wasted in the learning process which affects the amount of work accomplished.
      7. The mood or enthusiasm of the person affects the work performed.

3. Equipment (13)
   a. Bicycle jig saw
   b. Platforms of various heights
   c. Holding devices—special clamps, vices or other apparatus which will hold work materials
   d. Variable height work bench
   e. Blocks and wedges—used to change the angle or height of the pedals on the bicycle jig saw

    f. Tool handles
      1. Build up handle—increase or decrease the difficulty of grasp
      2. Angulation of handle—bend handles to ease range of motion required to reach
      3. Shovel type handle—used to assist limited pronation or supination
      4. Length of handle—extending or shortening the handle increases efficiency and comfort
      5. Rotation of lever—changing the lever on the axis may bring the handle into the person's range of motion.
    g. Seat variation—the seat can be moved closer or further away or can be raised or lowered to change the range of motion and muscle contraction.
    h. Incline plane—controls the grading of energy, especially for upper extremities.
  4. Prerequisites and precautions
    a. Status of bony union
    b. Tissue continuity
    c. Paresis
    d. Fatigue
    e. Impaired circulation

SUMMARY

Licht attempted to organize the practice of occupational therapy in physical disabilities into three major categories: kinetic, metric and tonic. Kinetic or functional treatment includes muscles strengthening, increasing range of motion and improving coordination. Metric or graded exercise involved improving work tolerance. Tonic or diversional treatment included maintaining muscle and mental tone. Licht also categorized the objectives for psychiatric occupational therapy but did not promote them. A complete outline is included in Table 12.1.

Licht was instrumental also in promoting the use of activity analysis of craft motions and tool use. He provided good documentation of some adaptations to equipment although he did not invent or create the adaptations himself.

Analysis and Critique of Biomechanical or Kinesiological Models
FRAME OF REFERENCE

The biomechanical models are based on the mechanistic, reductionistic medical rehabilitation philosophies. Man's activities are controlled by forces such as disease or trauma acting on the musculoskeletal parts which can be analyzed into individual muscles and joints with specific actions. The development of the biomechanical models is the result of pressure on the profession to adopt the scientific method of analyzing the internal structures and functions of man in order to control change (10). The pressure did result in more knowledge about the application of occupations to specific muscle and joint groups. However, the internally directed focus decreased the awareness of the total environment in which

Table 12.1
Objectives of Occupational Therapy[a]

I. Kinetic (old word—functional) used to restore or improve
   a. Muscle strength
   b. Joint mobilization
   c. Coordination
II. Metric (old word—graded) used to
   a. Improve work tolerance
   b. Measure progress of tolerance
III. Tonic (old word—diversional) used to improve and maintain
   a. Muscle tone
   b. Mental tone
IV. Psychiatric used to favorably influence
   a. Psychomotor activity
      1. Stimulation
         a. Arouse interest
         b. Improve concentration
      2. Sedation
         a. Energy release
         b. Lessen destructive tendencies
            1. Aggression outlet
   b. Emotional disturbance
      1. Emotional stability (contentment)
      2. Mood
   c. Behavior
      1. Behavior (habit) training
   d. Abnormal mental content
      1. Guilt complex
      2. Paranoid trends
         a. Crowd out delusions
   e. Psychosocial activity
      1. Socialization
         a. Interpersonal relations
         b. Attitude
            1. Self-respect
            2. Confidence
            3. Self-control
      2. Provide obtainable objective
         a. Gratify narcissism
   f. Diagnosis
      1. Reaction to situation in clinic
      2. Identification of problem (in psychodrama)
      3. Determine limit of intellectual work capacity
      4. Prevocational exploration
   g. Mental hygiene
      1. Overcome restlessness
      2. Promote good work and play habits

[a] Reprinted from S. Licht (9), with permission from Williams & Wilkins.

the person must function. The direction of change was individual. Little demand was made upon the external environment.

CLARITY

The belief that man can influence change in the environment as well as in the self is lost under biomechanical models. Also lost is the concept of balance between activities in a person's life. The focus is on enabling the person to become productive so that the individual can contribute to society. Self maintenance and leisure occupations are not stressed. Independence really meant financial independence. Another loss is the emphasis on total performance including intra- and interpersonal skills which meet the needs of self-esteem and self actualization as a person, not just as a worker. Occupational therapy under the biomechanical models uses art and craft occupations to promote therapeutic exercise and thus is an extension of concepts of physical therapy. The primary differences other than media were slight. Licht (10) says occupational therapy does a better job of improving coordination and promoting interest to combat fatigue.

On the positive side is the increased knowledge the profession gained about the effects of activity on muscles and joints which are recovering from changes produced by disease or trauma. Another useful outcome is the increased skill in analyzing occupations into patterns of motion and tasks. A third outcome is the increased knowledge of methods to adapt equipment to facilitate performance.

UNIQUENESS

The biomechanical models have not added to the understanding or advancement of occupational therapy as a unique discipline. Instead the models increased the confusion between physical and occupational therapy by suggesting that both provide therapeutic exercise as a primary objective.

RESEARCH GUIDE

The biomechanical models have fostered some research in occupational therapy, although the primary results have been of a descriptive rather than experimental nature. The primary difficulty has been the reductionistic focus which means the results seem to support physical therapy more than occupational therapy.

SPECIALIZATION

As a guide for specialization, the biomechanical models are not very successful. Each model tends to derail or misguide the use of occupational therapy as an approach to helping people achieve or regain health function, and a sense of well-being. The models if used at all should be observed in practice to avoid losing the essence of occupational therapy as a profession.

ELABORATION AND REFINEMENT

Improved methods of analyzing occupations and of analzying the needs of people for certain types of occupations or subskills are useful, regardless of the philosophic problems in assumptions and concepts. Also useful are more effective methods and more adaptive equipment to facilitate performance skills for use in fulfilling occupational needs and demands. The biomechanical models have contributed in these areas of assessment and intervention and may continue to do so.

EXPLANATORY USEFULNESS

The biomechanical models do not provide much useful information in explaining what occupational therapy is from a philosophic framework. Likewise, some of the assumptions are inadequate and the concepts misleading. The process of intervention, however, is basically the same, although the choice of methods for assessment and intervention tend to be different because of a dichotomy of view concerning locus of control. The organismic orientation includes the person as an integral part of the process, whereas the mechanistic view does not depend on person-therapist interaction as a critical variable in performance acquisition and maintenance.

COMMONALITY

The biomechanical models do have more in common with medicine and physical therapy. However, there is less in common with nursing and education. Commonality at the expense of philosophy seems a poor choice. Occupational therapy has much to offer people in its own right without following the coattails of medicine and physical therapy. Occupational therapy uses occupations and tasks to promote integrated function and facilitate interrelatedness and interdependence with the human and nonhuman environment. Occupational therapy is not primarily concerned with the physical properties of physical agents and therapeutic exercises as the primary method. Occupational therapy is not just another form of noninvasive surgery or noningested drug.

PRACTICE MODELS

As the previous sections of the critique suggest, the biomechanical models do not provide the best source of information and data for practice model and theory development. Although some aspects of the models may be useful, such as the analysis of media, the application must be observed closely to avoid practicing physical therapy and not occupational therapy.

SUMMARY

A summary of the biomechanical models is provided in Table 12.2. In general, such models are not very successful in meeting the requirements for models of practice in occupational therapy. Failure to meet criteria for practice models, however, should not necessarily eliminate the models from consideration as research models to evaluate effectiveness of certain techniques. As stated previously, techniques may be used in either organismically or mechanistically based models. The caution with the biomechanical model is to recognize that all techniques must be reevaluated carefully before including the techniques in an intervention pro-

Table 12.2
Biomechanical Models Summary Critique

Evaluation Criteria	Very Good 1	Moderately Good 2	3	4	Very Poor 5
Frame of reference					X
Clarity	X				
Uniqueness				X	
Research guide				X	
Specialization				X	
Elaboration/refinement			X		
Explanatory usefulness				X	
Commonality			X		
Practice model				X	

gram so that the locus of control is shifted from the therapist to the person.

Compensatory Model

FRAME OF REFERENCE

The compensatory model is appropriate for persons whose disability is temporary or permanent. The model focuses on the use of remaining abilities and strengths. This focus on remaining abilities may be necessary in the short run to permit a part of the body to heal. An example is a broken arm. The person uses the "good" arm and hand alone until the broken arm is healed. On the other hand, a person may lose the use of the arm permanently through amputation, for example. Now the use of one-handed techniques is a valuable backup skill whenever the prosthetic arm needs service.

There are no specific models of compensation written by occupational therapists which the author could locate. Rather, this section is drawn from general occupational therapy references which include extensions of some of the biomechanical models.

Some assumptions of the compensatory model are as follows:

1. Devices external to the individual can be devised to substitute for motions not available to the individual, *i.e.*, a wheelchair or prosthetic limb.
2. Muscles and joints can be used on one side of the body to substitute for motions not available, *i.e.*, substitute one-handed shoe lace tying for two-handed (one-handed techniques).
3. Devices external to the individual can be devised which reduce the demand for skills (fine motor activity, *i.e.*, substitute for lack of range and strength, such as enlarged handles which use cylindrical grasp for three jawed chuck grasp; incoordination, limited range of motion and decreased strength).
4. The external environment can be modified to reduce or eliminate

the need for certain motions, *i.e.*, build a ramp to eliminate stairs (architectual barriers).

5. Other parts of the body may be used to substitute for motions not available, such as using the teeth to tear open a package instead of the hands.
6. Other parts of the sensory system may be used to substitute for sensory loss, *i.e.*, substitute tactile sense for visual sense.

CONCEPTS

Orthosis—a device applied to the exoskeleton to limit or assist motion of any given segment of the human body (*see also* splint)

Splint—a device used to assist (dynamic) or prevent (static) motion of joint (*see also* orthosis)

Sling—a band suspended from the neck or from overhead to support an arm or hand. Related terms include suspension or overhead sling

Prosthesis—an artificial device used to replace a missing limb or bodily part

Architectual barrier—structural design in the environment which prevents or hinders a person from using that environment

Adapted/assistive device or equipment—the altering of a tool, utensil, or machine to permit the item to be used by a person who is handicapped or to improve the use by a normal person

Self-help devices or equipment—utensils which have been altered to facilitate the performance of daily living tasks.

EXPECTED RESULTS

The person will be able to:

1. Use the specialized equipment to substitute for lost motions.
2. Learn and use one-handed techniques.
3. Use adapted devices to overcome the problems of incoordination and decreased strength.
4. Eliminate or reduce the limitations caused by architectual barriers.
5. Learn to substitute other parts of the body to perform certain motions.
6. Learn to use other sensory modalities to substitute for sensory loss.

ASSESSMENT INSTRUMENTS

The most common form of assessment is a checklist on which a list of tasks is given. The therapist asks the person to perform the task and notes the quality of the performance given. If an adapted device orthosis or prosthesis is needed, the equipment is secured and another checklist is used to determine the effectiveness of performnce with the device. If a structural modification is needed, another assessment is completed after the modification is completed. Examples include a prosthetic checklist, wheelchair checklist, self-care checklist, homemaking checklist or aritectual barriers checklist.

INTERVENTION STRATEGIES

1. Media
   a. Orthotic devices and splints
   b. Prosthetic devices and braces
   c. Wheelchairs
   d. Self-care devices for feeding, bathing, grooming, brushing teeth, dressing
   e. Self-help devices, such as reachers, grab bars, elevated chairs
   f. Reconstructed structures such as kitchens
   g. Braille typewriters and labels in braille on equipment
2. Methods
   a. Standard teaching methods such as demonstration and practice
   b. Specialized teaching methods such as backwards chaining to learn the use of self-care devices (performing steps of task in reverse order)
3. Equipment—covered under media
4. Prerequisites and precautions
   a. Do not use compensatory media unless necessary.
   b. Be sure training is complete for proper use.
   c. Beware of "gadget tolerance." Too many devices may be more difficult for the person to use than not enough.
   d. Include instructions on washing, maintaining and repairing devices if appropriate.

SUMMARY

The compensatory model is based on the assumption that the person needs assistance from external or artificial devices, equipment or structural modifications to facilitate the process of regaining maximum function. Such devices, equipment or structural changes may be temporary or permanent. The devices and equipment range from simple items such as button hooks to a complete prosthesis. Structural modifications may be minor, such as installing a grab bar to remodeling a kitchen.

Assessment usually involves a checklist observation and recheck if modifications are needed. Intervention occurs to demonstrate how the device or equipment is used or to explain what modifications in structure or furnishings are needed. Major prerequisites and precautions included providing sufficient training to ensure proper and safe use and an awareness that some people have a limited tolerance or acceptance of "gadgets" no matter how useful.

Analysis and Critique of the Compensatory Model
FRAME OF REFERENCE

The compensatory model as developed in the United States is an extension of the biomechanical models. A biomechanical model is tried first when the individual is encouraged to redevelop strength, range of motion and coordination within the person's body. Compensatory methods are employed as a second choice when the person is unable to accomplish tasks unaided or may be able to perform sooner with external assistance. Inability to perform also includes unsafe to perform and probability of potential nonperformance (preventive splinting).

As an extension of the biomechanical model, the philosophy of the compensatory model is the same. The model is based on the mechanistic, reductionistic and rehabilitative approach. The dysfunctional part is analyzed, and an appropriate substitute or extension is prescribed.

CLARITY

The assumptions and concepts have not been clarified by the profession. However, most therapists learn the concepts at one time or another during their education and practice experience. As a single source, the textbook by Trombly (14) presents most of the concepts.

Of more concern is the apparent lack of understanding by many clients in or out of the hospital. There are repeated examples of splints not being worn and devices not being used. Sometimes prostheses and wheelchairs are abandoned likewise. Somewhere in the compensatory model there is a breakdown between theory and application. Clients either do not learn to use the appliances satisfactorily or fail to find a reason for incorporating the use into their daily lives. Could the problem be related to locus of control? If given a free choice could it be that the client would choose not to have the appliance in the first place? Perhaps clients should be permitted to choose those devices they wish to use instead of having them recommended.

UNIQUENESS

The development of splints and adapted devices has been a trademark of occupational therapy. However, occupational therapists rarely have pressed to gain control over the making of temporary splints or of recommending the use of adapted devices for daily use.

As a general model, compensation does not offer much that is unique to occupational therapy. Prosthetics is a field in itself. Architectual barriers are a social problem. Physical therapists train clients in the use of wheelchairs as often as occupational therapists. Teachers of the blind use many adapted devices.

RESEARCH GUIDE

The compensatory model could offer some interesting subjects for studies. A few studies have been done comparing different types of splints, but more could be done (15, 16). The long-term effects of wearing joint protection splints could be evaluated. The use of devices in prolonging or facilitating independent living could be explored.

SPECIALIZATION

The use of the compensatory model as a basis for specialization does not appear in the occupational therapy literature, except perhaps in the area of splinting. As developed under the medical rehabilitation model, compensatory techniques have had only moderate success. Using the concepts of compensation but reorienting the philosophy to a more organismic view could provide the basis for specialization.

ELABORATION AND REFINEMENT

The compensatory model needs elaboration and refinement to account for client acceptance and use of compensatory devices, equipment and modifications. The client is a missing focal point in the compensatory approach.

EXPLANATORY USEFULNESS

The compensatory model does explain a part of the rationale for working with clients who have physical dysfunction. The rationale is that therapists attempt to provide assistive or substitute device equipment and modifications when a person is unable to function through individual efforts or when such efforts cost too much energy. The rationale is not specific to occupational therapy but is used as part of a general rationale for relating to clients in occupational therapy. What is not explained is the role of the client in determining which, if any, of the recommendations made by the occupational therapist will be accepted by the client.

COMMONALITY

The compensatory model does have rationale and techniques in common with other discplines, as discussed under the section on Uniqueness. Compensatory techniques can be used as a basis for discussing the interdependence of professions and the necessity of working together. For example, if a splint is to be used properly the instructions for wearing and caring for the splint must be observed by the nursing staff and any other professional which the client encounters. Likewise, if adapted utensils are to be used at mealtime, they should be available and not lost in the dishwasher in the kitchen. Communication and understanding of the compensatory model among professionals can facilitate the acceptance by clients.

PRACTICE MODELS

Any practice model or theory built on the compensatory model must be careful to avoid the mechanistic aspects which appear in the development of the compensatory model. Although the compensatory techniques have a place in the total sphere of occupational therapy practice, their use should be consistent in application with other approaches. Of particular concern is the philosophical issue of locus of control so that the person, not the therapist, is the central focus. Thus, in order to build a strong practice model based on the compensatory model, the first step should be to restructure the compensatory model into an organismic framework.

SUMMARY

The compensatory model presents many of the same problems in application to practice as the biomechanical model. A summary is provided in Table 12.3.

NEUROBIOLOGICAL MODELS

The neurobiological models developed during the 1950s and 1960s in response to (a) better knowledge about human function and control of the nervous system and (b) increased numbers of clients being referred with central nervous system problems (cerebral palsy and hemiplegia) as opposed to peripheral nervous system problems (peripheral nerve injuries and poliomyelitis). Emphasis in the neurobiological models is on the normal development of the nervous system as an intact unit. Thus the focus of treatment is to normalize the nervous system which has been injured or damaged. The normalizing techniques vary according to the model being presented based on the modeler's collection of assumptions and concepts.

Neurobehavioral Model—Banus

FRAME OF REFERENCE

The neurobehavioral model is the organizing theme of the text *The Developmental Therapist*, second edition by Banus and others (17). The model is based primarily on the works of Piaget and Gesell with additional material from the neurobiological sciences. Piaget's developmental stages of cognition have been used in toto. Gesell's assumptions regarding the role of maturation and reciprocal interweaving are adopted. Also extensive use of neurobiological assumptions regarding the organization of the nervous system are incorporated through the writings of Norton, an occupational therapist.

ASSUMPTIONS (17)

1. There is a wide range in the rate of normal development among all children in even single culture (based on Piaget) (p. 7).

Table 12.3
Compensatory Model Criteria Summary

Evaluation of Criteria	Very Good 1	Moderately Good		Very Poor 5
		2	3	4	
Frame of reference				X	
Clarity				X	
Uniqueness			X		
Research guide			X		
Specialization				X	
Elaboration/refinement				X	
Explanatory usefulness			X		
Commonality			X		
Practice model				X	

2. Different behaviors develop at different rates in the same child (based on Piaget) (p. 9).
3. Development can be analyzed horizontally be evaluating a number of different functions or longitudinally by tracking developmental progress sequentially over time (based on Piaget) (p. 9).
4. Awareness and attention span increase in response to adequate stimulation (based on Piaget and Norton) (p. 65).
5. Subcortical activity of the newborn and infant is gradually replaced with cortical activity (p. 65).
6. Content of thought is less influenced by sensorimotor experience and more dependent on abstract psychological process over time (p. 66).
7. Psychological structures functionally emerge from the biological-environmental interaction (p. 67).
8. Schemes are the structures on which behavior is based and which develop progressively from the overt physical acts of the newborn to the covert knowing behavior of the adolescent (p. 67).
9. Psychosocial development is an ongoing process from birth until death (p. 69).
10. An individual inherits a genotypic potential for the organism to develop in response to its environment (the geneticoenvironment law borrowed from Dobzhansky) (p. 71).
11. Maturation tends to proceed in a descending direction from head to tail (direction of development, borrowed from Gesell) (p. 71).
12. There is a fluctuating dominance of counterbalance such as agonists and antagonist, right and left limbs, ipsilateral and contralateral segments until a balanced mature stage is achieved (reciprocal interweaving, borrowed from Gesell) (p. 71).
13. Man tends to develop hand, eye, foot, and ear preferences (laterally or functional asymmetry) (p. 71).
14. Man reflects and is the product of his evolutionary heritage (phylogenetic development) (p. 71).
15. Reflexive muscular activity provides the supporting framework within which volitional or voluntary movement operates (p. 72).
16. Skilled movement is a product of the integration of willed movement and postural reflexes and reactions (p. 72).
17. There are degrees of volition of movements from "least automatic" to "most automatic" (p. 72).
18. There is a transition in development from an excitatory organism to a more inhibited organism (p. 72).
19. There is a trend of refinement of the early gross uncoordinated movements, the increased ability to localize stimuli and toward localization of reflexes (p. 72).

CONCEPTS

Growth—the increase in size of an individual or his body parts as measured by increased weight volume or linear dimensions (p. 6)

Maturation—refers primarily to the maturity of the central nervous system (p. 6)

Phylogenetic development—structural and behavioral change that replicates the evolutionary development of the individual's species (p. 7)

Ontogenetic development—the progressive behavioral change that occurs between birth and the adult state (p. 7)

Developmental evaluation—assesses a cross-section of the child's behavior (p. 12)

Developmental stimulation—the activities which promote typical development behaviors in children with or without problems (p. 13)

Developmental specialist—a person who has mastered the knowledge of the total developmental process (p. 15)

Developmental therapy—a planned program designed to meet specifically a child's individual developmental and learning needs based on his rate of progress (p. 14)

Developmental therapist—anyone who analyzes the child's development, recognizes the discrepancies between his development and the norm, plans an appropriate program of maintenance, correction or prevention and provides therapy for the child.

Developmental task—the functions which an individual is expected to perform successfully with a given range of time according to the standards of his culture (p. 9)

Biological structures—includes physical and behavioral structures which are variant and invariant (p. 66)

Physical structures—structures which are inherited and predetermined by the species (p. 66)

Behavioral responses—responses which dominate, such as reflexes, at birth to ensure survival of the neonate prior to the development of automatic and spontaneous movement (p. 66)

Biological functions—includes the biological aspects of organization and adaptation (p. 66)

Organization—tendency for all species to systematize or organize their processes into coherent systems such as physical or psychological (p. 66)

Adaptation—balanced interaction between the body and the world around it (p. 66)

Accommodation—the process an individual uses biologically to adapt himself to the environment through physiological changes (p. 66)

Assimilation—the process an individual uses to adapt the environment to meet his own biological needs (p. 66)

Schemes—the logical and repeated behavioral or mental actions (p. 67)

Psychological functions—includes the psychological aspects of organization and adaptation (p. 67)

Sensorimotor stage—devoted to inner self programming, largely structured by organization and increasingly modified by his actions, and the practical "knowing" of the child's limited environment by his actions upon it and it upon him (from Norton) (p. 68)

Preoperational stage—general coordination of the sensorimotor systems through better developed feedback and neural integration (from Piaget) (p. 68)

Concrete stage—implies an understanding of classification, of the interrelation among categories and of seriation and number (from Piaget) (p. 68)

Formal operations—utilizes abstract abilities that have developed out of earlier stages of "knowing" and organization (from Piaget) (p. 68)

Psychosocial—refers to those aspects of man which involve his sense of self and his interactions with others in his life space (p. 69)

Neuromotor development—refers to that portion of the human nervous system which implements or carries out the actual response (p. 70)

EXPECTED RESULTS

Assist the child to acquire the phyloontogenetic developmental substrate which is basic to learning.

ASSESSMENT INSTRUMENTS

1. Types
   a. Interview schedule—play, development or sensorimotor history
   b. Denver Developmental Screening Test—Frankenburg
   c. Southern California Sensory Integration Tests—Ayres
   d. Bayley Scale of Infant Development—Bayley
   e. Task Analysis—What sensory systems are activated, what are the adaptive responses, is the task compatible with developmental capacities, is the task compatible with needs, what are the cortical and subcortical components of the task, relationship of structure to creativity, central indications?
2. Assessment procedures
   a. Informal evaluation—casual, nonorganized observation of behavior (p. 173)
   b. Formal evaluation—organized, preplanned observation that entails interaction with the child (p. 174)
   c. Standardized tests—provide normative data on specific behavior of a specific population (p. 175)
   d. Nonstandardized—not defined
   e. Group evaluation—not defined
   g. Screening test—cursory examination of some portion of a child's behavior (p. 176)
   h. Probing or comprehensive test—follow screening test to verify the existence of the problem, define the problem or dismiss the results as spurious (p. 176)
   i. Pre- and posttesting—a means of measuring process over time (p. 176)

INTERVENTION STRATEGIES

1. Media—not discussed although toys and games are mentioned.
2. Methods
   a. Consideration for the effects of general stimuli such as lighting, temperature, background sounds, smells, time of day, relation to other events, and color
   b. Consideration of instructions as to whether subcortical (nonverbal) or cortical (verbal) input is required and the effect of directions on the integration of the nervous system
   c. Consideration of the effects of the task, the people and the equipment on the child's responses
   d. Consideration of the types of feedback and their effects on adaptation—sensory, biofeedback and reinforcement
   e. Types of treatment include home treatment, activity treatment, individual or group treatment
3. Equipment—not discussed. Some photographs show equipment, but use is not discussed.
4. Prerequisites or precautions
   a. Punishment, time out and extinction are generally not recommended.
   b. Tactile and vestibular input should be used with caution with a young or seizure-prone child.

SUMMARY

The neurobehavioral model is based on the assumption that the nervous system is responsible for the development and organization of sensorimotor, cognitive and psychological behavior. Influences on the nervous system are both biologically inherited and environmentally controlled so that there is a constant interaction between the biological and environmental forces.

Assessment involves the analysis and synthesis of data based on standardized tests of normal developmental progression and on interviews regarding specific aspects of development. Further information is gained through observation.

Intervention is based on consideration of the general stimuli in a given environment, the effect of verbal or nonverbal instruction, the influence of a given task, person or equipment on responses and the type of feedback which may be used to change the nervous system and facilitate an adaptive response (Fig. 12.1). Specific media and equipment are not discussed. Precautions are limited to various types of punishment or extinction and to the possible negative effects of tactile and vestibular stimuli.

Reflex Development—Fiorentino

FRAME OF REFERENCE

Fiorentino's model of reflex development is based primarily on the work of Karl and Bertha Bobath, a neurologist and physical therapist, respectively, who developed the treatment approach known as neuro-

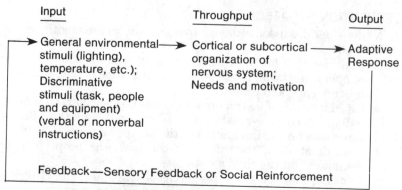

Figure 12.1. Neurobiological model.

developmental therapy or NDT. The primary assumptions of the Bobaths which Fiorentino borrowed are that (a) motor developmental tasks emerge as a function of reflexive maturation and (b) motor task assimilation depends on the establishment of certain higher chain synaptic arrangements (18). Fiorentino's (19) identification and organization of reflexes seem to be one of the earliest attempts to outline postural reflexes into an objective framework; the first edition of her book on reflex testing appeared in 1963. Although some attempts to categorize reflexes do appear earlier, there is little evidence that a systematic assessment instrument was used widely prior to Fiorentino's first edition.

ASSUMPTIONS

View of Man

1. Movement is an essential characteristic of living organisms (20).
2. The basic elements of movement activities include tone, control and strength (20).
3. The elements underlie the specific functions such as movement, postural stability, balance and coordination (20).
4. The integration of functions leads to the development of skill (20).
5. The total postural behavior of an individual is the result of the interaction of all reflexes and the relative strength of each one of them (20).
6. Postural reflexes and their interaction and integration form the background of normal voluntary movement and skill (20).
7. Integration occurs from mass excitation to controlled voluntary, cortical movements in cephalocaudal, proximal-distal and gross fine sequence (20).
8. Maturation and integration of the lower centers contributes to the development of the higher center (20).
9. With more inhibitory control from the higher centers, the mass movements are integrated, and goal-directed movements are developed (20).

10. At birth the body responds mechanically and automatically (20).
11. The primitive, postural reflexes primarily involve changes in tone and distribution which affect posture and movement (20).
12. There are four basic components which are necessary for the acquisition of motor skills: (a) head control, (b) extensor tone, (c) rotation within the body axis and (d) equilibrium reaction (20).
13. Postural reflexes supply the basic balance of tone (20).
14. The labyrinths are the most important organs concerned with the development of antigravity posture and balance (20).
15. As the head rights, extensor tone develops in the upper limbs (20).
16. Postural reflexes determine the strength and distribution of muscle tone and regulate it during movement (20).
17. Normal motor development proceeds in an orderly sequence of events from the apedal, to the quadrupedal, to the bipedal level of maturation (21).
18. Muscles are grouped in coordinated action patterns (21).
19. The normal child changes and modifies the sensorimotor patterns of early primitive movements and adapts them gradually to more complex functions as prehension and walking (21).
20. The learning of movements is entirely dependent upon sensory experience, sensory input which not only initiates but also guides motor input (21).
21. Human behavior follows a pattern of maturation which assists the normal child to develop in a well ordered sequence of events (21)

View of Health
22. When inhibitory control of higher centers is disrupted or delayed, primitive patterns dominate to the exclusion of higher integrated sensorimotor activities (19).
23. The more primitive reflexes result in abnormalities manifested by phylogenetically older posture and movements and abnormal muscle tone (19).

View of the Profession
24. The basic aim of occupational therapy is purposeful function, the development and/or restoration of such function to the maximum ability of the child (22).

CONCEPT
Reflex—a specific, automatic, patterned response that is elicited by a particular stimulus and does not involve any conscious control (20)

Apedel—predominance of primitive spinal and brainstem reflexes with motor development of a prone or supine lying creature (19)

Quadrupedal—predominance of midbrain development with righting reactions and motor development of those of a child who can right himself, turn over, assume crawling and sitting positions (19)

Bipedal—at cortical level of development reveals equilibrium reactions with motor development that of a child who can assume the standing position and ambulate (19)

Spinal reflexes—are "phasic" or movement reflexes which coordinate muscle of the extremities in patterns of either total flexion or extension (19)

Brainstem reflexes—are "static" postural reflexes and effect changes in distribution of muscle tone throughout the body, either in response to a change of the position of head and body to space (by stimulation of the labyrinths) or in the head in relation to the body (by stimulation of proprioceptors of the neck muscles (19)

Righting reactions—are integrated at the midbrain level and interact with each other and work toward establishment of normal head and body relationship in space as well as in relation to each other (19)

Automatic movement reactions—are not strictly righting reflexes but are reactions produced by changes in the position of the head (19)

Cortical level reactions—are mediated by the efficient interactions of the cortex basal ganglia and cerebellum to provide body adaptation in response to change of center of gravity in the body (19)

Normal muscle tone—is the result of the total integration of postural reflex activity at all levels of the CNS (20)

Postural reflexes—form the background of normal voluntary movement and skills through interaction and integration (20)

Disassociation—movement of one part(s) from another part(s) as limb movements separate from trunk (20)

Control—not defined—used in connection with facilitatory or inhibitory control and with voluntary or involuntary control

Strength—not defined—used in connection with reflexes and related to predominant or diminished response of a reflex to stimuli

Postural stability—not defined—used in connection with descriptions of maintaining a given position of the body, such as prone on elbows or standing

Balance—not defined—used in connection with maintaining an upright posture for sitting, standing and walking and in connection with the relative amount for time on the flexor, adductor and internal rotator muscles as opposed to the extensor, abductor and external rotator muscles

Coordination—not defined—used in connection with alternating patterns of involvement such as flexion and extension and in connection with use of parts of body together, such as hand and eyes

Tone—not defined—is used in connection with muscle tension as a result of reflex action

EXPECTED RESULTS

1. Normalize tone
2. Change abnormal patterns of movements by:

a. Integrating primitive reflexes
b. Enhancing higher reactions and
c. Facilitating sequential development

ASSESSMENT

1. Reflex Testing Chart
   The chart records the positive or negative reactions to 24 different reflexes which have been divided into the four levels: spinal, brainstem, midbrain and cortical, plus a category for automatic movement reactions (19).
2. Motor Development Chart
   The chart includes 21 developmental behaviors associated with head raising, turning, crawling, sitting, and standing, plus 19 developmental behaviors associated with hand and forearm development (19).
3. Questions for analysis of chart data:
   a. What is the basic tone?
   b. What is its reaction under various conditions?
   c. Are there primitive and/or postural reflexes persisting?
   d. How do these postural reactions interfere with balanced tone in the flexors and extensors?
   e. How do these postural reactions influence the distribution of tone?
   f. How does this interfere with the development of higher reactions, such as the righting and equilibrium reactions?
   g. How does the total sum relate to skill and/or functional abilities?
   Also consider:
   h. If there is failure of integration of postural reflexes, how much will this prevent sensorimotor development?
   i. To what degree will abnormal distribution of tone prevent or maintain asymmetry or symmetry of movement?
   j. How will abnormal tone or lack of balance between agonist and antagonist muscle groups?
   k. How are various parts of the body involved and how does the patient compensate?

INTERVENTION STRATEGIES (20)

1. Media and modalities—no specific mention.
2. Methods and techniques
   a. Meaningful input
   b. Active participation
   c. Repetition with change (so the system does not habituate)
3. Equipment—none mentioned.
4. Prerequisite skills
   The model is based on a hierarchical system in which each previous level of skills is prerequisite to the next level.

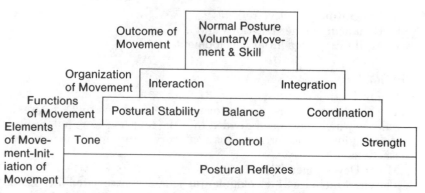

Figure 12.2. Development of posture movement and skill.

SUMMARY

The model of postural reflex development is based on the assumptions that tone, control and strength are the basic elements of the movement activities known as postural stability, balance and coordination which in turn form the background for normal posture, voluntary movement and skill through the processes of interaction and integration (Fig. 12.2). Reflex development with the nervous system is refined through the process of inhibition as higher centers in the brain gain control and integrate lower center reflexes.

Motor skills and complex functions also depend on the acquisition of key components organized from the postural reflexes, including head control, extensor tone, rotation within the body axis and equilibrium reactions (Fig. 12.3). These components facilitate the development of sensorimotor patterns which lead to prehension and walking.

Assessment is designed to determine the level of reflex integration. Intervention is directed toward facilitating the integration of higher level

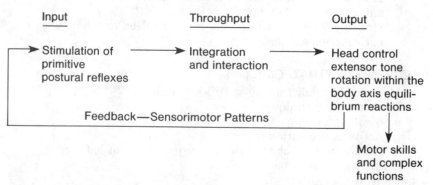

Figure 12.3. Refinement of motor skills and complex functions.

reflexes and promoting the development of sensorimotor patterns into more complex and purposeful function.

Analysis and Critique of the Neurobiological Models
FRAME OF REFERENCE

The frame of reference is based on the organismic and developmental sequence models. However, the focus is primarily on the development of the nervous system in relation to the sensorimotor system with secondary concerns for cognitive and psychological development. This narrow focus provides an in depth focus on early development of the brain and nervous system but limits the breadth of focus on other aspects of development and on the acquisition of complex tasks beyond basic motor functions.

CLARITY

Neurobiological models stress the acquisition of motor behavior as the basic component in the development of human behavior and adaptation. However, one of the difficulties in translating from basic models to practice models is in assessment. The basic model suggests that neurobiological development is an open and spiralling process, but assessment measures closed processes such as reflexes or developmental milestones. Open processes lead to other neurobiological behavior, while closed processes only reinforce the same behavior.

The problem of closed vs. open loops depends on an assumption regarding neurobiological development. At issue is the heredity vs. environment controversy. How much of neurobiological behavior is inherited and thus wired into the nervous system and how much neurobiological behavior is influenced by environmental factors and thus subject to external stimuli and learning?

Milani Comparetti (23) has suggested that there are three types of motor patterns: (a) primary motor patterns, (b) primary automatisms and (c) secondary automatisms. The three patterns have two functions: neuromotor and psychomotor. The neuromotor function provides the movement or motor pattern, while the psychomotor function affects how, if or for what purpose the motor pattern will be used.

Primary motor patterns can only be evaluated through ultrasound. However, primary automatisms can be assessed. Traditionally, they have been called reflexes or primitive reactions. The problem with measuring them is that they are an extension of the primary motor patterns and thus are modified very little by the outside environment. As a result, primary automatisms are static indicators of the nervous system's performance. Such reflexes, reactions or development milestones indicate where the nervous system has been but do not really indicate what the potential is for future progress.

Instead developmental assessment should attempt to measure dynamic indications which are open looped behaviors and which are the outcomes of actual purposeful use. Milani Comparetti suggests the most useful motor behaviors would be those that permit recognition of the rules of the game.

UNIQUENESS

Neurobiological models do not provide much information on the unique aspects or focus on occupational therapy in relation to dysfunction, deficits or limitations. The stress tends to be on interdisciplinary actions in which several types of therapists are doing basically the same thing in promoting normal acquisition of motor functions and integration of postural reflexes. Although occupational therapy can provide such services, the unique aspects of occupational therapy in providing approaches to increase the repertoire of useful behaviors is rarely utilized.

RESEARCH GUIDE

The neurodevelopmental approach of the Bobaths has fostered some research, although not to a significant degree. The neurobehavioral model is an organizational tool primarily. Research is needed to support the assumptions. Of special concern is the relation of sensorimotor skills to cognitive and social development. Does neuromotor behavior form the basis of cognitive behavior or simply facilitate the expression of behavior but not control the basic ability to think and feel?

SPECIALIZATION

The neurobiological models have lead to the specialization in pediatric practice mostly with young children. Many of the children have brain dysfunction which is evident through observation or delays in development and movement abnormalities. Extensions of the neurobiological techniques have been used with adults whose nervous systems have been injured by a stroke or other upper neuron problem.

ELABORATION AND REFINEMENT

Elaboration is needed to include open looped and learning behavior instead of focusing only on closed looped and genetically controlled neuromotor behavior. Refinement is needed to explain the sequence of learned motor acts in relation to cognitive and social learning.

EXPLANATORY USEFULNESS

The focus on neurobiology has facilitated the explanation of occupational therapy services to insurance carriers. However, the problem has been the interest in facilitating the return or development of neuromotor function without necessarily integrating the functional capacity into the performance of daily occupations.

COMMONALITY

The focus on brain function and early development facilitates communication among disciplines but does not necessarily increase the understanding of occupational therapy. Occupational therapists need to communicate both the similarities of occupational therapy to other disciplines as well as the differences.

PRACTICE MODEL
The neurobiological model has not lead to the development of practice models and submodels at this time.

SUMMARY
The neurobiological models are moderately successful as practice models in occupational therapy. Strengths are in specialization, explanatory usefulness and commonality. Weaknesses are in clarity of assumptions, uniqueness and research guidance. A summary is provided in Table 12.4.

Sensorimotor Model—Rood

FRAME OF REFERENCE
Margaret S. Rood, M.A., O.T.R., R.P.T., was one of the first occupational therapists to explore the literature in neurophysiology in an attempt to understand the development and function of the nervous system and dysfunction in relation to cerebral palsy and hemiplegia. Her early writings reflect the influence of H. Kabat and his work in neuromuscular education at Kaiser Permanente Foundation in California. Other early influences were Temple Fay and W. K. Phelps. Later her work is based on her analysis of the literature in neurophysiology. Analysis of normal growth and development is based on the works of Gesell.

Only Rood's writings are reviewed for this model. Her work has been continued by other physical and occupational therapists. Also, the neurophysiologic information has been limited to the concepts associated with the model. Specific textbook-type neurophysiology has been omitted, since there has been considerable revision after Rood's last article appeared in 1967.

Table 12.4
Neurobiological Models Criteria Summary

Evaluation Criteria	Very Good 1	Moderately Good			Very Poor 5
		2	3	4	
Frame of reference		X			
Clarity			X		
Uniqueness				X	
Research guide			X		
Specialization		X			
Elaboration/refinement		X			
Explanatory usefulness		X			
Commonality		X			
Practice model				X	

ASSUMPTIONS ABOUT SENSORY INPUT

1. The sensory end organ is the basic unit for bringing information about the body and its environment to the brain, and learned motor action is the response to sensory stimuli (24).
2. Input affects all levels of the nervous system for physical, somatic, automatic and emotional responses (25).
3. Sensory postural reception changes with position of the body in relation to gravity and is affected by higher postural receptors associated with the eye, ear and its labyrinthine mechanism (24).
4. Motor engrams, available for reproduction in motor action initiated at the control level, are based on the summation of many sensory impressions arising within the physical structures of the past (24).
5. Reflexes are the basis for later voluntary action (26).
6. The activation and inhibition of reflex action proceeds in the orderly manner as seen in the normal developmental sequence (25).
7. Cutaneous reflexes are for light work patterns for reciprocal inhibition, whereas deep receptors are for activating antigravity muscles which participate in heavy work postural or synergistic stabilizing patterns (26).
8. The effect of the labyrinth and/or the tonic neck reflex may assist or retard the effect of pressure, stretch or stroking (first principle) (24).

ASSUMPTIONS ABOUT MOTOR DEVELOPMENT AND OUTPUT

1. Motor patterns are developed from fundamental reflex patterns present at birth which are utilized and gradually modified through sensory stimuli until the highest control is gained on the conscious cortical level (24).
2. There are two developmental sequences, one for the vital functions and one for skeletal muscle function (26).
3. Developmental sequence of muscle action patterns (25, 26)
   1. A shortening and lengthening range with their antagonists (reciprocal inhibition with no distal demands)
   2. A cocontraction team work pattern for static posture
   3. A heavy work movement pattern superimposed on cocontraction with distal end fixed
   4. Skill patterns using cocontraction and movement for light work demands in distal part of extremity.
4. If one of a pair of muscles does not function in reciprocal innervation, eventually the normal one will be seriously affected (27).
5. Cocontraction or static support positions are essential before heavy work movement is effective (28).
6. Gravity or stress is essential for the stimulation of the heavier work muscles and for bone growth.
7. Muscles have different duties, such as heavy work, light work or a combination (third principle) (24).

8. Heavy work should precede light work except in the case of speech and feeding muscles (fourth principle) (24).
9. Heavy work stimuli lead to relaxation and renewal of the body (28).
10. Light work patterns of skill require cortical or voluntary attention (28).
11. Cortical control, the highest level of somatic activation, requires the greatest effort, is the least efficient, and the most fatiguing method of motor control (25).

ASSUMPTIONS ABOUT SENSORY INPUT IN THERAPY

1. Stimulation of specific receptors will give specific reactions which are meant for maintaining, protecting and developing the skills of the body (second principle) (24).
2. In a patient in whom there is imbalance in reflexes or a high threshold for sensory receptors, there is a need to intensify the stimuli over what is normally received (26).
3. Cutaneous and deeper proprioceptive receptors can be used to activate or inhibit muscle action in the sequence in which these receptors are stimulated in the stages of normal development (26).
4. Cutaneous receptors give bilateral effects, are slow to initiate but have a long after-discharge which facilitates for voluntary use (26).
5. Thermal receptors are for automatic nervous system reaction (26).
6. Fast brushing activates (2 to 5 times per second with 10 strokes); slow brushing inhibits (26).
7. In general, quickly applied stimuli cause a quick reaction followed by a rebound tonic in the opposite direction (27).
8. Repetitive, rhythmical patterns will release top level control after patterns have been learned (27).

ASSUMPTIONS ABOUT MOTOR OUTPUT IN THERAPY

1. It may be possible to reactivate muscles if the cause is physiological discontinuity and not anatomical destruction (28).
2. Activation of muscles proceeds from reflex or involuntary stimulation to voluntary control (28).
3. The developmental sequence of patterns of action of muscles is the key to order of application of stimuli (25).
4. Activation is from the head on down, muscle by muscle, from cervical segments down to the sacral. Flexors are stimulated first, extensors next, adductors third and abductors fourth (fifth principle) (24).
5. Flexors, adductors, internal rotators and multiarthrodial muscles are activated by both primary and secondary stretch and inhibit their antagonists (29).
6. The joint extensors, abductors and external rotators are activated by primary stretch but inhibited by the more numerous endings of secondary stretch (29) (Table 12.5).

Table 12.5[a]
Muscles and Their Responses

Multiarthrodal Muscles and Flexors and Adductors	Stimulus	One Joint Extensors and Abductors
Activates muscle stretched and inhibits antagonist.	Stretch	Lengthens muscle stretched and activates antagonistic flexor and/or adductor in shortened range.
Inhibits muscle contracting and activates antagonist. Difficult to maintain in contraction voluntarily.	Contraction	Few contraction receptors. Less effect on antagonist and not as difficult to maintain in contraction voluntarily.
Major facilitation to muscle being resisted. Slight stimulation to antagonist from contraction receptor.	Contraction plus stretch or outside resistance	Contraction of antagonists if short lever arm favors muscle being resisted. If longer lever arm greater activation of antagonistic muscle. If distal extremity fixed, different pattern from distal extremity free.
Body weight only inhibits muscle action.	Joint compression	Cocontraction with greatest facilitation to one joint extensor at intermediate joint and lengthening of antagonistic flexor, *i.e.*, vastus medialis and anconeus.

[a] Reprinted from M. S. Rood (25), with permission from The American Occupational Therapy Association.

CONCEPTS

Two development sequences:
  a. *Vital functions developmental sequence* (26)
    1. Inspiration
    2. Expiration
    3. Sucking
    4. Swallowing fluids
    5. Phonation
    6. Chewing
    7. Swallowing solids
    8. Articulation
  b. *Skeletal muscle function developmental sequence* (25, 26) (Fig. 12.4).
    1. Withdrawal in the supine position (total flexion pattern)
    2. Roll over (flexion of half the body)

Ontogenetic Motor Patterns According to Rood

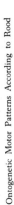
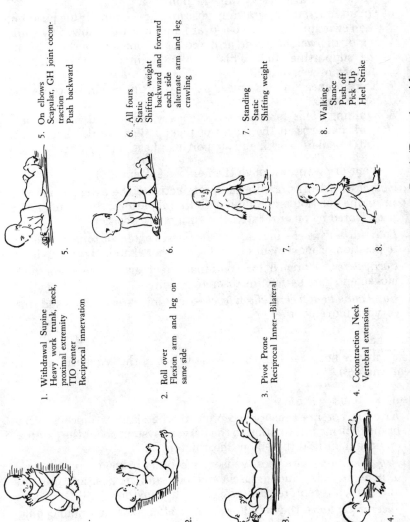

1. Withdrawal Supine
   Heavy work trunk, neck, proximal extremity
   TIO center
   Reciprocal innervation

2. Roll over
   Flexion arm and leg on same side

3. Pivot Prone
   Reciprocal Inner—Bilateral

4. Cocontraction Neck
   Vertebral extension

5. On elbows
   Scapular, GH joint cocontraction
   Push backward

6. All fours
   Static
   Shifting weight backward and forward
   each side
   alternate arm and leg
   crawling

7. Standing
   Static
   Shifting weight

8. Walking
   Stance
   Push off
   Pick Up
   Heel Strike

Figure 12.4. Ontogenetic motor patterns according to Rood. (Reproduced from M. S. Rood (25), with permission from The American Occupational Therapy Association.)

3. Pivot prone
4. Neck cocontraction
5. On elbows, prone, beginning with static, maintained positions and progressing to the heavy work movement of pushing the truck backward (heavy work flexion)
6. On all fours, in the crawling position, first maintaining position, then swinging the body backward and forward followed by shifting of the weight to the arm and leg of one side without lifting the supporting limb. This is followed in turn by a diagonal pattern of weight shift.
7. Erect stance. In this stage, weight shifting again precedes the next stage.
8. Walking. This is composed of heavy, light, and intermediate work patterns in the stages of pickup (light work), heel strike (intermediate work), and supporting phase (heavy work).

Development of posture through the nervous system (24)

a. *Spinal level*—(a) pressure receptors activate the extensor muscles in supine position and inhibit withdrawal pattern; (b) stretch reflex is activated by postural stress or antigravity position
b. *Labyrinthine level*—increases or decreases extensor tone in relation to position or movement of the head rather than body to gravity
c. *Cortical level*—area 8 for coordination of eyes, area 6 for body movements, area 4 for fine discrete action
d. *Basal ganglia and cerebellum level*—rhythmical repetitious and stereotyped movement

Functional use

The way the body calls on the muscle to act in the sequential pattern of learning (26)

Sensory systems:

a. *Exteroreceptors*—sensory receptors in the skull or mucous membrane to bring information to the nervous system about the external environment (25) (based on Sherrington)
b. *Proprioceptors*—are those sensory receptors in the deep structures of bone, muscle, tendon, fascia and joint and are position, pressure and stretch receptors (26) (based on Sherrington)
c. *Viceroreceptors*—the receptors which affect the autonomic functions of the body (25) (based on Sherrington)

Primitive reflexes (26)

a. *Labyrinth, static and accelerating reflexes*—activated by the position of the head in relation to gravity or its movements
b. *Tonic neck reflexes*—activated by the head in relation to the neck

Autonomic nervous system (28)

    a. *Parasympathetic*—for maintenance of the individual and race. Responsive to rhythmical movement, light, repetitious sounds or cutaneous stimuli

    b. *Sympathetic*—for protection of the individual. Responsive to extremes in emotion, temperature and cutaneous stimuli

Voluntary nervous system (28)

    a. *Heavy work (postural work) muscles*—respond to specific sensory receptors of pressure for muscle, joint and bone. Are found in the postural surfaces of the body such as palm and sole, at the midline and at the proximal ends of the extremity (Table 12.6)

    b. *Light work (fine coordination) muscles*—the stimulus for light work is primarily stroking (Table 12.6)

Dermatone—specific areas of sensory representation of the skin which correspond to the segmental representation of the motor innervation of the desired muscle (26)

Types of location of sensory receptors

Cutaneous receptors—pain, light touch, pressure, hair cells and thermal receptors (26)

Stretch receptors—found in heavy work muscles in the muscle spindle for facilitation, in the tendon for inhibition (26)

Pressure receptors—found on the postural (volar) surface of hands and feet in the fascia between the muscle layers, under insertion of muscle on bone (26)

Therapeutic techniques

Fast stroking or brushing—use of soft brush at the rate of 5/second for at least 10 strokes to very specific areas of sensory representation on the skin which correspond to the segemental representation of the motor innervation of the desired muscle (26)

Slow brushing, tapping, joint traction, and joint compression—not described

Icing—ice administration (ice cubes) to parts of the body such as the abdomen to increase rate and depth of breathing (28)

Neutral warmth—body temperature of the individual (25)

EXPECTED RESULTS

1. Greater skill return (26)
2. Normalizing the mechanics of living such as feeding, dressing and writing (30)
3. Increasing play time and motivation (30)
4. Facilitating educational tasks (30)
5. Promoting prevocational training (30)

Table 12.6
Voluntary Nervous System[a,b]

	Patterns of Action	
	Light Work	Heavy Work
Neck and trunk Extremities	Erect Distal extremity free to move. Muscle moving insertion end which is smaller segment.	Horizontal to gravity Supporting the trunk against gravity. The distal end of extremity is fixed. On elbows, on hands and knees, standing. Muscle acting on origin end.
	Muscles	
	Light Work	Heavy Work
	Long muscles for range and speed. Tendinous origin and insertion. More range in contraction, less to stretch. Flexors and two-joint muscles	One joint deep muscles. Greater number of fibers. More power. Less range in contraction, more in stretch. Wide attachment at origin end. One joint extensors and abductors.
	Cortical Representation	
	Somatomotor—Sensory Area I	Somatomotor—Sensory Area II

	Rolandic fissure
	  From opposite side of body
	  To opposite side of body
	Somatic or willed
	
	Area 4, 6,
	  primary and supplementary
	  motor areas.
		Sylvian fissure
		  Ipsilateral and bilateral
		
		Branchial motor system and
		  autonomic
		Lies at base of Area 4 with
		  overlap of head region.

[a] Reprinted from M. S. Rood (25), with permission from The American Occupational Therapy Association.
[b] Special Comment: If pyramidal tract intact, but reticular formation injured, voluntary activation is not possible.

ASSESSMENT INSTRUMENTS

1. Analyzed according to abilities in the sequential stages of a normal baby's development (26)
2. Performance of both holding and movement patterns of normal development is analyzed (26)
3. Development stages are used for analysis of the patient's needs and a guide to treatment (26)

INTERVENTION STRATEGIES

  I. Media

    A. General (30)

    1. Woodworking (planing, sawing)
    2. Toys
    3. Games (bean bag or ball throwing)
    4. Writing
    5. Weaving
    6. Block printing
    7. Feeding
    8. Dressing

B. For all fours positions (sample) (26)
    1. Gardening, cleaning or polishing of floors in the kneeling or squatting position with body weight supported on the affected arm.
    2. Sawing in which the affected arm holds the work in position.
    3. Add (from beater to front supports) rubber resistance on loom to require pushing against the beater while the shuttle is passed through the shed.
    4. Archery. The bow should be horizontal and in front of the body to give internal rotation of shoulder and pronation of forearm.
    5. Relay games may be adapted to be played in the static all fours position, such as passing bits of paper from child to child by suction through a straw.
    6. Other heavy grip activities include cake decorating with a plastic bag: ceramic decoration done in the same way, rolling pin pressures for cookies or pastry, spatter printing using a squeeze bulb and ratchwheel toys for sound and action.

II. Techniques (samples only)

A. Levels

1. Cranial nerves V VII, IX and X	Light touch stimulus fast brushing or stroking (25)
2. C2	Place head on pillow to activate neck flexors. Extensors do not usually need therapy (avoid stroking chin which increases drooling) (28)
3. C3 and 4	Raise head against gravity for flexors (sternocleidomastoid). Stroking, squeezing muscle belly and giving resistance to extensors (upper trapezius (avoid stroking hypoglossal root triangle which is for swallowing) (28)
4. T 7–10	Icing of dermatone representation of diaphragm to in-

	crease rate and depth of breathing (24)
5. L 1,2	Brushing or icing to facilitate voiding (25)
6. S 2 3 4	Fast brushing for control of incontinence (25)

B. Cocontraction of the shoulder girdle in the all fours position (26)
  1. Brush the isolated radial innervation and remainder of the radial distribution and the webs of the fingers on the dorsum of the hand to stimulate extensor pollicis longus and dorsal interossei.
  2. Brush over the thenar eminence which has its greatest effect on the abductor pollicis brevis. Avoid brushing the flexor tendons of the wrist.
  3. Brush posterior brachial cutaneous nerve over the triceps: the intercostobrachial over the tendon of pectoralis major; in the axilla for the serratus anterior (avoid latissimus dorsi).
  4. Brush anterior and posterior neck over the bellies of upper trapezius and sternocleidomastoid and from below the ear to the hyoid for the short neck flexors which flatten the physiological curve of the back of the neck.

C. Stimulation for normal arm raising (26)

1. Pressure for upper trapezius and levator scapulae	Apply pressure at the insertion followed by resisted shrugging of the shoulders.
2. Pressure to lower trapezius, serratus and rhomboids	Apply pressure to area between the vertebral border of the scapula. Use manual or sponge rubber ball to apply.
3. Pressure for supraspinatus and upper infraspinatus	Pressure is given above and below the spine of the scapula followed by pressure to the insertion on the humerus.
4. Pressure for pectoralis major	Compress near the insertion
5. Pressure for medial arm and triceps	With the elbow flexed, the upper arm may be repeatedly slapped against a firm surface
6. Stretch for 3rd and 4th dorsal interossei and lumbricles	Attempt to separate 4th and 5th and 3rd and 4th fingers at the metacarpophalangeal joint

7. Pressure for flexor carpi ulnaris — Apply pressure to the pisiform bone

D. Fast brushing — To back of ears on the pinna seems to minimize the force of phonation with less effort (25)

Of the forehead seems to be particularly effective for control of startle reflex (25)

E. Slow stroking — Slow rhythmic hand over hand stroking for 3 minutes down the posterior primary division of the skin representation causes muscularskeletal relaxation (29)

F. Joint pressure
1. Body weight — Releases flexors at ankle and wrist, knee and elbow (29)

2. Greater than body weight — Causes contraction in the shortened range of the dorsiflexors and knee and elbow extensors (29)

3. Pressure to muscle insertion — Inhibits muscle such as a hard object used in the hand of a spastic (29)

4. Tapping — Activates time anterior horn cells from primary stretch (29)

G. Work patterns
1. Light work — Stroking at 2/second times 10 repeat 3 to 5 times; request voluntary action. Also can use the head of a pin over some area (24)

2. Heavy work on joint muscles (soleus and vastus) — Slow knee bends with heels flat—will get both lengthening and shortening reaction (squatting) (28)

3. Postural cocontraction — Dental dam rubber—resistance to top of head or over each shoulder following appropriate stimulation (28)

H. Specific disorders
1. Spastic CP — Fast brush and briefly maintain ice to the weak antagonists. Followed by isometric hold in the shortened range

                                        with resistance, tapping to
                                        antagonists and release the
                                        stretch reflex (29)
    2. Athetoid   Fast brush and ice one joint
                                        extensors, abductors and ex-
                                        ternal rotators (29)

III. Equipment
   a. Woodworking tools
   b. Treadle sewing machine
   c. Foot power jig saw
   d. Mats
   e. Sponge rubber ball
   f. Camel hair brushes
IV. Prerequisites and precautions—important to know areas which
    should not be stimulated

SUMMARY

The sensorimotor model is based on the "utilization of the cutaneous (exteroceptors) and deeper proprioceptive receptors to activate or inhibit muscle actions in the sequence in which these receptors are stimulated in the stages of normal development" (26). Exteroceptors, proprioceptors and viceroceptors are used also to activate or inhibit the autonomic nervous system as well as the voluntary system.

Therapy for the voluntary muscle system is based on an analysis of the normal sequence of heavy and light muscle function development and the specific response patterns to different stimuli, such as stretch, pressure, ice, and warmth. Muscle function is coordinated with the developmental milestones as the child develops from flexion withdrawal to standing and walking.

Therapy for the autonomic nervous system is concerned with promoting the activities which provide maintenance and protection to the person; of special concern are the sucking, swallowing and inspiration patterns which facilitate feeding and breathing.

Analysis and Critique of the Sensorimotor Model
FRAME OF REFERENCE

The frame of reference of the sensorimotor model is consistent with the organismic and developmental sequence models. The maturation and sequence of the autonomic and voluntary nervous systems are the central focus.

CLARITY

The sensorimotor model has been developed over many years through analysis of the literature and careful clinical observation. Unfortunately, Rood has written very few articles stating her own model. Instead, she has lectured and left the writing to others, such as Stockmeyer (31, 32) and Huss (33, 34). Furthermore, the model keeps changing as new information is gleaned from the literature or Rood modifies existing ideas. Tables 12.7, 12.8, 12.9 and 12.10 illustrate changes and interpretations in the four stages of motor control. The step sequence within the categories is slightly different in each table. Some variation may be to do different interpreters, but other changes are modifications of Rood's ideas. These changes are difficult to follow chronologically because publication dates do not necessarily reflect Rood's changing thoughts and in most cases the date of the table is not given.

UNIQUENESS

The uniqueness of the sensorimotor model is the developmental sequence related to neuromuscular development. Although other models have been created, the sensorimotor model is the earliest involving an occupational therapist. The Bobaths, Kabat, Knott and Voss, Fay and Doman, and Brunnstrum are either physical therapists or physicians. Thus Rood is the first occupational therapist to document in print a model of development based on neurophysiologic and neurodevelopmental principles.

The sensorimotor model and related models established a new basis for program intervention with upper neuron disorders which attempted to change the organization of the nervous system (throughput) rather than simply increasing learned responses (output). In other words, within the intervention program, the quality of the response is more important than mere practice or repetition. The rationale is as follows: if the sensory input is controlled to maximize throughput organization then the response will be of good quality and the feedback will be positive (24) (Fig. 12.5).

Another basic change in the intervention program was the emphasis on organizing lower centers of the brain such as the brainstem before organizing higher centers. The rationale is as follows: if the different stimuli are organized as the input is received through the lower centers of the brain, there is an increased chance of the higher centers organizing the input effectively and an increased chance of producing effective output (24) (Fig. 12.6).

RESEARCH GUIDE

Research using the sensorimotor model itself has been limited. However, a few studies have been done. Carlsen (35) found that children with cerebral palsy receiving facilitation techniques based on Bobath, Rood and Ayres showed significant improvement in developmental age over those receiving intervention in fine motor and self-care skills. Rider (36) found a significant increase in muscle strength in both normal children and children with cerebral palsy when facilitation techniques based on Rood were used. In addition, there was cross-transfer to the nonfacilitated arm.

Both the Carlsen and Rider studies used variations of the experimental research design. The sensorimotor model has not affected the research

**Table 12.7
Stages of Control: Framework for Progression of Treatment[a,b]**

Mobility		Stability		Combined Mobility and Stability Weight-bearing		Combined Mobility and Stability Non-Weight-bearing Movement	
Stage 1: Neonate Responses, Extreme Positions, Movement with Much Range	Stage 2: Early Modification of Neonate Patterns	Stage 3: Tonic Extensors in Nonweight-Bearing, Midline Holding	Stage 4: Bilateral Weight Bearing, Cocontraction	Stage 5: Movement with Bilateral Weight Bearing	Stage 6: Maintained Unilateral Weight Bearing	Stage 7: Controlled Placement of Distal Part	Stage 8: Precision of Distal Movements
Nonweight-Bearing Movement, Phasic Responses				Axial and Proximal Limb Stabilization for Distal Mobility			
Protective responses—withdrawal and avoidance	Righting reflexes give rise to chain reflexes	Deep atlanto-occipital extensors on a stretch, cocontraction holding weight of head		On elbows rocking push backward	Weight shift to unilateral weight bearing on one elbow with unilateral reaching Equilibrium responses		
Moro reflex	Supine flexion	Tonic extensors on stretch in elbow weight bearing					
Traction response	Prone extension	Bilateral weight bearing on hands					
Stepping, placing	Rolling						

Hold semisquat and squat

Up to standing from squat

Bilateral weight bearing on hands and knees

Rocking in quadruped

Weight shift to unilateral weight bearing on one upper extremity— the other exremity reaches forward or advances in creeping

Unilateral weight bearing on one knee— other extremity advances in creeping

Bilateral weight bearing on hands and feet, plantigrade position

Bilateral weight bearing on feet

Rock back to semisquat, up to standing

Bounce in standing

Step in place
Side step holding on

Step forward, upper extremities held forward, in readiness to catch weight

Step forward, upper extremities at sides

Heel-toe gait, base smaller,
Fine manipulation by hands

ᵃ Based on the Ontogenetic Motor Patterns according to Rood (1962). Reprinted from P. H. Pearson and C. E. Williams: Physical Therapy Services in the Developmental Disabilities. Springfield, Ill., 1972, pp. 218–219, with permission from Charles C Thomas.

Table 12.8
Integration of Ontogenetic Motor Patterns with Levels of Motor Control[a,b]

Level I: Mobility (31)		Level II: Stability		Level III: Mobility on Stability (31)		Level IV: Skill	
Skeletal	Vital	Skeletal	Vital	Skeletal	Vital	Skeletal	Vital
1. Supine withdrawal	1. Inspiration	4. Pivot prone (held)	5. Phonation[c]	6. Neck cocontraction (orient head in space)	4. Swallow fluids	9. Prone-on-elbows, head is doing skilled movement and one arm is free for skilled use. Belly crawling.)	5. Phonation
2. Roll over	2. Expiration	5. Neck cocontraction	3. Sucking	8. Prone-on-elbows, (shift from side to side, push backward and pull forward, unilateral weight bearing)	6. Chewing	12. Quadruped (one arm free for skilled use. Creeping, trunk rotation and reciprocal movement, crossed diagonal.)	8. Speech
3. Pivot prone (assume the position)		7. Prone-on-elbows		11. Quadruped (rocking, shifting, unilateral weight bearing)	7 Swallow soilds	15. Standing and walking	
		10. Quadruped		14. Standing (weight shift, unilateral weight bearing)			
		13. Standing					

[a] Reprinted with permission from C. A. Trombly and A. E. Scott (14).
[b] The steps are numbered sequentially, but they blend together, i.e., one step is not completely mastered before the next begins at the most basic level.
[c] Although out of sequence, phonation is facilitated in the pivot prone position (31).

Table 12.9
Developmental Sequence[a]

Reciprocal Innervation	Stability or Coinnervation	Movement Superimposed on Stability	Skill
Skeletal developmental sequences			
1. Withdrawal: total flexion in supine	4. Cocontraction of neck with vertebral extension	6. Push back	8. Belly crawling
2. Roll over: flexion top side, extension bottom side	5. Prone on elbows static holding with cocontraction neck and shoulder	7. Pull forward	11. Creeping: homologous, homolateral, reciprocal
3. Pivot prone: total extension in prone except for elbows, which are flexed with arms adducted	9. All-fours: static holding	10. Shifting weight backward-forward, side-to-side, alternate arm-leg	14. Walking: must analyze stance, push off, pick up, and heel strike
	12. Standing: static	13. Shifting weight backward-forward, side-to-side	
Vital function developmental sequences			
1. Inspiration	3. Sucking	4. Swallowing fluids	5. Phonation
2. Expiration		6. Chewing	8. Speech
		7. Swallowing solids	

[a] Reprinted from H. Hopkins and H. Smith (38), with permission from Lippincott.

Table 12.10
Neurophysiological Sensorimotor Approach to Treatment[a]

Progression of Motor Development

Reciprocal Innervation: Mobility	Coinnervation: Stability	Heavy Work Movement: Combined Mobility and Stability in Weight Bearing	Skill: Combined Mobility and Stability in Nonweight Bearing

Withdrawal from stimulus
→

Flexion pattern → Extension pattern → Neck cocontraction → Head oriented to vertical → Speech articulation eye control
toward stimulus   pattern   plane (rotation available)
→
Roll

Prone on elbows:
→
Prone on extended
arms   Weight shifting backward, → Unilateral upper extremity weight bearing and reaching
All fours   → forward, side to side
→   Weight shifting forward
                           and backward

Bilateral lower
extremity weight → side to side → Unilateral reaching during creeping
bearing

                   Weight shifting in standing
Hold semisquat and   → Cruising
squat   →
                   Squat to stand   → Walking
                                                 →
                                              Hands free for prehension

[a] Compiled by Becky Porter, MS, RPT, Indiana University Physical Therapy Program, 1978. Reprinted from S. Farber (40), with permission from Saunders.

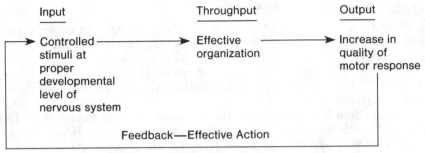

Figure 12.5.   Intervention rationale—one.

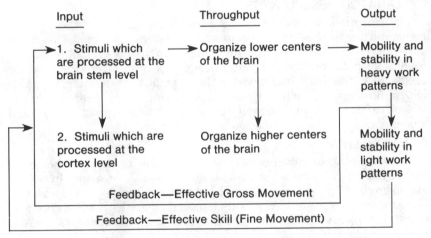

Figure 12.6.   Intervention rationale—two.

designs used in studies involving the model at this point. Perhaps later studies will suggest the need for different emphasis in research design.

SPECIALIZATION

If the sensorimotor model is taken by itself the effect of specialization has not been impressive. However, as an example of a broader category of facilitation models the effects on practice have been substantial. Most of the major textbooks related to occupational therapy for persons with physical disabilities include a section on Rood and the sensorimotor model (14, 37, 38). Other texts include Rood's methods of intervention (39, 40). Ayres' model of sensory integration is based on Rood (see next section). Thus, the impact of the sensorimotor model in the field has been considerable, even though specialization only within the model is not common.

ELABORATION AND REFINEMENT

Since Rood does not chose to write, elaboration and refinement will have to come from others. One area which would benefit from elaboration or refinement is the developmental sequence of activities within the ontogenetic motor patterns in relation to muscle actions (see previous Tables 12.7 to 12.10). A more stable presentation would be useful especially for research.

Another area for refinement is the organization of intervention methods and levels of the neuromuscular system. Charts or tables which organize the types of input, the level of the nervous system to be stimulated and the desired result would be useful to practitioners. Farber (40) has begun the process by organizing the sensory system stimuli and response patterns into a sensory system inventory.

EXPLANATORY USEFULNESS

The sensorimotor model provides a useful explanation of the development and function of the neuromuscular system. The model is useful particularly in explaining the problems seen in upper motor neuron lesions, such as cerebral palsy and hemiplegia from a cerebral vascular accident. A strength of the model is the attempt to correlate neurophysiologic findings with clinical observations. One major weakness is the lack of a textbook or common reference to which practitioners and students can turn for information and updating.

COMMONALITY

The sensorimotor model is most understandable to physical therapists and physicians who have the same basic knowledge of neurophysiology and neurodevelopment. Some speech pathologists also have had a biological science background. Most other professionals with whom occupational therapists work have not had the vocabulary and concepts to easily understand.

Educators, for example, would understand the concept of development but would have difficulty organizing the ideas of nerve transmission and its relation to mobility and stability. Thus, models such as the sensorimotor model are most useful to therapists in terms of improving intervention methods and not in terms of communicating with other disciplines.

PRACTICE MODEL

Although the potential for practice models and submodels exists, little evidence exists in the literature that specific theories or submodels exist. Perhaps the most significant impact has been in terms of splints and adapted equipment (40). Specific examples include the orthokinetic cuff, orthokinetic wrist splint for flexor spasticity, back and seat inserts for wheelchairs, dental dam or Theraband straps for truck stability, dynamic head support system, leg abductor devices, dynamic sling for hemiplegia and modified foot boards and shoes.

SUMMARY

Rood's sensorimotor model fulfills the criteria for a practice model in occupational therapy fairly well. Several problems could be improved upon with a little careful work. A summary is provided in Table 12.11.

Perceptual Motor Model

FRAME OF REFERENCE

A. Jean Ayres, Ph.D., O.T.R. (41), began studying the influences of perception on motor response in about 1958. Early references suggest the influences of Loretta Bender, a psychologist interested in children with psychiatric disorders, William Cruickshank, an educational psychologist interested in perceptual problems of children with cerebral palsy and A. A. Strauss, Newell Kephart and Marianne Frostig, all educational psychologists who were interested in perceptual problems of brain-injured children. Other sources of influence are from neurology, including the works of D. O. Hebb and V. B. Mountcastle, and Paul Schilder, a psychiatrist who was interested in proprioceptive influences on the concept and image of the body.

ASSUMPTIONS ABOUT PERCEPTUAL MOTOR DEVELOPMENT

1. Perceptual motor functions develop through specific steps of sequential maturation (42).
2. Purposeful motor experiences are the *sine qua non* of perceptual motor development (43).
3. There are identifiable areas of perceptual-motor dysfunction and by inference specific CNS mechanisms critical to the integrative process which enables perception (42).

ASSUMPTIONS ABOUT PERCEPTUAL DEVELOPMENT

1. Sequence of perceptual skills (41).
   a. Foreground, background—figure is seen as having shape which is determined by edges or boundaries. Background is less well defined.

Table 12.11
Sensorimotor Model Summary Critique

Evaluation Criteria	Very Good 1	Moderately Good 2	3	4	Very Poor 5
Frame of reference	x				
Clarity				x	
Uniqueness		x			
Research guide			x		
Specialization			x		
Elaboration/refinement		x			
Explanatory usefulness		x			
Commonality			x		
Practice model			x		

   b. Recognition of form—ability to identify.

   c. Concept formation—recognition that forms and objects belong to a certain category.

2. Much perceptual process is learned (44).

3. In order to respond to the environment purposefully and motor plan effectively in relation to it, one must first be able to interpret it (44).

4. Organizing and interpreting sensory information is the essence of perception (44).

5. Development of perceptual abilities is dependent upon obtaining some sensory feedback from the motor which was elicited by the perceptual process (44).

ASSUMPTIONS ABOUT TACTILE AND PROPRIOCEPTIVE INPUT

1. One of the directions of evolutionary development has been intersensory integration which enables us to associate information coming from the same source over more than one sensory modality (42).

2. The process of organizing tactile and proprioceptive impulses into meaningful perception is the most basic ontogenetic step in the developmental sequence (43).

3. Without adequate maturation in these (tactile and proprioceptive) areas, more highly adaptive behavior will not ensue (43).

4. Any part of the body surface which does not receive normal tactual stimulation will develop a protective as opposed to discriminative or perceptive type of response (43).

5. Touch, proprioception, and vestibular functions are usually elicited from movement or the part of the organism (44).

6. The spinothalamic system carries information for avoidance or withdrawal (protection and survival) (45).

7. Before an individual can obtain meaning from tactual stimuli, he must be able to inhibit the protective type of response (43).

8. When the protective system predominates the hyperactivity syndrome is aggravated, affect and somatic discomfort are heightened, and perceptual-motor development is retarded (45).

9. Activation of the discriminative system inhibits the protective system (42).

10. The medial-lemiscal system carries touch and proprioceptive impulses which are used for perceptual processes such as localization of a stimulus, two point tactual discrimination, direction of stimulus moving on the skin, and stereognosis (43).

ASSUMPTIONS ABOUT VESTIBULAR INPUT

1. The vestibular system is phylogenetically the oldest method by which animals have determined where they were in relation to the earth (through gravity) and whether or not they were moving (43).

2. The relationship between the vestibular system and the eyes, muscle tone, postural and fighting reactions also are involved in perceptual motor development (43).

ASSUMPTIONS ABOUT BODY SCHEME

1. Out of tactual, proprioceptive and visual stimulation evolves the body scheme (43).
2. Discriminatory interpretation of the spatial and temporal elements of tactile stimuli is essential to the development of the body scheme (42).
3. Body scheme is a neurological organization of previous tactile, kinesthetic and probably vestibular stimuli in association with planned movement (42).
4. Body scheme involves being able to visualize the anatomical elements of the body in movement and in different positional relationships (43).
5. Body scheme is acquired through the sensory receptors and through reinforcement from the results of purposeful movement (42).
6. All motions take place from the postural frame of reference of the body scheme (43).

ASSUMPTIONS ABOUT VISUAL PERCEPTION

1. Visual perception is partly dependent upon synthesizing visual information with that resulting from goal-directed movement (44).
2. Visual space perception is important to the direction of motor tasks (43).

ASSUMPTIONS ABOUT MOTOR PLANNING

1. The four major sensory modalities which contribute information which must be perceived for adequate, skilled motor planning and execution are touch, proprioception, vestibular functions and vision (44).
2. Motor planning is closely dependent upon and associated with the body scheme (43).
3. Planning requires a concept of the body scheme (41).

ASSUMPTIONS ABOUT THE RELATIONSHIP OF PERCEPTUAL MOTOR FUNCTIONS AND ACADEMIC PERFORMANCE

1. Reading and writing are dependent upon earlier development of visual and somesthetic (touch and proprioceptive) sensation (43).
2. Even as a child begins writing and reading, he is still improving his perception of visual, tactual and proprioceptive impulses (43).

ASSUMPTIONS ABOUT PERCEPTUAL MOTOR ACTIVITY AND OCCUPATIONAL THERAPY

1. Therapy should recapitulate the sequence of perceptual motor development (43).

2. Therapy should control sensory impact (43).
3. Therapy should evaluate, enhance and use skilled motor actions (46).

CONCEPTS

Perceptual motor function—described as consisting of knowing something about the environment and being able to act on the environment (42)

Sensory Input

a. *Proprioception*—refers to messages arising from muscles, joint-related structures and from the labyrinth (43) (Ayres separates the vestibular or labyrinth system beginning in 1964)

b. *Tactile perception*—described in terms of cutaneous receptors for touch concerned with protection (avoidance and withdrawal) and tactile impuses concerned with perception for tactual discrimination, direction of stimulous movement on the skin and stereognosis (43)

c. *Vestibular system*—the method by which man relates himself to space (43)

d. *Visual perception*—described as assisting in the orientation to space, motor planning and eye-hand coordination (43)

Perceptual and cognitive processes

a. *Perception*—refers to the use of sensations rather than to the raw sensations in themselves; a function of afferent neural interaction for the purpose of interpreting and organizing sensory stimuli for insight and use (41)

b. *Perceptual process*—concerned with the sources of sensation and how those sensations are integrated for use (44)

c. *Primitive or basic unity*—inherent human ability to recognize a form or object as simply existing and being separate or different from what is not part of it (41)

d. *Kinesthesia*—refers to the conscious proprioception arising from muscles and joints, particularly from the joints in terms of joint position and movement (43)

e. *Body scheme*—the knowledge we have of the construction and spatial relationship of the different anatomical elements, *e.g.*, fingers, legs, arms, that make up the body (43)

f. *Body image*—the emotional function as opposed to the neurological function of the construction and spatial relationships of the different anatomical elements of the body (43)

g. *Motor planning*—refers to the cortical determination of type and sequence of movements (43)

h. *Ideational apraxia*—inability to ideationally (put ideas together) plan the motor act (41)

i. *Ideokinetic apraxia*—interruption between ideation and crude motor function (41)

Factors related to perception (41)

a. *Time*—temporarily may be fundamental to proprioceptive and visual perception

b. *Relativity*—recognition of sizes, shapes and positions and relative direction

c. *Gestalt function*—perception of a pattern or an object as a whole

d. *Selectivity*—ability to attend to specific stimuli while ignoring or subordinating other stimuli

e. *Identity*—recognizing parts or the whole as having been in one's previous experience

f. *Relationships*—establishing the precept or concept of the part to the whole

Ayres' five syndromes

1. *Apraxia or developmental apraxia*—deficiency in the ability to motor plan in which the major perceptual deficiency is in the tactile functions, including finger identification, tactile perception, manual perception, kinesthesia and visual figure ground perception (47) (Fig. 12.7)

2. *Form and position in space perceptual dysfunction*—A deficit in perception of form and position in two-dimensional space which includes difficulties in manual perception of forms, kinesthesia and visual perception of form and space (47) (Fig. 12.8)

3. *Deficits of integration of function of the two sides of the body*—deficits in the ability to cross the midline of the body when engaged

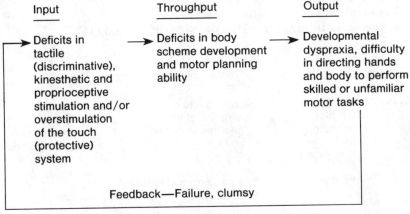

Figure 12.7.   Model of developmental disability.

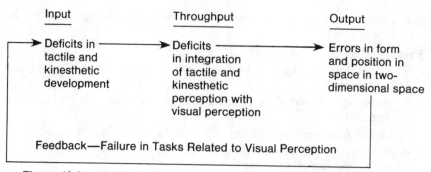

Figure 12.8. Model of perceptual dysfunction in form and position in space.

in motor tasks and difficulty in learning to discriminate and identify the right and left sides of the body (47) (Fig. 12.9)

4. *Visual figure ground perception dysfunction*—deficiency in visual figure ground perception (47) (Fig. 12.10)

5. *Tactile defensiveness*—Deficit in tactile perception, characterized by hyperactive, distractable behavior and by a defensive response to certain types of tactile stimuli (43). It consists of feelings of discomfort and a desire to escape the situation when certain types of tactile stimuli are experienced (45) (Fig. 12.11)

EXPECTED RESULTS

1. Increased foreground-background separation (41)
2. Improved form recognition (41)
3. Increased recognition of three-dimensional form and space (41)
4. Development of concept formation (41)
5. Improved motor planning skills (41)
6. Improved body scheme (43)
7. Decreased tactile defensiveness (47)
8. Increased integration of the two sides of the body (47)

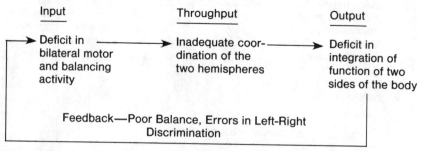

Figure 12.9. Model of deficit of integration of function of two sides of the body.

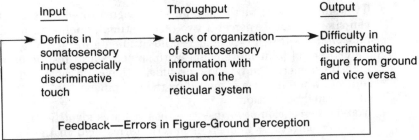

Figure 12.10. Model of perceptual dysfunction in visual figure ground.

ASSESSMENT INSTRUMENTS (48)

1. Tests of somatic perception
   a. Kinesthesia memory—with the working area hidden from view, the child is asked to place a stylus on a spot to which his hand, holding the stylus, previously had been passively taken. The score is determine by how close the child comes to the goal (Southern California Sensory Integration Tests (SCSIT—Kinesthesia)).
   b. Finger identification—the subject is required to identify fingers touched by the examiner (SCSIT—Finger Identification).
   c. Localization of tactile stimuli—the test ascertains the degree of accuracy with which a child can indicate with his finger tip at what part on his forearm or hand he had been touched with a pencil used by the examiner. Vision is occluded (SCSIT localization of tactile stimuli).
   d. Two point tactile discrimination—the standard test of two point discrimination is administered using the two points on a sewing gauge.
   e. Skin designs—after the examiner drew a simple design on the back of the child's hand, the child is asked to draw the same design with his finger on the back of the examiner's hand (SCSIT Graphesthesia).

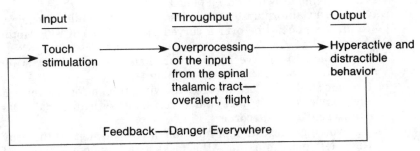

Figure 12.11. Model of tactile defensiveness.

f. Two simultaneous tactile stimuli—the degree to which a child can simultaneously perceive two tactile stimuli applied to hand and/or cheek (SCSIT Double Tactile Stimulation).

g. Perception of joint movement—with subject's arm resting on a kinesthesiometer and vision occluded, the child is asked to indicate when his arm is moved by the examiner.

2. Tests of visual perception

a. Manual perception of forms—the task requires identification of common objects or wooden geometric forms held in the hand and hidden from sight. The objects are identified verbally or the forms are identified by pointing to a chart of forms at which the child looks (SCSIT Manual Form Perception).

b. Embedded figures—simple outline drawings of common objects, superimposed on each other and occasionally embedded in superfluous lines (SCSIT Figure Ground).

c. Gestalt completion—the subject identifies the partial silhouette of an object.

d. Ayres Space Test—the subject selects a block to fit a formboard on the basis of perception of position in space and visualization of rotation of objects in space. Minimal motor activity was involved (SCSIT Space Visualization).

e. Marianne Frostig Spatial Relations—the task requires copying with a pencil patterns superimposed on a constellation of dots.

f. Marianne Frostig Figure Ground—the subjects draws around geometric forms which are superimposed or placed on a shaded background.

g. Visual perception of verticality—using a piece of apparatus which eliminated visual cues to verticality the subject adjusts a rod to his perceived visual vertical.

h. Marianne Frostig Form Constancy—test involves identifying circles and squares in a variety of visual contents.

i. Marianne Frostig Position in Space—subject differentiates mirror images from exact likenesses by pointing to his choice of figures.

3. Tests involving drawing with a pencil

a. Southern California Motor Accuracy Test—the child is required to draw a pencil line over a curved printed line (SCSIT Motor Accuracy).

b. Marianne Frostig Eye Motor Coordination—the subject is required to draw a line between two points.

c. Graphic skill—the task involves drawing, from a copy, a vertical line, circle, crossed lines and a rectangle with diagonal lines connecting opposite corners.

4. Tests involving integration of function of the two sides of the body

a. Right-left discrimination—the tasks requires identification of right and left on both examined and examiner.

  b. Crossing the midline of the body—the test attempts to evaluate the tendency to avoid crossing the midline of the body in picking up objects on placing the hands on various parts of the body (SCSIT Crossing Midline of Body).

  c. Bilateral Motor Integration—the test originally developed to evaluate time and rhythm, involves beating out a rhythm with one or two hands as demonstrated by the examiner (SCSIT Bilateral Motor Integration).

5. Tests for laterality

  a. Degree of agreement between eye and hand preference—the extent to which homologous eye and hand preference are demonstrated is the basis for the test.

  b. Strength of unilateral hand preference—the score is based on the frequency with which one hand is used for common tasks.

  c. Strength of unilateral preference of eye, hand and foot—the score is based on the frequency with which the subject prefers the eye and extremities on one side of the body for skilled activities.

  d. Hands test—plastic models of the hands are presented in different spatial orientations to the subject for right or left identification.

6. Tests of motor planning

  a. Fine motor planning—the instrument used consists of a twisted wire held in both hands by handles at end. By continuously changing the spatial orientation, a rubber grommet is manipulated from one handle to the other.

  b. Fine motor planning—the tasks involves the number of times the subject can wind a heavy string, making a figure eight around two bolts set 3 inches apart in a piece of plywood.

  c. Gross motor planning—subject was judged on the quickness and accuracy with which he could duplicate a posture assumed by the examiner (SCSIT Imitation of Postures).

7. Other tests

  a. Identification of body parts—the child is asked to point to a part of the body (such as knee or elbow) named by the examiner.

  b. Body visualization—the child is asked to respond to verbal questions regarding the spatial relations of the body such as "which is farther from your nose, your stomach or your feet?"

  c. Standing balance—the test score is dependent upon the length of the time the subject could stand on one foot, eyes open and then eyes closed (SCSIT Standing Balance).

  d. Eye pursuit—voluntary control of eye movements.

  e. Numbers concepts—the items involve counting objects, identifying numbers and coins, making numbers on paper with pencil on command and addition and subtraction problems.

  f. Freedom from tactile defensive behavior—a rating of the child's response to tactile tests in relation to motor and verbal responsess.

   g. Freedom from hyperactive and distractable behavior—a rating of the child's response to all tests in relation to motor and verbal responses.

INTERVENTION STRATEGIES

1. Media (41, 42)
   a. Manipulative toys
   b. Games especially in groups—relay races, ball games, Simon says
   c. Simple tools
   d. Weaving
   e. Jig-saw puzzles
   f. Obstacle courses
   g. Hand puppets
   h. Gross motor activities—rolling, crawling, jumping
   i. Rhythm band instruments
   j. Body stunts—elephant work, crab walk, duck walk, rabbit hop
   k. Balancing activities
2. Methods and techniques
   a. Follow the ontogentic sequence of gross motor skills before fine ones (42).
   b. Motor planning should be taught by taking the child passively through the motions (42).
   c. Enhance visual and kinesthetic perception through tactile stimulation and motor activity, especially that requiring strong muscular contraction and joint compression (42).
   d. Integration of the two sides of the body-use activities requiring reciprocal motion-bilateral activity (42).
   e. To enhance perception of any sensory modality, precede the specific perceptual task with general stimulation which will not cause overarousal and a protective type of response (42).
   f. Tactile defensiveness—use pressure applied along with cutaneous stimulation as in rubbing with a rough cloth or soft plastic scrub brush (45).
3. Equipment—no specific items mentioned except those related to media.
4. Precautions
   a. Avoid stimulation of tactile areas over spastic muscles.
   b. Stop activity if there is production of pallor, increased heart or respiration rate, strong negative reaction on the part of the person

SUMMARY

The perceptual motor model is based on the assumption that "motor performance is closely associated with perception, which, in turn, is strongly related to purposeful motor activity" (44). Perception involves attaching meaning to sensory input by organizing and interpreting the sensory information. Further information is obtained through feedback following a motor act.

Ayres assumes that the major sensory input channels for motor activity are touch, proprioception, vestibular functioning and vision. However, input from these modalities must be of the proper type. In particular, tactile input must be of the discriminative (epicretic) rather than the protective (protopathic) type. The discriminative tactile input provides information on the temporal and spatial aspects of the environment which are useful in developing body scheme and motor planning ability. Both body scheme and motor planning are part of the perceptual organization of the brain which are useful in preparing a motor act (Fig. 12.12).

In some children, and adults, the sensory input channels and processing mechanisms are not working properly which can be observed by careful testing of the quality and type of movement responses given to selected tasks, such as assuming a variety of postures demonstrated by an examiner. The problem may be illustrated by delayed responses, false starts, errors in responses or inability to perform the requested task at all.

Treatment is based on the analysis of the probable phyletic development of neuromuscular function. Generally the first task is to enhance tactile and kinesthetic discrimination through the control of sensory input. Next is to require the performance of purposeful movement which includes the need to plan and will provide feedback to the nervous system as to whether the action taken was successful. The motor planning begins with "gross motor equilibrium reactions and then proceeds to tasks that require finer skill" (44).

Analysis and Critique of the Perceptual Motor Model

FRAME OF REFERENCE

The frame of reference is consistent with the organismic meta model and developmental supermodel. Attention is focused on the maturational aspects of the perceptual motor functioning based on the assumption of ontogenetic development. Of significance is the assertion that motions

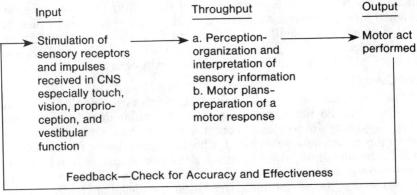

Figure 12.12. Model of perceptual motor function.

take place from the body scheme as a frame of reference. Thus, locus of control is within the individual.

CLARITY

Although there are definitions and descriptions of the sensory systems and the perceptual motor syndromes, there is not a definition of the term "perceptual motor." Godfrey and Kephart (50) define perceptual motor as the inseparable integration of perceptual and motor functions or activities as one interdependent and interrelated behavioral area.

One assumption which is difficult to follow is the role of sensory input in the development of body scheme. In one article (43) tactile, proprioceptive and visual input are said to contribute to body scheme, whereas in another article (42) body scheme is attributed to tactile, kinesthetic and possibly vestibular input. The problem is to clarify the role of vestibular input, vision, and proprioception in general, as opposed to the more limited aspects of kinesthesia.

UNIQUENESS

The interest in the study of perceptual motor development and dysfunction is not unique to occupational therapy. A number of educational psychologists have been interested in the subject also. What appears to be unique is the attempt to identify different types of perceptual motor dysfunction and to interpret the problems in relation to known facts about neurophysiology and assumed facts from phylogenetic neurobiology.

RESEARCH GUIDE

The perceptual motor model promoted interest in the field which was evident in the number of continuing education programs offered. However, there was not much research generated. One of few studies is by Llorens (51). She found that 9 to 11 of 12 emotionally disturbed children showed one or more of Ayres' five syndromes. A second study by Fox (52) found a correlation between the use of 5 minutes of cutaneous stimulation (pressure) and finger localization in adult subjects with hemiplegia. This study is an extension of the testing protocol, since the original information was collected on children. Another study by Sleeper (53) did not show significant differences in body balance and space perception in adult subjects with cerebral palsy using the Ayres Space Test (SCSIT Space Visualization) and Standing Balance Test.

SPECIALIZATION

The perceptual motor model started a trend toward specialization with children who did not have obvious neuromuscular disorders and who were frequently in regular classrooms rather than always in special education classrooms and special schools. Furthermore, the model focused attention on the role of neuromuscular development in relation to cognitive and academic performance. Evidence such as Lloren's findings suggested that emotional and psychosocial problems of children might also be related to neuromuscular deficits which did not appear evident by observation alone.

ELABORATION AND REFINEMENT

The development of the sensory integrative model from the perceptual motor model provided both elaboration and refinement. Therefore, discussion is not necessary in this section.

EXPLORATORY USEFULNESS

The perceptual motor model has been very useful in providing possible explanations for certain behavioral problems related to motor cognitive and social performances. Developmental apraxia provides an explanation for why some children appear to be clumsy and uncoordinated in performing everyday activities. Deficits in integration of the two sides of the body suggest a reason as to why some children cannot remember left from right. Tactile defensiveness can be used to explain why some children appear hostile and aggressive without obvious agitation. All of these examples are useful in explaining the role of occupational therapy in helping people to be able to perform those occupations and tasks which are necessary to meet basic needs and fulfill accepted values.

COMMONALITY

As mentioned under Uniqueness, the perceptual motor model is shared as a mutual area of interest by educational psychologists and physical education teachers. The focus, however, is a bit different. Psychologists seem to be interested in cognitive aspects of perception and educators are interested in the quality of motor response. Occupational therapists are interested also in the types of sensory input and subcortical organization. Thus, the interests in common exist, but differences also occur.

PRACTICE MODEL

Although the perceptual motor model has been superseded by the sensory integration model, the opportunity to develop practice models exists. Using the five syndromes as reference points a model of intervention could be developed for each.

SUMMARY

The perceptual motor model does a good job of meeting the criteria for a practice model in occupational therapy. The major weakness is in the uniqueness criteria. A summary of the criteria is given in Table 12.12.

Sensory Integration—Ayres

FRAME OF REFERENCE

Sensory integration was introduced by A. Jean Ayres, Ph.D., O.T.R. (54, 55), in 1968. The concepts had developed out of her earlier work in perceptual motor problems associated with visual and motor disorders (56, 57). The theory is based on the contributions to the developmental approach made by Gesell and Piaget, sensory stimulation and deprivation made by Harlow, Held and others and neurophysiologic concepts organized by Rood. The focus is on how the brain processes sensation and organizes a response. Although systems models are not identified, the influence is present in the descriptions of sensorimotor processing.

Table 12.12
Perceptual Motor Model Summary Critique

Evaluation Criteria	Very Good 1	Moderately Good 2	3	4	Very Poor 5
Frame of reference	x				
Clarity			x		
Uniqueness				x	
Research guide			x		
Specialization		x			
Elaboration/refinement		x			
Explanatory usefulness		x			
Commonality		x			
Practice model		x			

Sensory integrative dysfunction is Ayres' concept of the difficulty some children have in integrating sensory information. She assumes that the lack of sensory integration is associated with learning problems identified in education as learning disabilities. Although the frame of reference is similar to the models discussed under neurobiology, the special attention to sensory development and organization and the impact of the model on the profession require a separate discussion.

ASSUMPTIONS ABOUT BRAIN FUNCTION AND DYSFUNCTION

1. The brain is designed to follow an orderly, predictable, interrelated sequence of development (58, p. 4).
2. The early developmental steps have been "preprogrammed" into the human brain at conception, but ontogenetic experience is necessary for the full expression of the inherent development tendencies (58, p. 4).
3. Each developmental stage assimilates and builds upon part of the previous one (58, p. 5).
4. Higher intellectual functions are just as much a product of evolutionary development as lower functions (58, p. 5).
5. The more recently acquired evolutionary developments are more vulnerable to dysfunction (59).
6. When the development of the brain has deviated from the norm, the resultant behavior is often reminiscent of lower levels of the phyletic scale (58, p. 7).
7. Learning disorders reflect some deviation in neural function (58, p. 1).

ASSUMPTIONS ABOUT SENSORY INTEGRATION DEVELOPMENT AND FUNCTION

1. Intermodality convergence occurs at all levels of the brain (59).
2. The most commonly reported sensory modalities showing convergence are visual, auditory, tactile, vestibular and other proprioception (59, p. 317).

3. Sensory integrative processes result in perception and other types of synthesis of sensory data that enable man to interact effectively with the environment (58, p. 1).
4. The innate potential for development of sensory integration and related adaptive behavior is a substrate for individual development (58, p. 6).
5. Sensory integrative mechanisms mature in association with adaptive motor interaction with the environment (59, p. 323).
6. Adaptive motor responses impose organization upon sensory input (59, p. 323).
7. Effectiveness of response is partly dependent upon accuracy or precision of the sensory input and feedback from the response (59, p. 323).
8. It is the nature and sequence of sensory integration that is the *sine qua non* to understanding perception and the requirements of early academic learning (58, p. 5).

ASSUMPTIONS ABOUT VESTIBULAR AND POSTURAL INTEGRATION

1. Before an organism can relate itself to the environment it must have some concept of space (59, p. 333).
2. In man, the concept of space begins with the vestibular system, activated by gravity and motion (59).
3. The vestibular system is critical to the postural response system (59, p. 328).
4. Postural responses involve the body's dynamic relationship with the earth's gravitational force (59, p. 324).
5. Postural responses involve automatic or reflex-based reactions which are programmed into the nervous system, or patterns of motion which are basic to the developmental sequence (59).
6. Primitive postural reflexes must be integrated into the sensorimotor system before the ontogenetically more mature and normal postural reactions can develop (59, p. 326).
7. The vestibular system is the mediator of the tonic labyrinthine reflex (TLR) and many of the righting and equilibrium reactions (59).

ASSUMPTIONS ABOUT MOTOR PLANNING AND BODY SCHEME

1. As information from vestibular and other proprioceptors arises from moving about within the environment, a modular map develops of the environment to which the body relates (59, p. 318).
2. The body is the center of the environmental scheme, and the environmental plan exists only in relation to the body relating to the environment (59, p. 318).
3. Planning an unfamiliar task or one that never becomes automatic requires a sensorimotor awareness of the different anatomical elements of the body and their potential movements, especially in relation to each other (59).

4. Motor planning or praxis is dependent upon sensory integration (59).
5. Difficulty in formulating a motor plan is considered primarily a reflection of inadequate sensory integration, especially of tactile and kinesthetic input (59).
6. The body scheme is the neurophysiological substrate of which a person is generally only semiconscious and from which plans are formulated (59).
7. The body scheme is an end product of intersensory integration (59).
8. The body scheme provides an intact although constantly changing model from which any plan can be implemented (59).

ASSUMPTIONS REGARDING INTERHEMISPHERE FUNCTIONS—BRAINSTEM LEVEL

1. The brainstem interhemispheral integrating mechanism is functionally associated with the brainstem postural reflexes and reactions (59).
2. The innate neural connections serving the postural reflexes and centrally patterned responses provide a formation for the more critically planned motions (59).
3. The brainstem interhemispheral mechanism serves a critical role in the neural system, and it is frequently not functioning in the learning-disabled child (59).

ASSUMPTIONS REGARDING INTERHEMISPHERE FUNCTIONS—CORTEX LEVEL

1. In man bilateral symmetry at the neocortical level gives way to asymmetry in order to localize function for greater specialization and adaptiveness (59).
2. Optimizing cerebral function is enabled only when the two cerebral hemispheres are free to differentiate and specialize before information from one hemisphere is available to the other (59).
3. The capacity to specialize function in the cerebral hemispheres is generally considered an optimum neural basis for learning (59).
4. Interaction between the two hemispheres through the corpus callosum allows the two hemispheres to assist each other in somatosensory learning and resultant bilateral motor coordination, but at higher levels each hemisphere works independently (59).
5. Without the cross-integrational functions enabled by the corpus callosum, the facilities that suffer are those associated with cerebral dominance, such as lateral differentiation of higher mental processes, especially spatial orientation and abstract thinking (59).
6. Inadequate interhemispheral communication results in each hemisphere working independently which slows the process of certain types of learning, such as a visual or somatosensory task (59).
7. Lack of adequate integration of function includes difficulty in two-hand coordination, a tendency to avoid crossing the midline, use of one hand on one side of the body and the other hand on the other and difficulty in left-right discrimination (59).

ASSUMPTIONS ABOUT THE DEVELOPMENT AND FUNCTIONS OF THE VISUAL SYSTEMS

1. Learning to perceive the environmental scheme visually evolved over millions of years through association with the vestibular, locomotor and oculomotor processes (59, p. 319).
2. The evolution of visual perception began with perceiving gravity and the sense of movement, and using that information to make postural and locomotor responses relating self to environment, with the eye muscles providing an essential aspect of the musculoskeletal postural system (59, p. 319).
3. There are dual models of vision—ambient and focal (59, p. 319).
4. There is constant interaction among the extraocular muscles, vestibular system and the neck muscles (59).
5. Activation of the postural reflexes and contraction of the neck muscles against resistance help develop the extraocular muscle eye control (59).

ASSUMPTIONS ABOUT OCCUPATIONAL THERAPY

1. Occupational therapy was originally designed to help people with motor and behavioral handicaps form adaptive responses that enabled them to improve their own condition (60, p. 135).
2. Occupational therapists help the patient or client to perform some purposeful activity (60, p. 151).
3. Doing purposeful physical activities, rather than thinking or talking about them, is the best way to improve human functioning when the problem lies in the way the brain is working (60, p. 151).
4. One of the major reasons that movement is employed is for its sensory-producing effects (59).
5. Multisensory stimuli are more effective than messages from only one modality (59).

CONCEPTS

A. Basic

Integration—interaction and coordination of two or more functions or processes in a manner which enhances the adaptiveness of the brain's response (58, p. 26).

Sensory integration—the ability to organize sensory information for use (58).

Sensory integrative dysfunction—an irregularity or disorder in brain function that makes it difficult to integrate sensory input (60, p. 184).

Sensory integrative therapy—treatment involving sensory stimulation and adaptive responses to it according to the child's neurologic needs (60, p. 184).

Adaptive response—an appropriate action in which the individual responds successfully to some environmental demand (60, p. 181).

Occupational therapy—a profession that employs a purposeful activity to help the client form adaptive responses that enable the nervous system to work more efficiently (60).

B. Sensory systems

Vestibular system—the sensory program with receptors which respond to gravity and to accelerated or decelerated movement and all major neuronal mechanisms influenced by sensory input from those receptors (61).

Proprioception—the sensations from muscles and joints that tell the brain how the muscles are contracting or stretching and when and how the joints are bending, extending or being pulled or compressed (60).

Ambient vision—used to perceive the space to which the body is relating and is largely a function of the midbrain (59).

Focal vision—perceives a small area in great detail and is largely a function of the neocortex (59).

Tactile system—sensory input from the skin (58).

C. Methods of neural integration (55, 58)

Intersensory integration—the capacity to associate information from two or more different sensory modalities.

Centrifugal influences—the regulation of sensory input by control of the propagation of an impulse at the sensory receptor and at each major junction in the series of neurons conducting the impulse toward the cortex.

Regulation through feedback—reception of continuous information about the results of one's actions upon the environment.

Balancing excitatory and depressant neural activity—augmenting or suppressing the response to afferent flow.

D. Integrating mechanisms

Praxis or motor planning—the ability of the brain to conceive of, organize, and carry out a sequence of unfamiliar actions (60).

Body scheme—sensorimotor awareness of the different anatomical elements of the body, 1972 (58) (changed to body percept in 1979) (60).

E. Normal motor response

Postural Reactions—automatic muscle contractions that keep the body balanced. The ability to change position and move from one place to another without losing balance (60, p. 92).

Postural background movements—the subtle spontaneous body adjustments that make overt movements of the hands, such as reaching for a distant object, easier (60, p. 183).

Postrotary nystagmus—the horizontal reflex movement of the eyes following an abrupt stop after a series of rotations of the body at a constant velocity (61).

F. Sensory integration syndromes and problems

Vestibular-bilateral disorder—caused by underreactive vestibular responses and characterized by shortened duration nystagmus, poor integration of the two sides of the body and brain and difficulty in learning to read or compute (60, p. 185).

Overreactive or hyperactive vestibular disorder—described as a child who has a vestibular system which is overresponsive to vestibular input. The child responds by being insecure or intolerant to movement (60).

Developmental dyspraxia or apraxia—a brain dysfunction that hinders the organization of tactile, and sometimes vestibular and proprioceptive, sensations and interferes with the ability to motor plan (60).

Gravitational or Postural Insecurity—an abnormal anxiety and distress caused by inadequate modulation or inhibition of sensations that arise when the gravity receptors of the vestibular system are stimulated by head position or movement (60).

Tactile defensiveness—the tendency to react negatively and emotionally to touch sensations (60, p. 184).

Visual perception problem in space and form—described as difficulty in comprehending the dimensions of space and the relationship of the body to space (60).

Unilateral disregard and functions of the right hemisphere—described as the tendency of the child to avoid moving into the left side of space (in relation to the body) or incorporating the left side of the body space into the environmental scheme (58).

Auditory language disorder—described as involving problems in postural and bilateral integration, praxis, and visual perception (58).

EXPECTED RESULTS

1. Provide and control sensory input especially to vestibular system, muscles and joints.
2. Facilitate the formation of adaptive responses that integrate sensory sensations.
3. Develop a more accurate body percept.
4. Normalize the touch system of the tactilely defensive child.
5. Reduce hyperactivity and energize nervous system for more purposeful activity.
6. Increase flexor pattern of child with developmental dyspraxia.
7. Develop postural and equilibrium reactions.
8. Improve motor planning.
9. Improve visual perception through input to brainstem.
10. Provide a foundation for cerebral processes, such as language and reading and hand and finger movements for writing and tool use.

EVALUATION

Ayres has developed two standardized tests and a series of clinical observations. The standardized tests evaluate the following areas of function:

1. Somatosensory (62, 63)
   a. Double Tactile Stimuli: Two tactile stimuli are applied simulta-

neously to either or both the cheek and the hand of the child who then identifies where he was touched.
  b. Finger Identification: The child points to the finger on the hand which was touched previously by the examiner without the child watching.
  c. Graphesthesia: The child draws a simple design on the back of the hand, attempting to copy the design previously drawn by the examiner on the same surface of the hand.
  d. Kinesthesia: With vision occluded, the child attempts to place the finger on a point at which the finger previously has been placed by the examiner.
  e. Localization of Tactile Stimuli: The child is expected to place a finger on the spot on the hand or arm previously touched by the examiner.
2. Motor (62, 63)
  a. Bilateral Motor Coordination: Performing this test requires smoothly executed movements of and interaction between both upper extremities.
  b. Imitation of Postures: The child is required to assume a series of positions of postures demonstrated by the examiner.
  c. Motor Accuracy: A visual motor task requiring the child to draw a line over a printed line.
  d. Standing Balance Eyes Open and Closed: The test measures the ability of the child to balance while standing on one foot with eyes open and then with eyes closed.
3. Form and Space (62, 63)
  a. Design Copying: A visual motor task which involves duplicating a design on a dot grid.
  b. Figure Ground: Stimulus figures are superimposed and imbedded to require selection of a foreground figure from a rival background.
  c. Manual Form Perception: The test requires matching the visual counterpart of a geometric form held in the hand (may be included under somatosensory).
  d. Position in Space: Simple geometric forms are presented for recognition in different orientations and sequences.
  e. Space Visualization: Form boards are used to test the child's visual perception of form and space through mental manipulation of objects in space.
4. Nystagmus (63, 64)
  a. Postrotary nystagmus: The child is seated on a board which is turned 10 times in 20 seconds then stopped and the number of seconds nystagmus occurs are counted.
5. Other (62, 63)
  a. Crossing Midline of Body: The child imitates the examiner as the latter points either to one of the examiner's eyes or ears.
  b. Right-Left Discrimination: The child is asked to indicate right

from left on body of the examiner and relative to the location of an object.

Clinical observations include measurements of (a) hyperactivity or distractibility, (b) tactile defensiveness, (c) muscle tone, (d) eye preference, (e) eye movements across midline, pursuits, convergence and quick localization, (f) ability to perform slow motions, (g) forearm rotation, (h) thumb finger touching , (i) tongue to lip movement, (j) cocontraction of the arm, shoulder and neck, (k) postural insecurity in the supine position, (l) postural background movements, (m) equilibrium reactions in prone, quadruped and sitting, (n) protective extension, (o) Schilders arm extension posture, (p) prone extension posture, (q) symmetrical tonic neck reflex, (r) asymmetrical tonic neck reflex (s) flexed position in supine, (t) choreoathetoid-like movements and (u) space visualization contralateral use.

INTERVENTION STRATEGIES

1. Media and modalities
   a. Play activities
   b. Individual
   c. Dyad
2. Methods, techniques, approaches
   a. General (59)
      1. Permit child to select activity and amount of time
      2. Guide selection of activity and control time period
      3. Provide assistance in "hand on" or balancing on equipment and gradually withdraw support
      4. Suggest play themes such as "riding an airplane" to maintain interest
      5. Add to complexity of the activity to maintain interest
   b. Specific examples
      1. Activities for vestibular stimulation (59)
         a. Child spins self or have someone spin child sitting or lying in net hammock suspended from a common point
         b. Child lies on a scooter board and spins
         c. Rolling on the floor
      2. Activities for tactile stimulation (59)
         a. Rub skin with a terry cloth
         b. Fast brushing
         c. Lying on a rough or smooth carpet
      3. Extensor tone-inverted TLR prone flexion (59)
         a. Vibration to belly of extensor muscles
         b. Ride scooter down a ramp on belly.
      4. Inhibit TNR (59)
         a. All fours position, turn head, raise one leg to promote equilibrium reaction and flex arm on jaw side to promote positive supporting reaction.
         b. Vibration to extensors

    c. Rolling to promote neck righting

  5. Promoting the flexion synergy (59)

    a. Rocking back and forth—child should assist by holding on

    b. Riding the scooter board down a ramp and reaching up to touch an overhanging object as the child goes under

  6. Promoting protective extension (59)

    Roll crosswise over a barrel and catch self by placing both hands on the floor.

  7. Promoting the rotation synergy (59)

    Use piece of wood with two handles on top and three ball-bearing coasters on the bottom with child's knees on top, grasping handles and move in large figure eights

  8. Developing motor planning skills (59)

    a. Ride a scooter board down a ramp coasting under a strip of inner tube and catching the inner tube strip with one leg flexed at the knee

    b. Stand with one's back to a hanging ball and kick it

  9. Bilateral integration—integrate two sides of the body (59)

    a. Chalkboard exercises which require crossing midline

    b. Waving flags bilaterally and across the midline

c. Sequences

  1. Postural and bilateral integration of vestibular bilateral integration (58, p. 145)

    a. Normalize the tactile and vestibular systems in general

    b. Inhibit the primitive postural reflexes

    c. Develop equilibrium reactions

    d. Normalize ocular movements

    e. Enhance coordination of sensorimotor function of the two sides of the body

    f. Develop visual form and space perception

  2. Development of dyspraxia or apraxia (58, 60)

    a. Normalize the tactile and vestibular systems in general

    b. Inhibit the primitive postural reflexes

    c. Develop postural reactions, coordination and body percept

    d. Increase "library" of motor skills

    e. Increase opportunity to motor plan

  3. Tactile defensiveness (58, pp. 217–220)

    a. Inhibit or normalize the tactile protective response

    b. Promote a balance between the protective and discriminative tactile system

    c. Normalize the least defensive skin areas first

    d. Encourage adaptive responses

  4. Hemispheric specialization (58, pp. 232–234)

    a. Increase the tactile proprioceptive and vestibular input, especially to the involved side

    b. Facilitate postural adjustments and responses

    c. Increase the use of the orienting reflex on the involved side

      d. Promote the use of eye and hand coordination and other motor planning tasks.

  5. Development of visual perception (59, p. 344)

      a. Normalize the reticular mechanism through such stimuli as tactile, vestibular and other proprioceptive input

      b. Activate and bring to appropriate maturity for the age of the child postural and ocular mechanisms mediated by the brainstem

      c. Involve the neck musculature in contraction against resistance

      d. Engage in activities which relate the body to objects in space and provide extrasensory input from the body related to that activity.

      e. Eye-hand manipulatory activities involving form and space and space visualization

      f. Require differentiation of visual stimuli on the basis of a configuration or perception of a small focal area.

  3. Equipment (58)

      a. Scooter board

      b. Swing bolster

      c. Platform swing

      d. Ramp

      e. Net suspended from a hook

      f. Inflatable plastic shapes

      g. Buoy

      h. Jungle gym

      i. Mats

      j. Coaster board

  4. Prerequisites and precautions (59)

Any child receiving vestibular stimulations should be watched closely for:

      a. Flushing or blanching of the face

      b. Sweating

      c. Nausea

      d. A lower level of consciousness

      e. Indication of reduced respiration

      f. Decreased heart rate

SUMMARY

Sensory integration is based on development as a hierarchical process in which successive stages of sensation integrate the lower levels to promote adaptation to the environment (Figs. 12.13 and 12.14). The hierarchy of function applies to brain and nervous system functions as well as to physical maturation. Equally important is the emphasis on sensory physiology and the role of sensory input in promoting integration of function. It is the emphasis on organizing sensory input that separates the sensory motor models from the neurobiological models. Specifically,

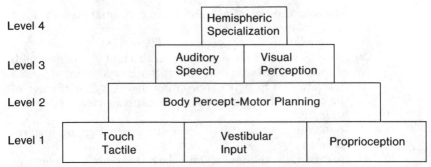

Figure 12.13. Levels of sensory integration. (Modified from A. J. Ayres (58, pp. 59–66).)

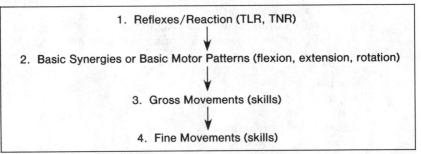

Figure 12.14. Developmental sequence of movement. (Adapted from A. J. Ayres (59).)

the sensory integrative model is organized around the assumption that sensory deprivation (lack of stimulation) contributes to the lack of development, regardless of whether the deprivation is the result of internal or external factors.

According to Ayres, the central idea of sensory integrative therapy is to "provide and control sensory input, especially the input from the vestibular system, muscles, joints and skin in such a way that the child spontaneously forms the adaptive responses that integrate those sensations" (60, p. 140) (Fig. 12.15). Thus, therapy usually involves total body movements that concentrate on providing vestibular proprioceptive and tactile stimulation. Such therapy does not use activities at a desk, speech training, reading lessions or training in a specific perceptual or motor skill. The goal of therapy is to improve the processing and organizing of sensations in the nervous system so that the end products will be effective in academic performance and other activities (Fig. 12.16).

Sensory Integration for Adult Schizophrenics—King
FRAME OF REFERENCE

King has classified schizophrenics into process and reactive types based on Harry S. Sullivan's classification and has cited a variety of authors in identifying characteristic behaviors; however, the primary treatment

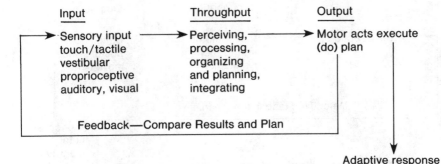

Figure 12.15. Sensory integration model.

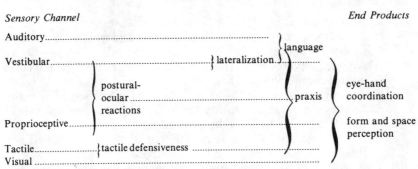

Figure 12.16. Goals of sensory integration therapy. (Reproduced from A. J. Ayres (63) with permission from Western Psychological Services.)

process is based on the work of A. Jean Ayres in sensory integration with some input from Margaret Rood concerning heavy work patterns. The model is described from King's (5) article "A Sensory-Integrative Approach to Schizophrenia."

ASSUMPTIONS

View of Man

1. Man is a single organism, highly complex and completely unified in mind and body.
2. Anything that affects the will inexorably affects the mind and vice versa.

View of Health

3. Some individuals have defective proprioceptive feedback mechanisms. The vestibular component in particular being first underreactive and second, underactive in its role in the sensorimotor integration process.
4. This defect, whether genetic, developmental, or the result of trauma, constitutes an important etiological or prodromal factor in process and reactive schizophrenia.
5. Chronic schizophrenics (nonparanoid) have several highly visible postural and movement features in common (Fig. 12.17).

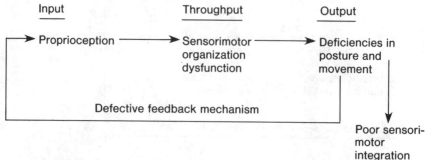

Input	Throughput	Output

Proprioception ⟶ Sensorimotor organization dysfunction ⟶ Deficiencies in posture and movement

Defective feedback mechanism

Poor sensori-motor integration

Figure 12.17. Disorganization of sensory information in posture and movement of schizophrenics (based on concepts 3, 4 and 5).

a. A pronounced head to toe "S" curve posture
b. A shuffling gait—inability to lift the feet and walk with a normal heel-toe pattern
c. An inability to raise the arms above the head to anything approaching a vertical line.
d. An immobility of the head and shoulder girdle which is manifested by an inability to rotate the head on the vertical axis or to roll the head to the side, forward and back
e. A tendency to hold arms and legs in a flexed, adducted and internally rotated position both sitting and standing
f. A lack of normal hand function that involves the thumb held in adduction, atrophy of the thenar eminence, ulnar deviation at the wrist, and also a weakness of grip.
6. Vestibular and tactile input are important in organizing and integrating sensory stimuli primarily at the brainstem level.
7. Integration of auditory, visual and other sensory input is essential to the development of visual size and form constancy, reliable localization of auditory stimuli and other sensory constancy.
8. Constancy and reliability of perceptual information are essential to all kinds of learning (Fig. 12.18).
9. The lack of perceptual constancy caused by faulty sensory integration may be the mechanism that produces hallucinations.
10. The reactive schizophrenic may lose perceptual constancy, whereas the process schizophrenic or autistic child may have never developed it.
11. Schizophrenic persons tend to have absent or underreactive vestibular response when light is present.
12. Such persons may be unable to process both visual and vestibular stimuli at the same time.
13. Abnormal vestibular reactivity may reflect defective brainstem processing which may be a cause of the lack of perceptual constancy in schizophrenic persons.
14. Chronic schizophrenics are unable to assume and hold the pivot-prone positon of hyperextension—counterposition to the tonic labyrinthine-prone reflex.

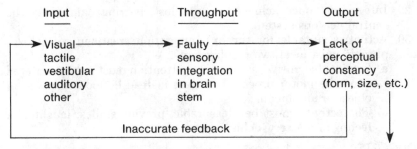

Figure 12.18. Disorganization of sensory information in perceptual constancy (based on concepts 6 to 9).

15. They have hypertension in the phasic muscle groups (flexors, adductors and internal rotators) and hypotonicity in the opposing tonic groups (extensors, abductors and external rotators).
16. Inadequacy of vestibular response may be part of a vicious cycle in which anxiety generalizes or is conditioned from man's innate fear of falling.
17. Lack of movement slows development of the vestibular system because of inadequacy of vestibular input which sequentially leads to inadequate development of perceptual constancy creating further anxiety and unsteadiness of movement.
18. A feeling of security is subject to the day to day dependability of what the senses tell us about the environment.
19. Vestibular stimulation is a basic and important source of pleasure to the normal human.
20. An important corollary of the schizophrenic's postulated lack of sensorimotor integration is corticalization of movement, *e.g.*, thinking about moving.
21. The attempt to think movement as a means of compensating for poor sensorimotor integration is costly in terms of energy expenditure.
22. The feedback stage of the perceptual act may be disrupted in the schizophrenic.
23. The lack of proprioceptive feedback may contribute to bizarre and insufficient associational processes and also to flattened or inappropriate affect.
24. Proprioceptive input has a tuning effect on the reticular activating system which produces a state of tension.
25. Without the tension or tone in the reticular system the associational process is slow or dull, and thinking tends to be limited to the concrete.
26. Movement and posture can affect emotion.
27. Movement behavior and thought processes can alter biochemical states.
28. Adults can benefit from treatment aimed at development of sensorimotor integration.

29. Integration, once achieved, is not lost, barring damage to the central nervous system.
30. Activities suitable for sensory integration treatment of schizophrenia must meet two requirements.:
    a. Cortical (cognitive or conscious) attention must not be centered upon the motor process but must instead be focused upon an object or an outcome.
    b. The activity must be pleasurable, provide smiles, laughter, a feeling of mastery, achievement, or pure fun.

CONCEPTS

Reactive schizophrenic—has functioned with at least marginal adequacy in life to a point where severe or recognizable stress was encountered.

Process schizophrenic—an individual, who from childhood has been *different*, and who gradually slips deeper into psychosis.

Paranoid schizophrenic—does not suffer the degree of personality disorganization and perceptual abnormality observed in reaction or process schizophrenia and is characterized chiefly by delusional patterns of a persecuting or grandiose nature.

Vestibular system, Vestibular stimulation—not defined

EXPECTED RESULTS

1. Extending range of motion
2. Increasing amount of spontaneous movement
3. Improvement in posture
4. Attempt to counteract or normalize patterns of excessive flexion, adduction and internal rotation

INTERVENTION STRATEGIES

1. Media and modalities
   a. Noncompetitive games
      1. Tossing a ball in a circle
      2. Kicking a ball
      3. Stepping over ropes
      4. Ducking under the volleyball net
      5. Passing a ball backward over one's head around the circle
      6. Jumping over a rope 2 to 3 inches off the ground
      7. Marching to music
      8. Scooter board
   b. Recreation—elements of skill, chance, surprise, incongruity and suspense
   c. Purposeful or task-oriented activities
      1. Digging
      2. Gardening
      3. Sweeping
      4. Folding sheets
      5. Gross motor activities
      6. Individual or group activities

2. Methods and techniques
   a. Tactile impact
   b. Heavy work patterns bilaterally
   c. Vestibular stimulation
   d. Integrate (counteract) primitive reflex pattern
   e. Touch pressure
   f. Proprioceptive feedback
   g. Eye pursuits
   h. Color
   i. Texture
   j. Rhythm
   k. Awareness of space and form
3. Equipment
   a. Parachute—for group activities
   b. Balloons—easy eye pursuit, do not hurt, have color, texture
   c. Beach balls—move faster, colorful, light-weight, harmless
   d. Bean bag chairs—learning to fall, proprioceptive input through crawling and rolling over a shifting surface
4. *Prerequisite skills*—not stated.

SUMMARY

King's model is based on the assumption that process and reactive schizophrenics have defects in the vestibular and proprioceptive systems that result in postural and movement disorders similar to problems seen in young children. These deficits are seen in "S" curve posture, shuffling gait, inability to raise arms above head, lack of head mobility, abnormal hand function with hypertonicity in the flexor muscles and hypotonicity in the extensor muscles. King has suggested that the same or similar management techniques are useful with the process and reactive schizophrenics as with children, including gross motor activities, noncompetitive games and task-oriented activities. The outcomes are extending the range of motion, improving posture, normalizing flexion and extension patterns and increasing spontaneous movement.

Analysis and Critique of the Sensory Integration Model

FRAME OF REFERENCE

The frame of reference for the sensory integration model is similar to the perceptual motor model. Development and maturation continue to be the dominant themes. These themes are supported by the belief that only the person can organize an individual's nervous system and frequently is able to select the best media and method to accomplish the task. Thus, the locus of control is maintained primarily within the individual.

CLARITY

One of the problems in understanding the sensory integration model is to comprehend the relationship to the perceptual-motor model (Table 12.13) in an attempt to illustrate some of the key differences. The Table illustrates that the differences are really a matter of degree of emphasis

Table 12.13
Differences in Emphasis between Perceptual Motor and Sensory Integration Models

Perceptual Motor Model	Sensory Integration Model
Focus more on the cortical aspects of perception	Focus more on the subcortical aspects of perception
More emphasis on the interpretation and organization of perception	More emphasis on the integration of sensory input
More emphasis on tactile perception	More emphasis on vestibular input
Less emphasis on reflexes and synergies	More emphasis on reflexes and synergies
Less emphasis on hemispheric specialization	More emphasis on hemispheric specialization

rather than being opposite thoughts or new ideas. Another problem is to remember which sensory modality does what and to relate the function to anatomical structures. Table 12.14 is a summary of the four sensory modalities mentioned most frequently by Ayres. These are vestibular touch/tactile, proprioception and visual receptors. A third problem is to understand how sensory integration as a technique differs from a perceptual motor technique. Sensory integration techniques are based on controlling input to facilitate intersensory association. Perceptual motor techniques tend to limit the input to one modality at a time in order to reduce the amount of information which reaches the brain. Thus, the environment suppresses the amount of input in a manner similar to the afferent suppression of centrifugal influences, instead of encouraging the individual's nervous system to establish control.

Table 12.14
Function and Structure of Four Major Sensory Modalities

Vestibular
  Static-otoliths
  Acceleration—linear-utricle and succule or deceleration—angular-semicircular canals
Tactile—cutaneous receptors
  Protective (light touch)—spinal thalamic tract
  Discriminative (deep touch pressure)—medial lemnescal tract
  Temperature—not used by Ayres
  Pain—discussed as a precaution
Proprioceptors (somatic)
  Flexion (abduction), TLR prone, flexion synergy, muscle spindles, and joint receptors
  Extension (abduction), TLR supine, extension synergy, muscle spindles and joint receptors
  Rotation, trunk reflex, rotation synergy, muscle spindles and joint receptors
Visual
  Ambient or peripheral vision—midbrain
  Focal or central vision—optic lobe

UNIQUENESS

The unique aspect of the sensory integration model is the focus on the importance of interaction and coordination of information from two or more different modalities to enhance the adaptiveness of the brain's response. Occupational therapists have been aware of the value in therapy of using multisensory input to facilitate responses. What the sensory integration model emphasizes is that use of multisensory input is a normal maturational sequence. Thus, multisensory input is not a special technique of therapy but a promotion of normal development which must be achieved by the person if a repertoire of useful adaptive behaviors is to be achieved. The ability to integrate multiple sensory input is therefore essential to enable a person to meet individual needs and values and social demands.

RESEARCH

The sensory integrative model has been very successful in promoting research. Ayres has stated that development of theory is at least as important, if not more important, than testing the theory. Many of the research articles have been addressed to enlarging the theoretical base of sensory integration.

Another research method used successfully has been the clinic-based research design which focuses on observation of changes occurring within a group of children receiving sensory integrating techniques as the major part of their intervention program. The focus is on whether the rate of change is significant rather than on the degree of change between an experimental and control group.

SPECIALIZATION

As a guide for specialization, the sensory integrative model has been successful. Sensory integration is the only theory and intervention program to have its own special interest section in the American Occupational Therapy Association. Therapists also can acquire a special certification in test administration of the Southern California Sensory Integration Tests. Furthermore there is a private organization devoted to activities related to the research in and practice of sensory integration called the Center for the Study of Sensory Integrative Dysfunction.

ELABORATION AND REFINEMENT

The sensory integration model could be expanded or refined by adding knowledge about any of the following questions.

1. What rate of motion and head position are most excitatory and which are most inhibitory (66)?
2. What rate of motion and head position are optimum for activating the orienting reflex unilaterally (65)?
3. What rate of motion and oscillation (excursion) of vibration are most excitatory or inhibitory to children with sensory integrative dysfunction (67)?
4. How much time should be spent in an intervention session or

normalizing sensory responses vs. engaging in gross or fine motor activities (68)?

5. What is the optimal age range (or is there any) for maximizing the effects of sensory integration intervention (68)?
6. Are there other types of sensory integrative disorders not yet identified (69)? These syndromes might be found in children or adults.
7. Is the order of test items in the SCSIT affecting the type of syndromes observed by artificially raising or lowering some scores (70)?
8. What is the correlation of the SCSIT which other development or intelligence tests such as the Bayley Scales of Infant Development or the Weschler Intelligence Scale for children (71)?

The sensory integrative model also could be expanded to respond to issues related to cognitive, intra- and interpersonal skills. For example:

1. Are there common thinking styles or difficulties in organizing cognitive processes that are common in sensory dysfunction in addition to basic academic difficulties?
2. Can sensory dysfunction be detected on the basis of psychological responses to questions related to self concept, competence or mastery?
3. Do people with sensory integrative dysfunction have different roles or values in their life space?

Figure 12.19 outlines the elaboration of the sensory integrative model to include the cognitive, intra- and interpersonal aspects.

EXPLANATORY USEFULNESS

As an explanatory tool, the sensory integration model is both helpful and limiting. The focus on basic development as a foundation for higher level skills such as academic learning is useful. However, the large amount of neurophysiologic and evolutionary theory incorporated into the model is not easy to understand and even less easy to explain to others. Explanation is particularly difficult with persons who lack knowledge of neurophysiologic and neuroanatomic terms. The best explanation is provided in *Sensory Integration and the Child* (60). However, the lack of graphic models reduces the effectiveness of the explanation for anyone who has difficulty with words alone.

COMMONALITY

The concept of following developmental sequences in organizing a program has been used by educators for many years. Thus, educators should understand the sensory integrative model as a developmental technique. However, educators are not familiar as a rule with the development of the nervous system. Thus, the commonality ends at the point of recognizing developmental relationships.

Some educators are familiar with the use of multisensory techniques to facilitate learning. For those teachers, the systematic presentation of sensory input is understandable. Nevertheless, there is a need to translate

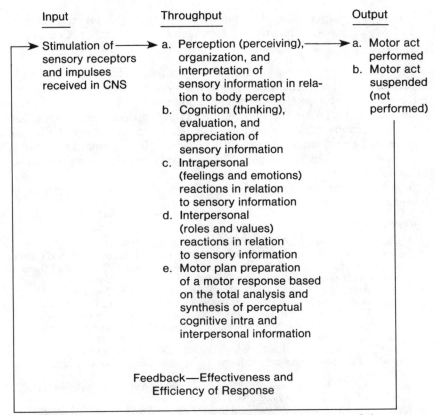

Input	Throughput	Output
Stimulation of sensory receptors and impulses received in CNS	a. Perception (perceiving), organization, and interpretation of sensory information in relation to body percept b. Cognition (thinking), evaluation, and appreciation of sensory information c. Intrapersonal (feelings and emotions) reactions in relation to sensory information d. Interpersonal (roles and values) reactions in relation to sensory information e. Motor plan preparation of a motor response based on the total analysis and synthesis of perceptual cognitive intra and interpersonal information	a. Motor act performed b. Motor act suspended (not performed)

Feedback—Effectiveness and
Efficiency of Response

Figure 12.19. The cognitive, intra- , and interpersonal aspects of the sensory integration model.

Table 12.15
Sensory Integration Model Summary Critique

Evaluation Criteria	Very Good 1	Moderately Good 2	3	4	Very Poor 5
Frame of reference	x				
Clarity			x		
Uniqueness		x			
Research guide	x				
Specialization	x				
Elaboration/refinement	x				
Explanatory usefulness		x			
Commonality			x		
Practice model	x				

much of the sensory integrative model into very simple language and to use common words as the primary approach to commonality of concepts.

PRACTICE MODEL

The sensory integration model has begun to develop practice models as evident by the delineation of specific syndromes and sequences of intervention techniques using specified equipment. Also, the model has been shown to be useful in evaluating and programming for other diagnosis groups besides learning-disabled children. Other diagnoses include emotional disturbance, autism, schizophrenia, mental retardation, brain injury and blindness. The age range also has been expanded to include adults.

A summary of the sensory integration model evaluation criteria is presented in Table 12.15.

References

1. Baldwin BT: Occupational therapy. *Am J Care Cripples* 8:447–451, 1919.
2. Baldwin BT: Helping the wounded soldier to "come back." *Mod Hosp* 12:370–374, 1919.
3. Baldwin BT: *Report of the Department of Occupational Therapy*, Walter Reed General Hospital, Takoma Park, Washington, DC, 1919.
4. Baldwin BT: *Occupational Therapy Applied to Restoration of Function of Disabled Joints.* Walter Reed General Hospital, Takoma Park, Washington, DC, 1919.
5. Taylor M: Anatomical considerations and techniques in using occupations as exercise for orthopedic disabilities: Introduction, and shoulder girdle and back. *Occup Ther Rehabil* 13:13–20, 1934.
6. Taylor M: The treatment of orthopedic conditions. *Can J Occup Ther* 2:1–8, 1934.
7. Taylor M: Precautions necessary with orthopedic cases. *Occup Ther Rehabil* 6:137–141, 1927.
8. Dunton WR, Licht S: *Occupational Therapy: Principles and Practice*, Springfield, Ill, Charles C Thomas, 1950, revised, 1957.
9. Licht S: The objectives of occupational therapy. *Occup Ther Rehabil* 26:17–22, 1947.
10. Licht S: Kinetic occupational therapy. In Dunton WR, Licht S: *Occupational Therapy: Principles and Practice.* Springfield, Ill, Charles C Thomas, 1957, pp 53–83.
11. Licht S: Kinetic analysis of crafts and occupations. *Occup Ther Rehabil* 26:75–78, 1947.
12. Licht S: Dosage in kinetic occupational therapy. *Occup Ther Rehabil* 26:167–171, 1947.
13. Licht S: Modifications of tools and activities in kinetic occupational therapy. *Occup Ther Rehabil* 26:240–247, 1947.
14. Trombly CA: *Occupational Therapy for Physical Dysfunction*, 2nd ed. Baltimore, Williams & Wilkins, 1983.
15. Charart SE: Comparison of volar and dorsal splinting of the hemiplegic hand. *Am J Occup Ther* 22:319–321, 1968.
16. Neuhaus BE, et al: A survey of rationales for and against hand splinting in hemiplegia. *Am J Occup Ther* 35:83–90, 1981.
17. Banus B, Kent CA, Norton YS, Sukiennicki DR, Becker ML: *The Developmental Therapist*, 2nd ed. Thorofare, NJ, Charles B. Slack, 1979.
18. Mysak ED, Fiorentino MR: Neurophysiological considerations in occupational therapy for the cerebral palsied. *Am J Occup Ther* 15:112–117, 1961.
19. Fiorentino MR: *Reflex Testing Methods for Evaluating CNS Development.* Springfield, Ill, Charles C Thomas, 1963, 1973.
20. Fiorentino MR: *A Basis for Sensorimotor Development, Normal and Abnormal.* Springfield, Ill, Charles C Thomas, 1981.
21. Fiorentino MR: *Normal and Abnormal Development: The Influences of Primitive Reflexes on Motor Development.* Springfield, Ill, Charles C Thomas, 1972.
22. Fiorentino M: The changing dimension of occupational therapy. *Am J Occup Ther* 20:251–252, 1966.

23. Milani Comparetti A: The neurophysiologic and clinical implications of studies on fetal motor behavior. *Semin Perinatol* 5:183–189, 1981.
24. Rood MS: Neurophysiological reactions as a basis for physical therapy. *Phys Ther Rev* 34:444–449, 1954.
25. Rood MS: The use of sensory receptors to activate, facilitate and inhibit motor response, automatic and somatic, in developmental sequence. In *Approaches to the Treatment of Patients with Neuromuscular Dysfunction.* Dubuque, Iowa, William C. Brown, 1964, pp 26–37.
26. Rood MS: Use of reflexes as an aid in occupational therapy. In *Occupational Therapy as a Link in Rehabilitation.* Copenhagen, Denmark, Proceedings of the Second International Congress of the World Federation of Occupational Therapy, 1958, pp 166–176.
27. Rood MS: Every one counts. *Am J Occup Ther* 12:326–329, 1958.
28. Rood MS: Neurophysiological mechanisms utilized in the treatment of neuromuscular dysfunction. *Am J Occup Ther* 10:220–225, 1956.
29. Rood MS: Proprioceptive neuromuscular facilitation and demonstration physiotherapy and occupational therapy. *South African Cerebral Palsy J* 13:12–15, 1969.
30. Rood MS: Occupational therapy in the treatment of the cerebral palsied. *Phys Ther Rev* 32:76–82, 1952.
31. Stockmeyer SA: An interpretation of the approach to Rood to the treatment of neuromuscular dysfunction. *Am J Phys Med* (NUSTEP Proceedings) 46:900–956, 1967.
32. Stockmeyer SA: A sensorimotor approach to treatment. In Pearson PH, Williams CE: *Physical Therapy Services in the Developmental Disabilities.* Springfield, Ill, Charles C Thomas, 1972, pp 186–222.
33. Huss J: Application of the Rood techniques to treatment of the physically handicapped child. In West W: *Occupational Therapy for the Multiply Handicapped Child.* Chicago, University of Chicago, 1965, pp 86–97.
34. Huss J: An introduction to treatment techniques developed by Margaret Rood. In Perlmutter S: *Neuroanatomy and Neurophysiology Underlying Current Treatment Techniques for Sensorimotor Dysfunction.* University of Illinois, Division of Services for Crippled Children, circa, 1970, pp 89–94.
35. Carlsen PN: Comparison of two occupational therapy approaches for treating the young cerebral palsied child. *Am J Occup Ther* 29:267–272, 1975.
36. Rider BA: Effects of neuromuscular facilitation on cross transfer. *Am J Occup Ther* 25:84–89, 1971.
37. Pedretti L: *Occupational Therapy, Practice Skills for Physical Dysfunction.* St. Louis, Mosby, 1981, pp 151–154.
38. Hopkins H, Smith H: *Willard and Spackman's Occupational Therapy,* 5th ed. Philadelphia, Lippincott, 1978, pp 127–130.
39. Abreau B: *Physical Disabilities Manual.* New York, Raven Press, 1981, pp 117–140.
40. Farber S: *Neurorehabilitation: A Multisensory Approach.* Philadelphia, Saunders, 1982, pp 115–177.
41. Ayres AJ: The visual-motor function. *Am J Occup Ther* 7:130–138, 155–156, 1958.
42. Ayres AJ: *Perceptual-Motor Dysfunction in Children.* The Greater Cincinnati District, Ohio Occupational Therapy Association, 1964 (monograph).
43. Ayres AJ: Perceptual-motor training for children. In Satteley C: *Approaches to the Treatment of Patients with Neuromuscular Dysfunction,* Third International Congress of the World Federation of Occupational Therapy. Dubuque, Iowa, W. C. Brown, 1964.
44. Ayres AJ: Interrelation of perceptual function, and treatment. *Phys Ther* 46:741–744, 1966.
45. Ayres AJ: Tactile functions. *Am J Occup Ther* 18:6–11, 1964.
46. Ayres AJ: Methods of evaluating perceptual motor dysfunction. In *Proceedings of the Third International Congress of the World Federation of Occupational Therapy.* Philadelphia, University of Pennsylvania, 1962.
47. Ayres AJ: The development of perceptual-motor abilities: a theoretical basis for treatment of dysfunction. *Am J Occup Ther* 17:221–225, 1963.
48. Ayres AJ: Patterns of perceptual-motor dysfunction in children: a factor analytic study. *Percep Mot Skills* 20:335–368, 1965.

49. Ayres AJ, Reid W: The self drawing as an expression of perceptual-motor dysfunction. *Cortex* 2:254–265, 1966.
50. Godfrey BB, Kephart NC: *Movement Patterns and Motor Education.* New York, Appleton-Century-Crofts, 1969, p 305.
51. Llorens LA: Identification of the Ayres' syndromes in emotionally disturbed children: an exploratory study. *Am J Occup Ther* 22:286–288, 1968.
52. Fox JVD: Cutaneous stimulation: effects on selected tests of perception. *Am J Occup Ther* 18:53–55, 1964.
53. Sleeper ML: Body balance and space perception. *Am J Occup Ther* 17:194–197, 1963.
54. Ayres AJ: Reading—a product of sensory integrative processes. In Smith HK: *Perception and Reading.* Newark, Del, International Reading Association, 1968, pp 77–82.
55. Ayres AJ: Sensory integrative processes and neuropsychological learning disabilities. In Hellmuth J: *Learning Disabilities,* Seattle, Wash, Special Child Publications, 1968, vol 3, pp 41–58.
56. Ayres AJ: Perceptual motor training for children. In Schnebly M: *Approaches to the Treatment of Patients with Neuromuscular Dysfunction.* Dubuque, Iowa, William C. Brown, 1964, pp 17–22.
57. Ayres AJ: Methods of evaluating perceptual motor dysfunction. In *Proceedings: World Federation of Occupational Therapists,* 3rd International Congress. New York, American Occupational Therapy Association, 1962, pp 113–117.
58. Ayres AJ: *Sensory Integration and Learning Disorders.* Los Angeles, Calif, Western Psychological Service, 1972.
59. Ayres AJ: Sensorimotor foundations of academic ability. In Cruckshank WM, Hallahan DP: *Perception and Learning Disabilities in Children, Volume 2.* Syracuse, NY, Syracuse University Press, 1975.
60. Ayres AJ: *Sensory Integration and the Child.* Los Angeles, Calif, Western Psychological Service, 1979.
61. Ayres AJ: Learning disabilities and the vestibular system. *J Learn Disabil* 11:18–29, 1978.
62. Ayres AJ: *Southern California Sensory Integration Tests.* Los Angeles, Calif, Western Psychological Service, 1972, revised 1980.
63. Ayres AJ: *Interpreting the Southern California Sensory Integration Tests.* Los Angeles, Calif, Western Psychological Service, 1976.
64. Ayres AJ: *Southern California Post Rotatory Nystamus Test.* Los Angeles, Calif, Western Psychological Service, 1975.
65. King LJ: A sensory-integrative approach to schizophrenia. *Am J Occup Ther* 28:529–536, 1974.
66. Ayres AJ: Research in sensory-integrative development: professional and theoretical implications. In Price A, Gilfoyle E, Myers C: *Research in Sensory-Integrative Development.* Rockville, Md, American Occupational Therapy Association, 1976, pp 107–109.
67. Danella EA: A study of tactile preference in multiply-handicapped children. *Am J Occup Ther* 27:457–462, 1973.
68. McKibbin EH: The effect of additional tactile stimulation in a perceptual-motor treatment program for school children. *Am J Occup Ther* 27:191–196, 1973.
69. Silberzahn M: Sensory-integrative function in child guidance clinic population. *Am J Occup Ther* 29:28–33, 1975.
70. Ward SE: Order effects on selected perceptual motor tests. *Am J Occup Ther* 27:321–325, 1973.
71. Ayres AJ: Relation between Gesell, developmental quotients and later perceptual motor performance. *Am J Occup Ther* 23:11–17, 1969.

CHAPTER 13

Descriptive Models: Intrapersonal and Interpersonal Performance Areas

PREOCCUPATIONAL THERAPY MODELS

From 1901 through 1916 a number of physicians, mostly psychiatrists, nurses and a few early therapists wrote about the effect of occupation on the insane. Their ideas were founded primarily on observation tempered with their knowledge of moral treatment. The theory of psychodynamics is not evidenced. Instead there is reference to the development of good habits to counteract faulty education while promoting proper methods of thinking.

The predominant frame of reference for the use of occupations with persons committed to mental institutions was two-fold. The first viewpoint stated that nature abhors a vacuum and will not tolerate total inactivity of the mind and body. Rather nature will fill the time and space with something. The expression that "idleness is the devil's playground" fits into this "vacuum approach." Thus, Thayer (1) states that "You cannot drive out morbid thoughts and keep them out, unless you fill their place with thoughts that are more healthy." In contrast the statement from the second point of view is that two thoughts cannot occupy the mind at the same time. Barrus (2) states that a "congenial occupation demanding one's attention furnishes a healthy channel for the thoughts and thus morbid fancies get crowded out." This point of view might be called the "substitution approach." Both viewpoints shared a common idea that idleness leads to excessive introspection, whereas occupation tends to direct attention toward activity occurring outside of the self.

The value of occupation according to these early writers can be summarized in the following assumptions:

1. Occupation is a normal part of living and is of value in maintaining health and well-being. According to Dercum who is quoted in Thayer (1), "The highest degree of health is constant, other things equal, with the highest degree of fun and activity." Van Nuys (3) says that "It is man's lot to work and in performance of the tasks has come his greatest degree of peace, happiness and contentment."

2. Occupations increase attention span. In 1902, Schwab (4) said "work (occupation) takes possession of attention and interest as well as sensory mechanisms." According to Atwood (5), through occupation the "power of attention and sense of perception is rendered acute."

3. Occupation exercises the mind and keeps it active. Sawyer (6) felt

the real purpose of work (occupation) therapy was "to exercise the mind just as massage exercises the muscles and to create new channels of thought." Haviland (7) suggests that the "use of hands means at least an elementary activity of the mind."

4. Occupation should have a definite object which the patient can appreciate. Haviland (7) states that "all occupation should have a definite object—should appeal to the patient."

5. Occupation should be selected according to the needs of the individual. Atwood (5) says that it is "always brightly deservable to fit the occupation to the individual case." Barrus (2) suggests that "each patient should be studied, his strength, his age, his nervous conditions and station in life, his tastes and capabilities before assigning an occupation." According to Ricksher (8), the "occupation selected for an individual should be suited to his intellectual ability, his normal as well as his present intellectual level."

6. Occupation should be an organized effort, and not haphazard. Cohn (9) suggested that the main feature of occupation is "a systematized schedule which satisfactorily accounts for every hour of the patient's day." According to Fields (10) "the best occupation is that of carefully trained and systematic effort with a definite purpose which demands self-control and concentration."

7. Occupation should be selected for the patient's recovery, not for the hospital's profit. Ricksher (8) states that "in the practical application of occupation, the improvement of the patient's condition should be the primary aim."

Suggestions for Intervention

There was little agreement among the authors as to what constituted an effective intervention program. The following statements summarize some of the approaches.

Thayer (1) suggests that "the best work is play. The best play is work and both are given recognition as means of cure." However, he does not elaborate.

Atwood (5) states that "occupations should correspond to those they would choose in their natural home life." He also felt that as a rule active methods of occupations and diversions were more valuable than passive.

Wade (11) felt that for the invalid, occupation should be of an outdoor character. On the other hand, Herring (12) indicates that different kinds of occupation and diversion should be furnished, both on the wards and elsewhere. He further states that special forms of occupation or diversion to be adapted should fit with the local conditions, needs and opportunities, as well as with the special interest, resourcefulness and ability of the leader.

Expected Results

Some general statements about the results of occupational treatment are provided. Moyer (13) says that as a result of employment, patients are less restless, sleep better, appetites improve and secretions become normal. Ricksher (8) claims that (a) patients are less introspective, (b) occupation gives hopes and ambition and (c) occupation reeducates as well as breaks up a day. Frost (14) felt that patients received therapeutic, recreational and economic values from occupation.

Evans and Mikels (15) summarized the effects of occupations as (a) reactivating apathetic patients, (b) attaining and retaining attention, (c) holding interest of patients and (d) reforming the behavior from destructiveness and vicious dominance to orderly personal conduct. Thus, it appears that the early writers were able to see the normalizing effect of occupation. Perhaps the evidence was easier to observe because the patient's degree of disorganization was greater prior to the use of drugs.

PSEUDOPHARMACEUTICAL MODELS

Historically, it is unclear who started the analysis of occupations according the their apparent pharmaceutical properties. Although Tracy and Dunton's models are reviewed, George Barton was writing about using occupations for their stimulating or sedating effects in 1915. His classic statement is that the "first thing to be done. . .is for occupational therapy to provide an occupation which will produce a *similar therapeutic effect to that of every drug in materia medica*" (16). Tracy stated a year earlier, in 1914, that occupations possess properties like remedies and can be classified according to their physiological effects (12). Dunton's statement does not appear until 1928 (18), but he may have accepted the idea earlier. Nevertheless, the organization of occupations in terms of properties attributed to drugs appears in an analysis of crafts during the 1920s (19).

Invalid Occupations—Tracy

FRAME OF REFERENCE

Susan Tracy seems to have drawn primarily from her own childhood experiences and from the observation of others in setting forth her ideas on occupational therapy. She does not mention reading the works of authors who practiced moral treatment or the reports of hospital superintendents. In her book *Studies in Invalid Occupations* (20), two chapters were written by hospital superintendents whom she knew personally. However, no mention is made of other writers, except a brief quote from John Dewey regarding the relationship of play to occupation.

Tracy was employed at a facility for psychiatric conditions. However, her illustrations in invalid occupations have more physical dysfunction problems than psychiatric. Her model is included in the subsection on psychosocial models because it focuses on psychological assumptions.

ASSUMPTIONS

1. There is a human impulse for activity (21, p. 398).
2. Just so surely as man is a motor animal, so surely will he turn to motor activities for the restoration of function (21, p. 397).
3. Whoever succeeds in making an invalid happy and in maintaining this same state of happiness has gone a long way toward making him well (22).

4. It is good to earn money. It is better to earn good health. Best of all is earning the love and respect of all (23, p. 403).
5. One should grasp first the patient's mental make-up to appreciate his point of view and to be able to deftly dovetail new thoughts of worth to the already existing interests (21, p. 173).
6. In working with patients, one must consider the case individually and find just the work indicated (24, p. 56).
7. Time, terms, methods, must all be determined by the individual ability of the teacher and the pupil (21, p. 397).
8. Occupations possess properties which can be classified according to their physiological effects (25, p. 386).
9. Stimulation by some carefully chosen occupation leaves the patient in better condition than does stimulation by drugs (25, p. 386).

CONCEPTS

Amusements—serve to pass time away (22, p. 172).

Occupations—treasure and redeem the time (22, p. 172).

Occupational therapy—the treatment of disease by occupation (26, p. 120).

EXPECTED RESULTS

1. Reduced pain and suffering.
2. Reduced self-mutilation and self-destructive behavior.

ASSESSMENT INSTRUMENTS

Tracy indicates that the following tests were developed along the lines of certain mental tests such as the Binet or Binet-Simon, the Yerkes, Bridges and the Healey which were all early intelligence tests (27). She does not elaborate on the scoring of the tests or the use of the tests in evaluating patients' ability to perform occupations. Also, some of the instructions are vague. The purpose seems to have been to confirm or refute the findings of the intelligence tests.

1. Judgment in estimating distances test. Given a bit of leather and a pencil, the subject is required to make a line of dots at equal distances around the margin and at a uniform distance from the edge.
2. Simple coordination test. Given a leather punch, the subject is to punch a hole at each dot.
3. Aesthetic coordination and rhythm test. Given two pieces of punched leather and a thong, the subject is told to lace the two pieces together, arranging the thong so that a regular slope forms an attractive border.
4. Differentiation of Form and Size-Purposeful Relation Test. Given four different pieces of metal, the subject is to select, fit together and fasten to the leather, a clasp. (Note: Numbers 1 to 4 make a purse).
5. Opposites (rough and smooth) and Coarse Coordination Test.

Given a rough board, the subject is to smooth the board by sandpapering.

6. Aim Test (Also equilibrium and steadiness). Given a needle and thread, the subject is to thread the needle.

7. Contrast Movement (forward and backward). Given a large wooden crochet hook and strips of rag, the subject is to crochet a rug.

8. Differences and Similarities Test. Given a string and round and long beads, the subject is to form a necklace by alternating stringing the round and long beads.

9. Opposites Test (different textures). Given a piece of cotton flannel, the subject is to describe the two sides and tell which way the nap runs.

10. Reproduce by Pattern Test. Given a simple animal pattern, the subject is to cut out the animal from the cloth used in number 9.

11. Relations of Parts to Whole. Given a needle and thread, the subject is directed to baste together the pieces that were cut in number 10.

12. Opposites (hard and soft, smooth and lumpy). Given the stuffing material, the subject is to stuff the cloth case. (Numbers 9 to 12 make a stuffed animal.)

13. Relative Position, Sense of Rhythm and Purposeful Repetition. Given a small frame with tape wound in one direction, the subject is to weave in the transverse tape or flat reed as in chairseating.

14. Analytical Test. Given an unfinished reed basket, the subject is required to ravel and describe its parts.

15. Sense of Quality, Weight, Form, Differences and Similarities and Arithmetic Test. Given a large lump of salt bead mixture, the subject is instructed to mold 24 beads of like size.

16. Sense of Form, Rhythm, Size, Practical Judgment, Efficiency and the Deduction of Value from Work Test. Given a skein of yarn, the subject is to wind the yarn into a ball.

17. Sense of Free Association of Ideas, Flow of Thought, Relation of Parts to Whole, Differences and Similarities of Color and Color (organization) Test. Given colored papers, the subject is to build (make) an original picture.

18. Trial and Success Learning Test. Given the directions to the sailor's knots, the subject is to tie successfully the knots.

19. Stimulation of Attention by Element of Surprise Test. Given the ink and a stencil, the subject is to apply the color over the stencil.

20. Same as no. 19. Given a piece of paper the subject is required to fold the paper in half, quarters and eighths. Then to tear or cut irregular openings on the edges of the folds which are opened up to reveal the design created.

21. Visualization Test (Similar to #20). Given a piece of paper, the subject is instructed to fold it in half, quarters and eighths. Before tearing and cutting the subject is instructed to consider the shape of the opening and is then required to draw or verbally describe the object thus made.

22. Series of Acts Test for Memory. Given instructions for folding paper, the subject is to make the object. No indication is given as to how many steps the subject must do from memory.
23. Color sense and Practical Judgment Test. Given two primary colors such as blue and yellow, the subject is to mix them while naming the colors in order of handling and the result.
24. Logical Sequence. Given a small box of freshly mixed plaster of paris, a half walnut shell and some Vaseline, the subject is instructed to cover the outside of the shell with the vaseline and press it into the plaster. When set remove the shell and mix a little more plaster. Instruct the subject to fill in the cavity made by the shell.
25. Recognize and Rectify Error Test. Given a torn page from a book, thin paper, scissors and paste, the subject is instructed to mend the book.

INTERVENTION TECHNIQUES

1. Media
See Table 13.1 for a list of 171 activities included in *Studies of Invalid Occupations* (20).
2. Methods
Tracy's methods probably were based on what is known as "common sense." Thus, she did not seem to feel the need to elaborate. However, analysis of her case histories suggests that she used some of the following approaches. (a) Select occupations which are of interest to the individual or familiar to the person. (b) Projects should be simple and quick for those with short attention span. (c) If possible the occupation should have an economic value. (d) Projects should teach useful skills.
3. Equipment
   a. A good sized room, well lighted with heater
   b. Two long tables
   c. Closets for storage
   d. Blackboard
   e. Couch
   f. Bed table or bench
   g. Scissors, needle and thread
   h. Pen, knife and paste brush
   i. Ruler
   j. Pliers, awl and hammer
4. Precautions
   a. Watch for eye strain.
   b. Watch for signs of fatigue.
   c. Do not aggravate symptoms.
   d. Do not overspend the family's income.

SUMMARY

Tracy viewed occupations as having the same attributes as drugs. She felt that occupations could have the effects of a stimulant, depressant,

Table 13.1
List of Occupations[a]

Afghan, rake-work, 48
Animals
Cloth, 50, 133
Cut paper, 24
Fruit and vegetable, 46, 77
Apple-seed mousetraps, 41

Baby's handkerchief cap, 136
Bags
Bean, 82
Braid, 144
Leather, 143
Raffia, 54
Basketry, 91, 128, 147
Baskets
May, 41, 43
Raffia, 92
Strong, 128
Beads, sealing wax, 64
Beadwork, 91, 148
Bed-desk, 48
Bed puffs, 149
Belts, tape, 61
Birch-bark frames, 125
Bird, flying, 35
Birthday cake board, 122
Blackberries, 90
Black cat balls, 56
Black Dinah Emeries, 86
Block printing, 120
Blue prints, 79
Bookbinding, 24, 112
Books
Scrap, 56
Story, 24
Buckles, sealing wax, 63

Cake board birthday, 122
Calendar quilt, 97
Candle penwiper, 56
Cards, dinner, 69
Chair caning, 145
Chair, grandmother's, 99
Charcoal drawing, 70
Charlotte Russe cases, 57
Chatelaine pinballs, 82
Chinese junk, 31
Christmas stockings, 60
Cloth animals, 50, 133
Clothespin dolls, 45
Coloring photographs, 68
Cook stove, paper box, 45
Cork and pin furniture, 46

Cottages, paper box, 44
Cozy, egg, 101
Crocheted dolls, 52
Cross-stitch embroidery, 72
Cupboard, paper-box, 45
Cut out pictures, 59

Designing toilets, 71
Desk, bed, 48
Dinner cards, 69
Dishes
Eggshell, 45
Leather, 45
Dolls
Clothespin, 45
Crocheted, 52
Nature, 45
Nut, 52
Rag, 52, 103
String, 45
Dory, 27, 28
Drawing, 74
Dyeing, 66

Egg cozy, 101
Eggshell dishes, 45
Embroidery, cross-stich, 72
Emery
Black Dinah, 86
Heart-shaped, 86
Envelope sachets, 70
Eyeglass cords, 127

Fans, turkey feather, 107
Fish pinball, 87
Flowers, ribbon, 88
Flying bird, 35
Frames, picture, 57, 125
Frieze, cut paper, 24, 59, 134
Frog, Japanese, 38
Fruit and vegetable animals, 46, 77
Furnishing, house, 26
Furniture
Cork and pin, 46
Paper-box, 44

Gardening, 110
Go-cart, 44
Gondola, 30
Grandmother's chair, 99

Hammock, doll's, 55
Heart-shaped emery, 86
Holders, 100
House furnishing, 26

Table 13.1—Continued

Spatterflies, 78	Tooling, leather, 71
Stencil, 65, 77	Turkey feather fans, 107
Stockings, Christmas, 60	Turtle penwiper, 57
Stories, picture, 24	
Stove, 45	Vegetable animals, 46, 77
Straw braiding, 126	Violets, ribbon, 88
Street car signs, 77	Watch cords, 127
String doll, 45	Water color painting, 70
Sweet peas, ribbon, 89	Wax, sealing, 63
	Weaving, 53, 74, 143
Table mats, 66	Whittling, 125
Tape belts, 61	Wishbone Indian, 80
Toilets, designing, 71	Writing for the blind, 141

[a] Reprinted from S. E. Tracy (20), pp. 171–173, with permission from Arno Press.

or anesthetic. Furthermore, she felt that nurses were the most competent to administer the occupations and encouraged schools of nursing to include training in occupations in the curriculum.

Intervention was based on an analysis of each individual person. Although Tracy does not outline her evaluation criteria her case examples suggest consideration of age, sex, disorder, occupation, general temperament and socioeconomic status. The assessment tests listed under assessment techniques were developed in response to suggestions that occupational therapy could be used to assess intellectual capacity. Tracy does not indicate she used them for initial evaluation purposes.

Intervention techniques were based primarily on distracting the person from confining or limiting situations over time. None of the techniques appears to be used to remediate any specific physical motor problem. Most of the techniques are organized to deal with feelings or emotions by changing the mood or affect, whether the problem was of physical, sensory or psychological origin.

Therapeutic Occupation Model—Dunton

FRAME OF REFERENCE

William Rush Dunton, Jr., M.D., began his work in occupational therapy in 1911 when he gave a short course to nurses on occupations for mental diseases (28). His interest had been aroused by Edward N. Brush, M.D., who was Superintendent of the Sheppard and Enoch Pratt Hospital where Dr. Dunton was Assistant Physician.

Dunton's great grandfather was a woodcarver, his father had a number of tools and his mother did needlework. His own interests had been in woodworking and printing. In medical school he had made scenery for the drama club. Later, Dr. Dunton read many of the articles in the *American Journal of Insanity (American Journal of Psychiatry)* regarding moral treatment, work cure and diversion. However, many of his basic ideas seem to have been formulated already through his own experience regarding the therapeutic value of occupations.

ASSUMPTIONS ABOUT PLAY, WORK AND OCCUPATION

1. The play instinct, which exists in all of us, is too often suppressed and frequently with disastrous consequences, as many mental breakdowns may be attributed to the fact that the patient leads a one-sided existence (29).
2. Many individuals do not know how to play and must be taught (29).
3. Work of some sort has a very definite value in the reeducation of our patients (29).
4. The man who has nothing to do but amuse himself is usually one of the most unhappy and the man who is most happy and for whom we have the greatest respect is the one who is always busy with something and doing it well (30).
5. The desire for occupation seems to be almost instinctive in man and plays a major role in his existence (31).
6. A desire for occupation persists even in the sick, until they have lost interest in living (31).

ASSUMPTIONS ABOUT ATTENTION AND INTEREST

1. But one idea can occupy the focus of the attention at a given time (29).
2. We can frequently best help our patients by training the attention (29).
3. The power of attention is dependent upon emotion (29).
4. The patient's attention must be engrossed (30).
5. The occupation selected should be within the patient's estimated interest and capacity (32).
6. The work must be interesting (33).
7. Occupational therapy can give patients broader interests, make them less self-centered and stimulate the cultivation of a hobby (34).

ASSUMPTIONS ABOUT THE CLASSIFICATION OF OCCUPATIONS

1. Categories of amusement (29)
   a. Large groups
   b. Small groups
   c. Individual
2. Occupation is not restricted to crafts alone. Games, exercises, music, reading etc., are quite as important (29).
3. Occupations may be grouped or classified into stimulating, sedative, active or passive (32).
4. All handwork or craft activities are grouped around six materials: wood, metal, paper, textiles, clay and leather (32).

ASSUMPTIONS ABOUT THE USE OF OCCUPATION WITH TYPES OF PSYCHIATRIC DIAGNOSIS

1. In the case of mild excitement occupation will keep the patient's mind more continuously on one subject than is possible if he does not have stimulus (29).

2. In case of marked excitement, it is usually impossible to use occupation in treatment (29).
3. In case of dementia, the purpose may be to reeducate, to train the patient to develop the mental process by educating the hands, eye muscles, etc. (29).

ASSUMPTIONS ABOUT THE PURPOSES OF OCCUPATIONAL THERAPY

1. The primary purpose of occupation may be said to be to divert the patient's attention from unpleasant subjects (29).
2. The mechanism by means of which a recovery is brought about may be summed up by the words *substitution* or *replacement* (29).
3. Any means, such as occupation, which helps to keep our patients in a cheerful frame of mind is of undoubted value (30).
4. Patients are much less apt to be restless (30).
5. Another purpose of occupation may be to give the patient a hobby (29).
6. The person who has a hobby has a safety valve which enables him to escape worries which the more idle person cannot (30).
7. Another purpose is that of giving the patient a means of livelihood (29).
8. Regular occupation should partake more of the quality of labor than of amusement, as such is a more normal way of living (29).

ASSUMPTIONS ABOUT THE TYPES OF OCCUPATIONAL THERAPY

1. The subject of occupational therapy may be divided into three parts (33).
   a. Invalid occupation
   b. Occupational therapy
   c. Vocational education
2. Invalid occupation is chiefly diversional (33).
3. The term occupational therapy should be reserved for the instances in which work or occupation is given with the primary object of function (33).
4. Vocational training or education when given to reestablish function or to give a more normal view of life may be classed as a form of occupational therapy (33).

ASSUMPTIONS ABOUT IMPLEMENTING THE OCCUPATIONAL THERAPY PROGRAM

1. The treatment should be prescribed and administered under constant medical advice and supervision and correlated with other treatment of the patient (32).
2. The treatment should, in each case, be specifically directed to the needs of the individual patient (32).
3. As the patient's strength and capability increase, the type and extent of the occupation should be regulated and graded accordingly (32).
4. As a rule, the effort should be directed to arouse the patient in something with which he is unfamiliar (29).

5. Novelty, variety, individuality and utility of the product enhances the value of occupation as a treatment measure (32).
6. The object of treatment to be attained should be kept in mind, and treatment should not degenerate into mere diversion (32).
7. The only reliable measurement of the treatment is the effect on the patient (32).

Assumptions about the Fundamental Principles of Occupational Therapy According to Dunton (33)

1. That work should be carried on with cure as a main object.
2. The work must be interesting.
3. The patient should be carefully studied.
4. That one form of occupation should not be carried to the point of fatigue.
5. That it should have some useful end.
6. That it preferably should lead to an increase in the patient's knowledge.
7. That it should be carried on with others.
8. That all possible encouragement should be given the worker.
9. That work resulting in a poor or useless product is better than idleness.

CONCEPTS

Occupational therapy—the use of any occupation for remedial purposes (35)

Interest—the state of consciousness in which the attention is attracted to a task, accompanied by a more or less pleasurable emotional state (32)

Attention—described as attraction to a task without emotional content or accomplishment (32)

Stimulating occupation—one which is varied in character and requires active correlation to direct the various motor processes connected with it (32)

Sedative occupation—one which requires repetition of similar (stereotyped) movements and thoughts (32)

Active occupation—one which requires active physical exercise (32)

Passive occupation—one in which the patient takes no active part, but passively observes or listens (32)

EXPECTED RESULTS (32)

1. Exercise body and mind in healthy activity.
2. Arouse interest, courage and confidence in overcoming disability.
3. Reestablish capacity for industrial and social usefulness.
4. Reestablish health.
5. Training in orderly habits of thought.
6. Concentration of attention.
7. Better contact with reality.
8. Functional training of muscles and joints.

ASSESSMENT PROCEDURES

Dunton did not use any specific assessment procedures except to observe and ask questions about possible interests.

INTERVENTION STRATEGIES

1. Media (28)—the media first used by Dunton is listed.
   a. Games—cribbage, euchre, whist; bridge, fan-tan, solitaire, baker's dozen, klondike, rainbow, dominoes, sniff and checkers
   b. String work—braid, flat or round, tie square, crown and wall knots
   c. Paper folding—envelope, a cup, a fish's mouth, a frame and a box
   d. Paper cutting—a star, string of dolls
   e. Binding
   f. Crepe paper work
   g. Reed basketry
   h. Embroidery—cross stitch
   i. Leather work—carving and hammering
   j. Woodwork—wood carving, paper knives, canes, trays, bird houses, wind toys, stools
   k. Metal work—venetian iron work, hammering copper, making copper ornaments, initials, paper cutters
2. Methods
   a. Develop a regular schedule (36).
   b. Select activities with which the patient is unfamiliar (28).
3. Equipment—no special equipment except those needed to complete the crafts listed.
4. Precautions—avoid fatigue.

SUMMARY

The therapeutic occupations model is based on Dunton's belief that occupations such as crafts and games could be used to divert the attention of a person with psychiatric symptoms to think about the occupation rather than the unpleasant subjects. Dunton suggests that the process is one of substituting or replacing one thought for another on the assumption that only one thought can occupy the mind at one time.

A second belief of Dunton's was that everyone should have a hobby in which to engage as a means of escaping from the worries of the regular job and daily living. He felt that many persons with psychiatric symptoms did not know how to play and had not developed broad interests as a child. Through occupations he felt that play skills could be developed.

Dunton was concerned always that people be questioned and observed regarding their interests. He felt that occupations should be selected on the basis of interest and that occupational therapy could benefit people by broadening their interests. At the same time, he also felt that occupations had properties similar to drugs and could be used to stimulate or calm people when necessary. Thus, by observing a person's interests one could expand knowledge, while simultaneously effecting a cure through the selection of an occupation for its properties in relation to the symptoms presented.

Analysis and Critique of the Pseudopharmaceutical Model
FRAME OF REFERENCE

The invalid occupations model appears to be consistent with the organismic and humanistic philosophies. References to the individual turning to activity as a means for restoring function and to the value of appreciating the person's point of view in developing intervention plans suggest that the locus of control was maintained by the individual. The occupation worker was a facilitator not a controller of change.

Dunton's model of therapeutic occupations continues the theme of individual control by focusing on personal interest as a key to the selection of occupations. Interest is seen as internal mechanism expressed by positive feelings and emotions and by focusing attention on the object of interest. Such a focus on internal mechanisms is consistent with the organismic philosophy. The major difficulty with assessing the frame of reference is the lack of information. A few phrases are repeated but not expanded.

CLARITY

Neither Tracy nor Dunton explain in any detail their source of belief in the value of play, work, occupation or activity. Each accepts the value as self apparent. Likewise the need to individualize an intervention program also seems to be self-evident. However, their approach to the selection of an occupation differs somewhat. Tracy suggests the new thoughts of worth in occupations should be diverted to already existing interests (22), while Dunton suggests that the arousal should be through something with which the person is unfamiliar (36). Both seem to agree that diversion of the mind to an improved state is a major outcome (Fig. 13.1).

UNIQUENESS

To the model builders, the concepts of diversion and substitution seem to be the unique aspect. Perhaps if there were documentation that hospitalized persons recovered faster and required less medication, the concept of diversion would not have acquired a negative image of a nice but not necessary service. Apparently, the uniqueness was acceptable in

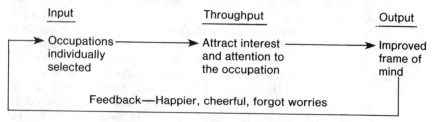

Figure 13.1. Diversional model.

the early years, but by today's standards such a statement of uniqueness is simply not enough.

RESEARCH GUIDE

The pseudopharmaceutical models probably contributed to the interest in activity analysis which could be classified as descriptive research. Although not accepted today in research there were many testimonials by therapists as to the effectiveness of occupations in improving the frame of mind and aiding recovery.

SPECIALIZATION

At the time the pseudopharmaceutical models were developed being an occupational therapist was a specialty in itself. Possibly, the only specialization might have been in psychiatric cases, physical cases and tuberculosis cases. Both Tracy and Dunton began their interest in occupational therapy through their work in psychiatric institutions which had a long history of using occupations. Thus, occupational therapy in psychiatry may be called the first specialization in the profession of occupational therapy. Nevertheless, the models do not seem to have been major influences beyond the first years.

ELABORATION AND REFINEMENT

Elaboration of the concepts of play and work and the role of occupation or activity in promoting health would have been helpful. Although Dunton knew Adolph Meyer well, he did not choose to elaborate on Meyer's ideas. Instead, Dunton's focus was on interest and attention. Perhaps Dunton saw the cognitive aspects as more important than the feelings, rhythms and balance that characterized Meyer's work. Dunton did elaborate on his concept of interest in 1951 (37). However, little attention was attracted in the occupational therapy community until Matsutsuya developed her checklist in 1969 (38).

EXPLANATORY USEFULNESS

The concept of substitution and its assumption that only one thought could occupy the mind at a time was widely accepted in the early days as a useful explanation to both professional and nonprofessional people. Unfortunately, the explanations fall short today. Diversion is not enough. There must be direction toward observant change as the primary target. Likewise, the assumption that occupations can substitute for drugs apparently was acceptable in the early years but would melt with skepticism today. Occupations may change moods, but the emphasis is on changing functional ability. Thus the pseudopharmaceutical models do not provide a useful explanation.

COMMONALITY

The pseudopharmaceutical model is the only one which suggests that pharmacists and occupational therapists may be meeting similar objectives for people, especially those with mental health problems. Certainly, today close coordination between pharmacy and occupational therapy

Table 13.2
Pseudopharmaceutical Model Summary Criteria

Evaluation Criteria	Very Good 1	Moderately Good			Very Poor 5
		2	3	4	
Frame of reference	x				
Clarity		x			
Uniqueness		x			
Research guide			x		
Specialization			x		
Elaboration/refinement			x		
Explanatory usefulness				x	
Commonality					x
Practice model				x	

seems to miss the mark. Thus, the pseudopharmaceutical model does not seem to suggest a commonality which is useful today.

PRACTICE MODEL

The major impact of the pseudopharmaceutical model seems to be on early activity analysis formats. Neither Tracy's or Dunton's models seem to have been widely developed in the literature beyond the descriptive stage, although some examples may never have been recorded. Most therapists seem to have preferred to follow the Meyer-Slagle models in actual practice.

SUMMARY

A summary of the evaluation criteria appears in Table 13.2.

Object Relations Model—the Azimas

FRAME OF REFERENCE

Object relations was developed because Wittkower (39), an associate of the Azimas, felt that occupational therapy in its present form (a) was of little value for the treatment of chronic psychotic patients, (b) excluded grossly disturbed patients, (c) offered media which were not in keeping with the regressed state of many of the patients and (d) was aimed at predominantly diversional activity. Azima (40) felt that occupational therapists did not understand that (a) a patient's ego system might be unable to control impulses, thus limiting normal living, (b) the symbolic significance of an object could be an important aspect of media and (c) an adequate theory could explain the use of occupational therapy and serve as a guide for selecting activities. Azima (40) suggested that the theory should be based on psychodynamic concepts related to instincts, mental structures and object relations.

ASSUMPTIONS

1. A partial libidinal regression to certain fixation points is a feature of all psychopathological states (41, p. 60).

2. The main feature of schizophrenia process may be seen as a defense against the anxiety of contact with objects which are experienced as frustrating and perceived as dangerous through projective mechanisms (41, p. 60).
3. The dynamic structure may be understood as:
   a. Due to a tendency to return to the stage of psychosexual development when the primary frustrations were experienced in a vain hope of finding gratification.
   b. Due to a tendency to go beyond this stage with the unconscious aim of obviating the primary frustrations (41, p. 60).
4. The result is withdrawal from an abandonment of object-relationships and the adoption of a narcissistic manner of existence (41, p. 60).
5. By fostering regression beyond the fixation points and by gratification of originally frustrated basic needs the fixation point may be abandoned and desired progression may ensue (41, p. 60).
6. Both regression and progression are facilitated if, for the gratification of needs and desires, appropriate primitive objects and substitute objects are offered (41, p. 60).
7. Created objects are the key phenomena representing the fantasy object relationships of the patient at the time (42, p. 177).
8. Created objects have a facilitatory effect on the uncovering of defenses, drives and transference relationships (42, p. 178).
9. Created objects may regressively evoke some early projections (42, p. 178).
10. The created object can become, by its continuous presence, an impetus for evoking associations and furthering the uncovering of unconscious processes (42, p. 179).
11. The created object may serve as means for (a) nonverbal discharge of needs, (b) nonverbal reorganization of needs (42, p. 179).
12. The created object may initiate the therapeutic process in the group (42, p. 179).
13. Fixation points and the regressive trends toward them are genetically initiated by frustration through inadequate gratification of basic object needs (40, p. 709).
14. Gratification should be fostered by offering of appropriate primitive objects (40, p. 709).
15. Projective material can provide data on the ego system, object relations, and body scheme (43, p. 216).
16. All needs are object needs, *i.e.*, there is a need for something which releases and gratifies that need (43, p. 219).
17. At different stages of development (oral, anal and genital), certain needs and their objects are emphasized more than others (43, p. 219).
18. Psychopathological states can be seen as persistence of unresolved infantile needs and related objects (fixation) (43, p. 219).

CONCEPTS

Withdrawal—a response to, and a defense against, anxiety arising from contact with objects (44, p. 121)

Anxiety—initiated and perpetuated by the expectancy of rejection and frustration and by the interplay of projected and introjected aggression in relation to external and internal objects (44, p. 121)

Primary organismic needs—oral and anal object needs associated and intermingled with the impulse to devour and destroy (44, p. 121)

Need—implies an appropriate object, at an appropriate time in an appropriate setting by an appropriate person (44, p. 121)

Ego Impairment (*ego disintegration, splitting*)—is the result of frustrations and fixations at the earliest stages of development (44, p. 121)

Sublimation—discharge of infantile drives in an inhibited, desexualized form (40, p. 709)

Projection—the visible nonverbal form of created objects may serve as a screen or a locality where fantasy object relationships may be projected with their associated drives and defenses erected against them (40, p. 709)

Free creation—patients are offered three media and are asked to make whatever comes to their mind (42, p. 177)

Free association—patients are asked to say what comes to their minds in regard to their own or others' creations (42, p. 177)

Projective group therapy—a group therapeutic situation in which some parts of the relating ego system and need system are sought in and through representation in an available external medium (42, p. 177)

Gratification—the offering of certain objects in an appropriate situation which will result in a decrease or discharge of dammed up tension due to the frustration and subsequent accumulation of drives in connection with controlling (superego) and integration (ego) systems (43, p. 218)

Projective material—material in which the patient is left to choose the object and the technique of manipulation (43, p. 216)

Projective tests—patient has to use the ready made materials which are always the same (43, p. 216)

Direct gratification—implies identical, similar or symbolically near primary; needed objects (breast, mother, milk, faces) are offered to the patient in a situation effectively similar to the primary mother-child state (43, p. 218)

Indirect gratification—implies essentially a social approach through superego reinforcement or atonement (43, p. 218-219)

Defense formation—the utilization of objects in such a way as to strengthen certain ego defenses and provide routes for sublimation of aggression and libidinal impulses (43)

Fantasy object relationship—during the different early stages of development, certain relationships with objects are made which remain unconscious but remain operative throughout life and influence later relationships (43, p. 220)

Projection—the mechanism by which a fantasy object relationship can be exteriorized (43, p. 220)

Introjection—Objects are endowed with characteristics which are derived from an inner necessity (43, p. 220)

Object situation or object field—objects are offered to the patient in a situation which evokes in the patient unconscious infantile prototypes which should be analyzed and understood if a therapeutic effect is expected (43, p. 220)

Symbolic readiness—the readiness to accept and respond to a symbol (43, p. 220)

Symbolic proximity—according to the degree of regression the objects should be farther or nearer, in form and in structure, to the primary objects (43, p. 220)

Object—an object is that which gratifies or frustrates a need in action or in fantasy, consciously or unconsciously (43, p. 219)

Object hierarchy—relates objects to the stages of development and unconscious need system operating at the time or having the greatest propensity to emerge (43, p. 220)

EXPECTED RESULTS

1. The therapeutic value of occupational therapy should be enhanced if the media offered are adapted to the regressive needs of the patients.
2. Provide gratification of basic needs which will (a) alleviate primitive feelings of anxiety, (b) lead to abandonment of fixation points, and (c) initiate a progression.

ASSESSMENT INSTRUMENT

The Azima battery (42, 43, 45) contains four steps (a) preparation, (b) production and completion, (c) association and (d) interpretation. Within the preparation phase the therapist should observe (a) the mode of approach of the patient to the object, (b) his selection of object, (c) his attitude toward the therapist and (d) his attitude toward other patients if in a group.

In the production and completion phase the patient is asked: (a) to do free drawing with a pencil, (b) to draw a whole person and a person of the opposite sex, (c) to make anything with clay, and (d) to do a finger painting. The association phase begins when the production is finished. The patient is asked to say what comes to mind, *i.e.*, to free associate about the object. In the interpretation phase, the general structural equilibrium of the mind is evaluated in terms of the status of drives, ego system and object relations. The specific assessment items are a determination of the degree to which the object ranges.

IMPLEMENTATION STRATEGIES

1. Media (39, 44)
   a. Oral objects—feeding milk in baby bottle, ball and bean bag throwing.
   b. Anal objects—mud, brown clay, cocoa power, cocoa paste, brown plasticine, finger paints, tearing paper, throwing darts.
   c. Structured activities—rope jumping, doll playing, listening to music and dancing, drawing on a blackboard, coloring, working with clay and making pots, playing games, such as badminton and ping pong.
   d. Making murals—depict childhood emotions.
2. Methods (39, 44)
   a. Offer objects to patients similar to those presented to babies in the oral or anal stage. Encourage smearing, tearing, and throwing.
   b. Decrease the resemblance and proximity to original objects as intervention proceeds.
   c. Attitude of permissive kindness.
3. Equipment—no specialized equipment.
4. Prerequisite skills—severely or moderately regressed behavior.

SUMMARY

Azima and his collaborators felt that there was too much emphasis on the diversional and occupational (work) aspects of occupational therapy rather than on the psychodynamic problems of diagnosis, especially schizophrenia. The model of object relations was an attempt to stress the dynamic value of occupational therapy rather than the traditional ego-strengthening function through the use of repression and suppression (Table 13.3). The focus of the object relations model is the object of the clinic environment and the symbolic interpretation of the meaning of objects. By helping people relate to objects at their level of psychodynamic development, the assumption is made that there will be a discharge of infantile drives, an uncovering of defense drives and transference relationships and a progression away from the regressed state of development.

Assessment involves having the person draw with a pencil, mold with clay and finger paint as projective techniques design to uncover the psychodynamic level of psychosexual development through interpretation of the object relationships. Intervention is begun at the lowest level, oral, and progresses through the anal, phallic and genital stages. Objects are selected which are characteristic or representative of each stage.

Analysis and Critique of the Object Relations Model
FRAME OF REFERENCE

The model of object relations is based on Freudian psychoanalysis which in turn is based on the mechanistic model. Locus of control is external to the individual. The environment, especially in childhood, provides or fails to provide for all basic needs. An infant is totally

Table 13.3
Comparison of Traditional and Dynamic
Occupational Therapy Outcomes[a]

Traditional	Dynamic
Purposes: 1. Divert attention from fantasy and inner preoccupation.	Purposes: 1. Provide objects which are representative of regressed fixated stages of psychosexual development
2. Produce a "normal" atmosphere for "pleasant occupation."	2. Encourage spontaneous free creation to uncover drives, defenses and transference.
3. Encourage socialization	3. Promote the free association of the objects by persons receiving intervention and interpretation by the therapist.
Mechanisms: 1. Repression 2. Suppression	Mechanisms: 1. Sublimation 2. Projection 3. Gratification

[a] Adapted from H. Azima and E. Wittkower: *American Journal of Occupational Therapy* 11:1–7, 1957 and H. Azima *et al.* (41).

dependent upon external objects, usually a mother or substitute. Psychiatric conditions are thus a result of the failure of the environment to meet basic needs. The role of the individual is that of passive reactive receiver and not active obtainer.

CLARITY

One major source of difficulty in understanding object relations or dynamic psychiatry is the concept of psychosexual stages of development. At first glance, such a concept appears to be based on the organismic model. The concept uses stages which are supposed to be qualitatively different from each other. However, if the stages were qualitatively different, they would not be subject to regression which is central to many of Freud's ideas about the causes of psychiatric disorders. In the organismic model, regression is not accepted because the attainment of a given stage in development is accompanied by a total reorganization of the whole. Development is unidirectional and not bidirectional in the organismic model. (Unidirectional development does not preclude the continuation of earlier skills which may be used from time to time.) Thus the term psychosexual stages of development is a misnomer. Change which is continuous and cumulative is not possible in developmental models which explain changes as discontinuous and discrete.

Another problem is that psychoanalysis offers intervention only for the first three types of problems: oral, anal and phallic. Latency and genital types largely are ignored. Apparently, there are no problems in latency or genital acquisition.

A third problem relates to the intervention process. If there are certain stages of development, why is the intervention approach the same for all stages? In each the intervention is simply to give the person objects associated with the level of fixation and wait for interaction to occur between the person and object. The primary role of the therapist is akin to that of a store manager who puts out the merchandise and observes whether the customer buys it. Occasionally, some remarks may be exchanged, but the primary interaction is between customer and goods or between client and object.

A fourth problem concerns the assessment instrument. There has never been an administration manual which outlines the procedures to be followed. As a result each article which addresses the battery has some major or minor changes in it which make for confusion on the part of anyone who might try to administer the battery according to Azima's rationale. Examples of changes have been the switch from plasticine to clay and the alteration of sequence from pencil, finger painting and clay to pencil, clay and finger painting (45).

A fifth problem is the recording of the information from the battery. The form is difficult to use without further directions and experience in watching the battery being administered. Some items on the form are not clear. For example, in the section entitled Organization of Mood (45), there is an item under the subsection on form related to the control of form. The range is from "controlled" to "symbolic." Does "controlled" mean "realistic" or something else? Another example appears under the section on Structure of the Object. The word "sytonicity" appears apparently as the opposite to culture. The writer has been unable to locate a printed definition for the word "sytonicity" in any dictionary of psychiatric terms or in any unabridged dictionary of the English and American language. Apparently, the word should be "syntonicity" or "syntonia" which is defined as a personality prone to manic depressive illness (46).

UNIQUENESS

The unique feature of the object relations model is the focus on the objects as real or symbolic sources of relationships which did not occur at the time and place expected in the person's chronological history. The use of objects is based on the assumption that the person has regressed to an earlier position in the individual's life history in an attempt to find gratification which was lacking (44).

Since object, not occupation, is the primary focus of the model, the Aximas suggest that the term "occupation" is neither the aim nor the mechanism of the profession (43). Such a view destroys the role of occupation as the means of interacting in a biopsychosocial world. Objects as used in the object relations model have meanings specific only to each individual. Occupations, on the other hand, have shared as well as individual meaning. Objects have a role limited to a certain point in the individual's history. Occupations continue to have a role throughout a person's history and society's history. Occupation as a part of the life process is much larger in scope than object relations.

RESEARCH GUIDE

The model of object relations has had a significant effect in promoting the development of projective evaluation instruments (47–56). However, the forms used to record data address questions related to the broader approach of a task as an occupation as observed through organization, dexterity and a level of independence rather than as a limited object which is associated with mood, drives and ego functions.

The Azimas can be credited with making occupational therapists aware that many craft activities could be used to analyze systematically a person's approach to handling and response to an unstructured, semistructured or totally structured task. In addition, the information obtained could be useful in pinpointing problems in skill attainment and functional performance. The emphasis on ability vs. disability, however, is a different assumption than drives vs. defenses. Although both are based on the Newtonian physics concept of equal and opposite forces (57), the transmission into psychology differs. Freud and Azimas used the concept of dynamics in terms of drives and instincts which strive for discharge and the forces which attempt to prevent discharge. Basically, the dynamics are between the unconscious vs. the conscious. Assessment and intervention are attempts to identify the instinctual energies and control their release in a manner which does not lead to self-destruction. Other psychologists such as Maslow and Rogers were more interested in the tendency to maintain the self rather than self-destruct. They reemphasized the old humanistic values of self-worth and growth potential which occupational therapy derived from the philosophy of moral treatment. Most of the so-called "activities batteries" initiated by the Azimas seem to follow the growth potentiating theme.

SPECIALIZATION

Although the literature in occupational therapy speaks to the issues of dynamics psychiatry, occupational therapists do not seem to have followed the regressive intervention model of object relations. Instead, the psychosexual stages of development have been employed more fully. West (58) suggests three aspects in which occupational therapy media can contribute to psychodynamic formulation: (a) the products are symbolic representations of the patient's basic conflicts; (b) the feelings the patient has about the product in terms of what is done with or said about the product and (c) the skills used in order to plan toward vocational rehabilitation. The Azimas used the first contribution only and then primarily in initial evaluation. Thus, occupational therapists enlarged upon the formulation of psychodynamics through object relations as used by the Azimas and rejected regressive intervention as a primary model for program development.

ELABORATION AND REFINEMENT

From the view of occupational therapy, the Azima's model of object relations seems to need elaboration and refinement in two major areas: (a) expansion to cover the five stages of psychosexual development and

(b) expansion of the creative or growth potential role of occupational therapy media.

Expanding the concern for psychosexual development would enlarge the scope of activities beyond those of a 5-year-old. Latency and genital psychosexual development are normal stages and complete the process of attaining adult level functioning. Objects continue to have significance in these latter two stages. The limitation of the object relations model to the first three stages only reinforces the regressive intervention approach. Regression to the genital stage would be impossible since it is the highest stage, and regression to latency perhaps does not reduce the behavioral effectiveness of the individual to the extent observed in the lower level regressions.

Expansion of the creative or growth potential area permits occupational therapy to contribute to the developmental process. The object relations model, however, does not stress the use of media for skill learning: only for psychodynamic conflict resolution. The stress on resolution is apparently a response to the selection of objects not commonly considered occupational therapy media, such as mud, cocoa powder and baby bottles. Other occupations such as leatherwork, wood working, mosaic tiles, basketry and needlepoint apparently did not fit the regressive scheme. Such media, however, do contribute to a creative or growth potentiation scheme.

EXPLANATORY USEFULNESS

As an explanation of occupational therapy, the model of object relations seems quite incomplete. The model does suggest that man relates to the objects in the environment and uses them to satisfy needs. However, the needs are restricted to those related to basic survival. Maslow calls such needs deficiency needs. Although occupational therapy can provide for deficiency needs the profession also can contribute to the growth needs, such as mastery, competence, recognition and self actualization. These needs require occupations as well as objects. The "doing" aspect of an occupation involves a process of learning a set of facts. Objects call forth an emotional or psychological reaction only. An occupation may include an object relation as well as a learning task at the cortical or subcortical level.

COMMONALITY

The object relations model appears to have been proposed primarily to increase the common concern for regressive behavior seen by psychiatrists and occupational therapists, and perhaps by other activity-focused professions who follow the strict Freudian interpretation of psychodynamics. For other psychiatrists, psychologists and therapists who follow other points of view, the model of object relations is of limited usefulness in conveying a common concern. A major concern the therapists have demonstrated in the occupational therapy literature is that the Azima model of object relations is too limited even within the profession of

Table 13.4
Object Relations Model Criteria Summary

Criteria	Very Good 1	Moderately Good			Very Poor 5
		2	3	4	
Frame of reference				X	
Clarity				X	
Uniqueness				X	
Research guide			X		
Specialization				X	
Elaboration/refinement			X		
Explanatory usefulness				X	
Commonality				X	
Practice model					X

occupational therapy. Object relations is an accepted concept, but the interpretation goes beyond the first three levels of psychosexual development as proposed by Freud and the limited interpretation of object relations used within the stages.

PRACTICE MODEL

The object relations model has had some effect on practice through the development of the projective testing procedures. However, there does not appear to be any specific practice model or theory which is based on the object relations model.

SUMMARY

The object relations model is not a very successful model on which to develop and expand the practice of occupational therapy. As a product of the mechanistic viewpoint there are too many problems in philosophy which are not reconcilable with the traditional view of occupational therapy. A summary is provided in Table 13.4.

Communication Process Model—Fidlers

FRAME OF REFERENCE

Although the Fidlers stated that the communication process model is not based on any specific school of thought the concepts and assumptions of Freudian psychoanalysis clearly are evident. The terms object relations, unconscious, ego, anxiety, oral and anal needs, transference and countertransference are from the psychoanalytic model.

Other influences are the interpersonal relations stressed by Harry Stack Sullivan, a milieu approach which is based on learning theory, the use of group techniques as advocated by S. R. Slavson, and the role of disturbed communication based on Jurgen Ruesch's work. Many additional references are cited throughout the text and in the bibliography. However, Freud, Sullivan, Slavson, Ruesch and the concept of milieu therapy seem to be most predominant.

ASSUMPTIONS

Assumptions about Basic Needs (These needs are not totally consistent with the psychoanalytic frame of reference. See the critique.)

1. Certain basic needs are common to all men, and satisfaction of these needs is essential to existence (p. 134).
2. Basic needs include the:
   a. Need for love, acceptance and a sense of belonging.
   b. Need to perceive oneself as an individual distinct from others.
   c. Need to be self-determining, to exercise some free will.
   d. Need to experience a mutual sharing, collaborative relationship with one's fellowmen.
   e. Need to experience consensual validation.
   f. Need to perceive oneself as a productive contributing member of society (pp. 134–135).
3. The development of a realistic self concept and ego strength can occur only to the extent that one's primitive narcissistic needs are gratified (p. 87).
4. Many patients have a basic dependency need to be infantilized (p. 89).

Assumptions about the Role of Unconscious Mechanisms (59)

1. Comprehension of the unconscious and conscious mechanisms of action or behavior is essential to the understanding of the human being (19).
2. Acceptance of the phenomena of the unconscious commits one to the acceptance of the fact that action and words can be used to make feelings (p. 108).
3. Those ideas, attitudes and emotions that are acted out are much less likely to come under the scrutiny of one's more conscious intellectual repressing mechanisms (p. 81).
4. All mental mechanisms used to produce the pathology in the first place will be continued in the service of maintaining that pathology (p. 47).

Assumptions about Interpersonal Relationships (59)

1. The nature of one's self concept and personal identity is determined by one's early interpersonal relationships with the significant adult (p. 83).
2. Faulty or unsatisfying interpersonal relationships with the primary love object or significant person in one's early life experience result in the thwarting of basic ego needs (p. 95).
3. Interpersonal relationships are influenced by the patient, therapist, group and object (p. 72).
4. Relationships are held together by three mechanisms—rapport, transference and countertransference (p. 50).
5. Interpersonal difficulties in communication may stem from problems in:
   a. becoming aware of intrapsychic thinking

   b. organizing and translating this thinking into a thought
   c. selecting common, recognizable symbols to express the thought
     (p. 21).

Assumptions about Object Relationships (59)

1. Object relationships develop where there is instinctual gratification related to the object (p. 34).
2. Object loss produces a more or less standard reaction, including dejection, loss of interest, loss of capacity to love, inhibition of activity, self-reproach, and expectation of punishment (p. 34).
3. In schizophrenia object relationships are of a most primitive kind and identification is made rather crudely, so that one object is rather readily exchanged for another (p. 35).
4. For the person with very limited ego structure, experiences in handling and manipulating clearly defined and structured objects can be extremely helpful (p. 83).
5. Usually patients are able to express hostile aggressive impulses with less anxiety toward a symbolic object or through a symbolic act than toward a person (p. 91).
6. Working through problems in interpersonal relationships, hostility, dependency, etc., will create a growth awareness of the self and a personal identity and integrity (p. 83).

Assumptions about Activity (59)

1. The use of activities and objects has a psychodynamic impact on the performer (p. 75).
2. The use of activities as a psychotherapeutic measure requires a knowledge of the following.
   a. The phenomenon of the unconscious
   b. The nature and meaning of symbols
   c. Individual psychodynamics
   d. A sensitivity to the probable impact of each of the above on one another
   e. The inability to integrate such awareness into a therapeutic experience (pp. 75–76).
3. A patient's interest in an activity or choice should be viewed as a manifestation of needs, conflicts and the manner of dealing with these (p. 74).
4. Whether a patient should have an activity chosen or should be given a free choice in selection should be answered on the basis of what seems to offer the best therapeutic potentials (p. 74).

Assumptions about Intervention (59)

1. Treatment requires a body of scientific knowledge sufficient to enable one to perform the following.
   a. Delineate pathology
   b. Make reasonable predictions on the basis of the pathology
   c. Plan a course of treatment

    d. Recognize and understand what is occurring psychodynamically during treatment

    e. Be able to use and influence what occurs to the benefit of the patient (p. 117).

2. Therapeutic programs should achieve the following.

    a. Foster collaborative relationships wherein a person may explore concepts about the self

    b. Gratify some frustrated basic needs and devices

    c. Consolidate growth through continued experimentation and exploration (pp. 17–18)

3. A therapeutic milieu and the skills and techniques of implementation are essential (p. 26)

4. There is a recognizable correlation between the effectiveness of treatment procedures and the nature of the culture or milieu in which they occur (p. 26)

5. The therapeutic dyad is built on the basic human characteristics found in both partners of the helping relationship (problem areas include dependency, aggressiveness, gratification and integrity) (pp. 40–43)

Assumptions about Occupational Therapy as a Communication Process (59)

1. Occupational therapy in psychiatry is basically and primarily a communication process (p. 19)

2. Occupational therapy is in effect another language for communication with the patient (p. VI)

3. Occupational therapy is concerned with action, the meaning of action, its uses in communicating feelings and thoughts and the use of such nonverbal communications (p. 19)

4. Creative and structured activities in occupational therapy give opportunities to communicate problems and feelings (p. 94).

5. Those experiences in occupational therapy that focus on participative doing provide opportunities to (a) test new skills in living, (b) experiment and explore capacities in relationships, (c) learn more effective means of communication and (d) utilize insights gained (p. 97).

6. Occupational therapy knowledge and skill should be directed toward the following.

    a. Psychodynamics of action

    b. Real and symbolic meaning of objects

    c. Psychodynamics of interpersonal relationships (p. 22).

Assumptions about Occupational Therapy and Object Relations (59)

1. Utilization of the real and symbolic significance of object relationships and activities marks the major contribution of occupational therapy and differentiates it from interview psychotherapy (p. 118)

2. Occupational therapy encompasses thinking, feeling, and participating in a world of objects (p. 97)

Assumptions about Occupational Therapy and Activity (59)

1. The unique value of occupational therapy lies in the use of the psychodynamics of activities (p. 118).
2. In occupational therapy, the psychodynamics of activities are considered as catalytic agents giving impetus to the development of relationships and intrapsychic experiences (p. 118).
3. Many activities in occupational therapy provide opportunity for an agreement on the nature of reality because they (a) have easily understood and accepted values and purposes (b) have established standards and techniques and (c) may require varying degrees of communication (p. 94).
4. The structured activities in occupational therapy provide opportunity for reality testing since they offer sensory contact in a composition that is well defined (p. 93).
5. In occupational therapy, the nature of the process rather than the end product is of primary importance (p. 118).
6. Process includes the following.
   a. Real and symbolic meaning of an object or activity
   b. Intrapsychic responses of the person to such stimuli
   c. Pervading influence that such feeling, thinking and acting has an interpersonal relationship
   d. Collaborative efforts and communication between person and therapist (p. 118).
7. The occupational therapy experience constitutes:
   a. The action itself
   b. Those objects that are used in the action process, as well as those that result from the action
   c. Those interpersonal relationships that influence the action and are in turn influenced by it (p. 21).

CONCEPTS

Communication—the process of transforming inner private subjective experiences and thoughts into external public form accessible to recognition by people at large, where it can then acquire validity in the shared "real world." (Borrowed from Maria Lorenz.) (p. 21)

Treatment—the process that consciously applies a given body of knowledge and skill in an effort to change or correct pathology (p. 24)

Schools of thought in psychiatry
   a. *Psychoanalytic*—places primary emphasis on the unconscious, exploring unconscious needs, drives, and conflicts and resolving these by means of awareness and understanding (p. 25)
   b. *Supportive*—recognizes the significance of the unconscious phenomenon and helps to gratify basic needs by sublimation
   c. *Directive/repressive*—utilizes the existing ego integration to repress unacceptable feelings and behavior (p. 25)

Mental Health processes—those methodologies that are directed toward developing and sustaining an environment and culture base on the inherent worth and integrity of the human being (p. 26)

Rehabilitation—those efforts and procedures directed toward helping the patient learn to use more effectively existing integrative capacities, assets and abilities toward developing and refining skills that will enable the person to assume appropriate economic and social responsibilities outside the hospital (p. 27)

Object—a thing with which an instinctual impulse is gratified (p. 32)

Object relationship—perceived relationship between self and other (p. 32)

Rapport—is achieved when the interchange between people leads to an expectation of positive interest and good intentions toward each other (p. 50)

Transference—expressed as a reaction to another person based on past relationships rather than on the realistic observation of the present one (p. 51)

Countertransference—the unconscious reaction of the therapist to the transference behavior of the patient (p. 51)

Psychiatric occupational therapy—the use of psychodynamics of activities and concomitant relationships (p. 71)

Activity analysis—a guide to be used in evaluating one aspect of the activity experience (p. 75)

Dyadic relationship—term is used in relation to a therapist-patient interaction

Action—term is used but no definition is provided

Unconscious—term is used but no definition is provided

EXPECTED RESULTS (59)

1. Provide a means of expressing and uncovering unconscious needs, drives and feelings and of dealing with these in the indicated manner.
2. Provide a means of gratifying needs either directly or by sublimation.
3. Strengthen ego defenses by assisting the patient to reestablish previous defense mechanisms in a more constructive manner and to learn new satisfactory defenses.
4. Provide ego growth through opportunities to work through distortions in self concept and body image and to enhance the sense of personal identity and worth.
5. Provide reality testing through the opportunity to explore and test perceptions, to distinguish reality from fantasy and to experience consensual validation and agreement on the nature of reality.
6. Explore interpersonal relationships through opportunities to enter into one-to-one and group relationships to explore these, to work through interpersonal distortions, and to share and communicate with others on a verbal and nonverbal level.

7. Consolidate gains through continued experimentation, validation and communication in an environment of thinking, feeling, and action. Providing opportunity to test one's developing skills in living (p. 120)

ASSESSMENT INSTRUMENTS

1. Assessment considerations (p. 102)
   a. Objects, both real and symbolic
   b. Process of using objects
   c. Product itself
   d. Use of the product
   e. Relation to authority
   f. Relation to peers
2. Assessment areas (p. 103)
   a. Concept of self—assess how the person perceives the self and how the person functions within this concept. Includes body image, identification, self-esteem.
   b. Concept of others—how person perceives others and how the person may be expected to relate to others
   c. Ego organization—the nature and extent of the person's capacity for reality testing
   d. Unconscious conflicts—delineation of areas of unconscious conflicts
   e. Communication—the nature and manner of communicating feelings and thoughts
3. Outline for assessment (see Table 13.5, Outline for Evaluation)
   a. Relationship to the therapist
   b. Relationship to the group
   c. Relationship to the activity
4. Assessment questions
   a. What is the nature of the patient's pathology, including the difficulties in thinking, perceiving and functioning and unconscious needs and conflicts that seem to be causing the problem?
   b. Which problems are to be of primary concern at this time?
   c. Is the treatment process to be oriented toward uncovering, supporting or repression?
   d. What are the primary problems in the area of interpersonal relationships, including how does the patient behave in relation to others and what constitutes the nature and quality of the relationship?
   e. Which activities can be expected to meet treatment needs and elicit desired responses?
   f. What amount of support, reassurance, dependency, structure, or independent functioning and freedom is needed?
   g. To what extent should the patient be "left alone" to work by himself, included in a small group, introduced to a few or all patients, encouraged to share with others, etc.?
   h. What kind of activity and how should it be presented, such as

Table 13.5
Outline for Evaluation[a]

1. Relationship to the therapist
   a. What is the nature of the patient's overt behavior toward the therapist? (See Behavioral Characteristics) How is this manifested?
   b. What situations or experiences within the patient-therapist relationship increase or diminish such behavior?
   c. Does the patient succeed in communicating feelings and ideas? Is communication difficult to understand, incomprehensible, expressed in a bizarre or other abstruse manner? Describe.
   d. Is the patient's communication primarily verbal or nonverbal? Are actions (behavior) and verbal expressions coordinated, or is there a difference in how he behaves and what he says? What is the nature of this disparity?
   e. What defenses does the patient use in the relationship? (See Defense Mechanisms) How and under what circumstances are these defenses used?
   f. What unconscious conflicts concerning the relationship seem to exist—conflicting needs, drives, impulses, etc.? What is the nature of these and how are they indicated?
   g. What fears are manifested concerning the relationship? Under what circumstances does the patient seem to be most threatened? Most comfortable? To what extent and in what manner?
   h. How do you as a person seem to corroborate or refute some of his stereotyped role concepts? How is this responded to or handled by the patient? What does he seem to expect of you?
   i. How does the patient conceptualize himself in the relationship? What is the level of his self-esteem, feelings of adequacy, identification, etc.? How are these attitudes communicated to you?
   j. What is the patient's level of awareness of feelings, interaction, conflicts? What is the nature of his communication concerning this?
2. Relationship to the group
   a. What overt behavioral characteristics are evident in the patient's relationship to the group? (See Behavioral Characteristics)
   b. Is behavior in relation to the group fairly consistent or is there a marked difference in behavior toward certain group members? What is the nature of this difference?
   c. How do group members behave toward the patient? Describe the nature and quality of this behavior.
   d. What feelings does the patient elicit from the group? In what way and how is this handled by the group? By the patient?
   e. What fears and unconscious conflicts does the group seem to elicit in the patient? How does the patient express such conflicts and how does he handle them?
   f. What ego defenses does he use in the group? How and in what circumstances? How does the group respond? What is the extent of his control of feelings and impulses? What is the nature of this?
   g. What are the nature and level of the patient's communication within the group? (See paragraphs 1c and 1d.)
   h. What is the patient's role in the group?
   i. How does the patient see himself in relation to the group? To individual members of the group? How is this manifested?

Table 13.5—*Continued*

j. How does the patient feel about the group? About individual members? How are these feelings expressed?

k. What is his level of awareness of the group process, of feeling about the group, of the group's attitude toward him, of his interpersonal distortions, etc.? To what extent is he able to integrate such awareness?

3. Relationship to the activity

a. What are the characteristics of the activity the patient selects? What factors outside these characteristics seem to influence his choice—*i.e.*, to please or comply with the therapist, to gain the group's approval, to defy, etc.?

b. How does the patient respond to and deal with the realistic and/or symbolic characteristic of the activity? (See Activity Analysis)

c. What feelings are expressed in the content and in the way he handles the *material*, the *process*? Such as:

  (1) Use of form, movement, space.
  (2) Range and intensity of color.
  (3) Nature and use of symbols.
  (4) Quality of realism, distortions, fantasy.
  (5) Nature of his handling (stroking, rubbing, messing, tearing, beating, pushing, etc.).
  (6) Body response (muscle tension, facial expression, rigidity, etc.).
  (7) Content of form (animate, inanimate, human, animal, whole or part, etc.).
  (8) Nature of procedure (organized, meticulous, perfectionistic, decisive, persistent, sloppy, inaccurate, perseverating, etc.).

d. What needs and drives are expressed in his handling of *material*, of *process*, and in *content*? (See paragraphs 3b and 3c.) What is their nature?

e. To what extent does the patient seem to be aware of feeling? What is the nature of this awareness and how does he use it?

f. What ego defenses are manifested in the handling of material and objects? In the content? In what ways are these manifested?

g. What are the nature and quality of the patient's body image as it is manifested through performance and content?

h. What is the nature of the patient's self-identity? His concept of self, self-esteem, adequacy, sexual identification, worthlessness, etc.? How is this manifested through the use of the material, objects, content, and the process?

i. How does the patient handle abstraction, conceptualizations, concreteness?

j. What is the patient's level of organization, comprehension, perception, ability to predict as evidenced in performance and content?

k. Does the patient handle material and objects in a realistic or symbolic way? Is content realistic, symbolic, fantasy? In what way?

l. Are performance and content comprehensible? Can others understand what he is communicating? Is it idiosymbolic, bizarre, uncommunicative, or can it be consensually validated?

m. To what extent is the patient able to perceive his assets and limitations? How does he act on this? To what extent is he aware of what he can and cannot do?

---

[a] Reprinted from J. W. Fidler and G. S. Fidler (59), pp. 104–106, with permission from Macmillan.

Table 13.6
Outline for Activity Analysis

1. Motions
   a. Passive: Motions are considered passive when they do not involve active aggression, when the material or object moved against is pliable and nonresistive. Thus the motions in the use of clay are more passive than in stamping one's feet in a circle dance or punching holes in leather. Both the nature of the passivity and its frequency need to be evaluated.
   b. Aggressive: Motions such as striking, beating, hammering, throwing, etc., in which force is required. Nature and frequency.
   c. Destructive: An analysis of the nature and frequency of motions that lead to the destruction of the original object or material, such as sawing, tearing, cutting, carving, etc.
   d. Rhythm: Is a rhythm of motion required or possible? To what extent are motions repeated? Varied? Multiple?
   e. Size: What are the nature and extent of fine movement? Gross movement?
2. Procedures
   a. Motor and mental coordination: To what extent does the activity require cognitive motor skills? What is the nature of this requirement?
   b. What are the nature and extent of technical knowledge required?
   c. Is manual dexterity required or possible?
   d. Is there mechanical repetition of procedure? Are there few or multiple processes or steps? What is the extent of repetition of these?
   e. What is the frequency of new learning required within the procedure?
   f. Are there required delays or postponements in the process? Must or can completion be delayed and/or prolonged? To what extent?
3. Material and equipment
   a. Resistiveness: To what extent does the material or equipment resist the performer? What are the nature and extent of force necessary?
   b. Pliability: Do the material and equipment offer little or no resistance? Do they support or assist the doer? Does the material take form readily? Is it easily influenced?
   c. Controllability: Are the material and equipment readily controlled, *i.e.*, do they contain enough substance and/or form to provide some of their own control? Are they so unstructured and pliable as to make control difficult? Does the material tend to resist change?
4. Creativity and originality
   a. What is the extent of opportunity to express feelings and ideas freely?
   b. To what extent is performance or doing dependent on internal stimuli, creative thinking, planning, and implementation?
   c. What is the nature or characteristics of opportunity for invention, alteration, original planning, and action?
   d. What are the nature and extent of external limits and controls? To what extent does the nature of the equipment or material provide structure? To what extent does this structure inhibit or control creativity?
5. Symbols
   a. What symbols are inherent in methods of procedure, material, equipment, end product?
   b. What unconscious feelings, needs, drives may be represented by or symbolized in tools, equipment, motions, actions, etc.?

Table 13.6—*Continued*

   c. What is the potential for association?

6. Hostility and aggressiveness
   a. What are the nature and extent of hostile or aggressive expression directly and symbolically?
   b. What characteristics of motions, actions, procedures, material, and equipment provide opportunity for hostile or aggressive expression directly? Symbolically? What are the potentials for sublimation?

7. Destructiveness
   a. What are the nature and extent of actions or processes that destroy?
   b. Is such destruction controlled? What are the nature and extent of this control?
   c. What tools, equipment, actions, etc., may be considered symbolic of destruction? To what extent? What is the nature of this destruction?

8. Control
   a. What opportunities exist for the performer to be in control of the situation? See paragraphs 2, 3, 4, and 9 of the outline.
   b. To what extent is it possible for the performer to be in control of the learning experience? To what extent does participation require dependence on others for learning and/or performance?
   c. Does the process, equipment, or material provide control and/or set limits?
   d. What are the nature and extent of such limits and controls both symbolically and actually?

9. Predictability
   a. To what extent can "results" and the nature of these be predicted? What is the frequency of new learning experiences? Of repetitive performance?
   b. To what extent does the structure of equipment and material minimize chance of failure?
   c. What is the possible extent of or necessity for guides, aids, rules, etc.? What is the nature of their "assistance" and "assurance"?

10. Narcissism
   a. What opportunities exist for self-indulgence? Exhibitionism? Acquisition?
   b. What are the nature and extent of creative opportunity? Omnipotent endeavor?
   c. Is there an end product or demonstrable result? Does it have a monetary value?

11. Sexual identification
   a. What is the cultural frame of reference concerning the masculine or feminine connotation of the activity? Of the objects, actions, or motions used?
   b. What are the nature and extent of aggressive resistive media and performance?
   c. What are the nature and extent of passive, intricate, delicate media and performance?
   d. What symbolic associations exist?

12. Dependency
   a. What are the nature and extent of opportunities for being dependent on a person or existing structure (rules, patterns, etc.)?
   b. What is the frequency of change and new learning experiences that require dependency?
   c. To what extent are objects or processes symbolic of early infantile dependency? What are the characteristics of these?

Table 13.6—Continued

13. Infantilism
    a. What are the nature and extent of actual or symbolic oral activity, *i.e.*, eating, sucking, blowing, etc.?
    b. What are the nature and extent of anal activity, *i.e.*, smearing, excretory substitutes, possessiveness, retentiveness, collecting, washing, etc.?
    c. What are the nature and extent of opportunity for dependency?
14. Reality testing
    a. What are the nature and extent of sensory contact? Of well defined structure?
    b. To what extent is the process representational or reproductive rather than creative?
    c. To what extent does the structure and/or process provide opportunity for agreement on the nature of reality?
    d. Are there clearly established standards and techniques?
    e. To what extent can purpose be perceived and results predicted?
15. Self-identification
    a. What opportunities exist for the participant or doer to identify his contributions, efforts, and/or involvement?
    b. What are the opportunities for unique, individual performance?
    c. Is there an end product? To what extent can the end product or results provide personal identity?
    d. What are the nature and extent of the opportunity to test the reality of one's perceptions?
    e. What are the nature and extent of opportunity to deal with self-image and body distortions?
    f. What considerations in paragraphs 4, 5, 8, 9, 10, 11, and 14 may influence the nature and extent of self-identification?
16. Independence
    a. What are the opportunities for free and independent planning and performance? What is their nature?
    b. To what extent may processes be altered to allow for uniqueness or creative endeavor?
    c. What is the potential for successful competition?
    d. To what extent is individual responsibility possible? What is the nature of such responsibility?
17. Group relatedness
    a. To what extent can performance and planning be shared with others?
    b. Can processes be dependent on cooperation and mutual assistance from group members? What is the nature of this cooperation?
    c. To what extent do the materials, tools, and equipment offer possible shared experiences?
    d. To what extent can processes and the end product or results be adapted or varied to achieve social and/or cultural acceptability or commendation?

[a] Reprinted with permission from J. W. Fidler and G. S. Fidler (59), pp. 76–80.

the orientation to process, emphasis on performance, on the end product, or on minimizing these?
5. Categories of the activity analysis (see Table 13.6, Outline for Activity Analysis)
    1. Motions—passive, aggressive, destructive, rhythm
    2. Procedures

3. Material and equipment—resistiveness, probability, controllability
4. Creativity and originality
5. Symbols
6. Hostility and aggressiveness
7. Destructiveness
8. Control
9. Predictability
10. Narcissism
11. Sexual identification
12. Dependency
13. Infantilism
14. Reality testing
15. Self-identification
16. Independence
17. Group relatedness

INTERVENTION STRATEGIES (59)

1. Media
   a. Oral activities
      1. Sucking
      2. Drinking
      3. Eating
      4. Chewing
      5. Blowing
      6. Preparation of food
      7. Caring for and feeding animals
      8. Blowing musical instruments
   b. Anal activities
      1. Smearing or building with clay, paints or soil
      2. Collecting
      3. Filing
      4. Bookkeeping
      5. Gardening
      6. Doing laundry
   c. Hostile activities
      1. Sewing
      2. Cutting
      3. Hammering
   d. Gross muscular physical activity
      1. Ball tossing
      2. Marching
      3. Calesthenics
      4. Softball
      5. Soccer
      6. Relays
      7. Dance or circle games
   e. Passive table games

      1. Checkers
      2. Cards
      3. Dominoes
      4. Parcheesi
    f. Creative and structured arts and crafts
      1. Clay
      2. Painting
      3. Physical touching, tracing a part of the body, making a self-portrait
      4. Drama—plays
  2. Methods
    a. Use the features of activities such as (p. 36)
      (1.) amount of physical motion involved, large and vigorous aggression and hostility or small and controlled—not stated;
      (2.) degree of resilience, rigidity or fragility, pliability in the materials—permit more control.
    b. Offer food, help with dressing, washing and grooming to satisfy dependency needs.
    c. Use groups to develop awareness of feelings and behavior on others.
  3. Equipment—not discussed.
  4. Prerequisite skills—not discussed.

SUMMARY

The communication process model is based on the assumption that occupational therapy in psychiatry is primarily a communication process "which is concerned with action, the meaning of action, its use in communicating feelings and thoughts and the use of nonverbal communication" for the benefit of the person involved in treatment (59, p. 19). Furthermore, the Fidlers state that the unique value of occupational therapy is in the use of the psychodynamics of activities. In other words, the utilization of the real and symbolic significance of object relations and activities marks the major contribution of occupational therapy to the total intervention process and differentiates occupational therapy from interviewing psychotherapy which uses the methods of verbalization and association (59, p. 118).

Assessment involves the collection and analysis of information regarding a person's behavior in relating to the therapist, a group situation and to activities. Questions concern possible thoughts or feelings expressed verbally or nonverbally, defenses used and the level of awareness the person appears to have regarding self and situation.

Activities are analyzed in terms of their properties and characteristics related to psychodynamics. Analysis includes observing and recording the motion, procedures, use of symbols, destructive quality, sexual identification, potential to gratify dependency or infantile needs, amount of independence possible, potential for group interaction and other dimensions.

Intervention is directed toward providing gratification of infantile needs, assisting in reality testing, reestablishing defenses, providing opportunities for consensual validation and increasing ego support. Activities are selected for their properties and potential to meet one or more of the five objectives. Most of the activities are related to activities of daily living, creative arts and manual crafts.

Analysis and Critique of the Communication Process Model
FRAME OF REFERENCE

Although the Fidlers named their model a communication process, in many ways the model is an extension or parallel of the Azima's object relations model. The frame of reference remains that of psychoanalysis and a mechanistic viewpoint. The locus of control is external to the individual regardless of whether the intervention is classical psychoanalysis or a variation, such as the supportive or directive approach.

At the same time, the Fidlers (59) have introduced concepts related to mental health that are based on the organismic model, such as the need to be self-determining and to exercise some free will (p. 134). Such concepts are inconsistent with the philosophy of the communication model and cannot be integrated into the model. Thus, the suggestion regarding a therapeutic community and others are inconsistent with the approach to intervention through the psychodynamics of activities. Psychoanalysis is not concerned with the value or purpose of human life but only with the cause and effect of human events. The Fidlers discuss the inconsistent concepts under the title of Rehabilitation. Therefore, in the critique, the concepts and assumptions based on organismic views will be called the rehabilitation model.

CLARITY

The primary source of confusion is the attempt to integrate a model of practice based on mechanistic foundations into suggestions that the total intervention setting should be organized around organismic based concepts. There is a fundamental inconsistency in evaluating a person's behavior as the result of early environmental failure to provide for oral and anal needs (59, p. 87), which is a deterministic view, and then recommend that the person be encouraged to exercise free will (59, p. 134).

The confusion of philosophy is continued as discussion of the communication process model is completed, and a brief discussion of the rehabilitation model is begun (59, p. 49). Once again the outcomes of the rehabilitation model are based on organismic philosophy. Responsibility, exploration and interests become key elements. There appears to be a continuum of intervention suggested. Initially, the communication process model is followed, and after it has been completed at the anal, phallic stage of development, the rehabilitation model is begun. Thus, the problem of dealing with the latent and genital stages of development is solved. However, the philosophical issues have not been solved. Why is a person irresponsible and controlled by the environment until the age of 6 and then suddenly expected to become responsible and self-controlled thereafter?

UNIQUENESS

According to the Fidlers' communication model, the unique aspect of occupational therapy is the use of the psychodynamics of activity. Such an assumption is based in part on Freud's interpretation of psychodynamics which in turn was based on Newton's ideas of dynamics. The law of dynamics states that for every action there is an equal and opposite reaction. Thus, the psychodynamics of activity must be viewed as paired opposites in which one direction is positive while the other is negative. The activity analysis includes some aspects of the pairing but often does not complete the pairs. (59, pp. 76–80). For example, passive motions vs. active aggression motion is included, but constructiveness is not paired with destructiveness. Dependency and independence are both included but not together, while narcissism is discussed but altruism is not. Table 13.7 illustrates some opposite pairings which could be used in analyzing activities.

RESEARCH GUIDE

The communication process model does not seem to have led to much research in terms of experimental design. However, the model did provide a basis for activity analysis. In 1967, the clinical council of the Wisconsin Schools published a project on the therapeutic properties of activities which was based in part on the communication process model (60).

Also, the activity analysis form, evaluation form, progress report form and progress interpretation key have been widely adapted. The forms appear in a variety of sources with or without credit to the Fidlers.

Table 13.7
Activity Analysis by Opposite Pairs

Passive vs. aggressive motion
Destructive vs. constructive motions
Gross motor vs. fine motor movements
Monotonous vs. varied movements
Rhythmic repetitive vs. nonrhythmic, nonrepetitive movements
Immediate vs. delayed gratification
Resistive vs. probable material
Structured vs. unstructured material
Creative vs. stereotyped material
Symbolic vs. realistic association
Easily controlled vs. difficult to control material
Predictable vs. unpredictable material
Narcissism vs. altruism potential
Masculine vs. feminine identification
Dependent vs. independent potential
Reality vs. fantasy potential
Group vs. individual potential
Decorative vs. useful potential

SPECIALIZATION

The communication process model, rehabilitation model and the initial text (61) formed the basis of practice in psychiatric occupational therapy for many years. In 1959, West (62) reported that all schools were using the first edition of the Fidler and Fidler text (61, p. 120). Until 1970, when Mosey's text (63) appeared the Fidler text was the only comprehensive view of psychiatric occupational therapy. Thus, the communication process and rehabilitation models became the focus of specialization along with the Azima's object relations model. Both the communication process and object relations models were similar in focus and could be used together. As the primary models of the time, the influence of the three models on the specialization of psychiatric occupational therapy was considerable.

ELABORATION AND REFINEMENT

The communication process model requires even more expansion than the object relations model. Only the oral and anal stages are discussed in text. Phallic, latency and genital stages are ignored except in the chapter on rehabilitation. As stated in the section on clarity, the rehabilitation model constitutes a change in philosophy and thus may not be considered as an extension of the communication process model but as a separate model and frame of reference. If so, the communication process model includes only the ages of psychosexual development from 0 through about 3 years. Certainly, some psychosexual development and object relations to activities occur after age 3.

EXPLANATORY USEFULNESS

The limited scope of the communication process model constrains its usefulness in explaining psychiatric occupational therapy to others. Limiting intervention to the first 3 developmental years seems oversimplified as an approach to mental health problems and certainly limits the usefulness of occupational therapy as an intervention approach.

Furthermore, the focus on psychosexual development is a limited view of human potential which stresses determinism of environmental situations in early life as setting the course of a whole lifetime. If object relationships are nothing more than a constant repetition of early life experiences why do people bother with new objects? Why not just keep the same old familiar ones? The model of communication process does not seem to offer much growth potential in either object relations or in the use of occupations which involve objects.

The model of rehabilitation is more useful in explaining psychiatric occupational therapy. Developing skills in work, avocation pursuits and social situations is understandable by most people. Use of initiative, taking responsibility and relating to authority are accepted values in society. A discipline which fosters such skills and promotes such values through activities is comprehensible to both professionals and lay persons.

COMMONALITY

The primary point of commonality in the communication process model is the basis in psychoanalysis. Professionals who are knowledgeable about classical psychoanalysis likely would understand the model. Nurses and social workers should find some common themes if their experience includes regressive therapy as a means of intervention in mental health problems. The use of the psychodynamics of objects and object relations is a limited concept, however, and probably not easily translated to common terms.

The model of rehabilitation suggests more points in common with other disciplines and the family. Vocational counselors can relate to increasing work potential. Teachers can relate to increasing acceptance of instruction and criticism. The family can appreciate social skills and awareness of customs and norms.

PRACTICE MODELS

Because of the dual models which the Fidlers present, there is difficulty in determining whether practice models or theories have evolved. Furthermore, the Azimas' object relations model and the communication process model overlap.

Another problem is that the dual model reflected current practice in the early 1960s more than it projected a future direction. The dynamic approach to occupational therapy had been previously explored by the Azimas and by Weinroth (64). Use of the milieu setting had been described by Gratke and Lux (65). Rehabilitation concepts, however, did appear after the model was in print but did not credit the Fidlers for the ideas (66, 67).

As was mentioned under Specialization, the wide use of the book as a text means that most occupational therapists practicing in psychiatry were exposed to both the communication and rehabilitation models. Nevertheless, the impact on practice remains elusive. A summary of the critique is provided in Table 13.8.

Recapitulation of Ontogenesis—Mosey
FRAME OF REFERENCE

According to Anne C. Mosey, Ph.D. OTR, the model of recapitulation of ontogenesis is based primarily on the Fidlers' communication process model, Ayres' perceptual motor model, Marguerite Sechehaye's symbolic realization concept and H. Azima's object relations models. However, concepts of learning theory (behaviorism) and role theory also appear. The model was developed under a grant from the Vocational Rehabilitation Administration through the Massachusetts Department of Mental Health. The theory was first published in 1968 as a separate book (68) and as an article in the *American Journal of Occupational Therapy* (69). In 1970, it was included as part of the textbook on *Three Frames of Reference for Mental Health* (70). During the interval between 1968 and 1970, considerable revision in philosophy and concepts occurred. Because

Table 13.8
Communications Process Model Critique Summary[a]

Criteria	Very Good	Moderately Good			Very Poor
		2	3	4	5
Frame of reference	o			x	
Clarity			o	x	
Uniqueness			o	x	
Research guide			o	x	
Specialization			ox		
Elaboration/refinement			o	x	
Explanation			o	x	
Commonality			o	x	
Practice model			o	x	

[a] x, communication process model; o, rehabilitation model.

of the changes, the analysis of the model is based primarily on the 1970 version (70).

ASSUMPTIONS ABOUT MAN AND ADAPTIVE SKILLS (70)

1. An individual is able to interact effectively and with satisfaction to self and others through learning those adaptive skills which are characteristic of a mature well adjusted person (p. 133).
2. The development of an adaptive skill is hierarchical; the subskills acquired at a given time form the foundation or the capacity for acquisition of higher level skills (p. 138).
3. The learning of adaptive subskills is sequential and the sequence is considered to be invariant (p. 138).
4. Each adaptive skill is influenced by, and influences in turn, the development and use of other skills. Development is an interdependent process (p. 138).
5. Adaptive skills and subskills are learned through participating in growth-facilitating environments (pp. 141, 145).
6. Adaptive skills are universal and are not specific to a particular cultural group (p. 139).
7. Development and use of an adaptive skill is shaped to a greater or lesser extent by the (a) social and cultural environments in which the individual exists and (b) the individual's past and current biological composition (p. 138).
8. The level of development in each adaptive skill influences the social roles assigned to the individual (p. 139).
9. The individual is a willing being (active participant) in the acquisition of adaptive skills (p. 140).
10. Need for mastery serves as a motivational and regulating force in the development of adaptive skills (p. 145).
11. The mastery need motivates and facilitates subskill learning, i.e., gratification of the need for mastery reinforces learning.

12. There are seven adaptive skills: perceptual motor, cognitive, drive object, dyadic interaction, group interaction, self-identity, and sexual identity (p. 134).
13. Adaptive skills are composed of subskills which in turn are composed of components (p. 134).
14. It is through acquisition of adaptive skills that man is able to attain a true state of humanness and to find and give satisfaction and joy (p. 133).

ASSUMPTIONS ABOUT HEALTH (FUNCTION AND DYSFUNCTION)

1. Function and dysfunction are relative to the individual's expected environment and the social roles required of him with that environment (70, p. 143).
2. Dysfunction occurs when one or several adaptive skills have not been attained to a level typical of the person's age and/or the level needed for effective and satisfying interaction in the environment (70, p. 133).
3. Factors associated with dysfunction are:
   a. Abnormalities in physical structures
   b. Severe environmental stress
   c. Lack of "environmental elements" which are necessary for the development of various skill components
   d. Role-learned adaptive skills which are fragile and easily affected by stress (69, p. 428).
4. Marked deficiency in one adaptive skill is undesirable in that it usually inhibits complete learning of sequentially more advanced subskills in all of the adaptive skills (70, p. 138).
5. Behavior indicative of function and dysfunction includes (70, p. 144).
   a. The ability or inability to successfully participate in individual and shared tasks which require the use of various adaptive subskills
   b. Evidence of those inherent responses which occur when there are unconscious complexes
   c. Symbols produced by the individual
6. Lack of learning occurs when there is:
   a. Abnormality in the individual's physiological make-up or in the maturation process
   b. Environmental deficiency in providing environmental elements and learning integration necessary for the development of the various subskills (70, p. 143)

ASSUMPTIONS ABOUT OCCUPATIONAL THERAPY

1. Occupational therapy is an action-oriented doing process (68, p. 1).
2. Occupational therapy assists a person to develop those skills that will permit the individual to function more adequately in the environment with increased satisfaction to self and those around the self (68, p. 1).

3. The uniqueness of occupational therapy is its primary use of non-human objects as opposed to a subordinate use (68, p. 1).

CONCEPTS

Adaptive skills—learned patterns of behavior (70, p. 134)

Perceptual motor skill—ability to receive, integrate and organize stimuli in a manner which allows for the planning of purposeful movement (70, p. 134)

Cognitive skill—ability to perceive, represent, and organize objects, events and their relationship in a manner which is considered appropriate by one's cultural group (70, p. 134)

Drive object skill—ability to control drives and select objects in such a manner as to ensure adequate need satisfaction (70, p. 135)

Dyadic interaction skill—ability to participate in a variety of dyadic relationships (70, p. 135)

Group interaction skill—ability to be a productive member of a variety of primary groups (70, p. 136)

Self identity skill—ability to perceive the self as an autonomous, holistic and acceptable object which has permanence and continuity over time (70, p. 136)

Sexual identity skill—ability to perceive one's sexual nature as good and to participate in a heterosexual relationship which is oriented to the mutual satisfaction of sexual needs (70, p. 136)

Adaptive subskills—the sequentially ordered parts of an adaptive skill (70, p. 134)

Skill components—the various parts of a subskill which may not be sequentially ordered (70, p. 134)

Environmental elements—those objects and interactions which must be available to the individual for normal development to occur (70, p. 148)

Growth-facilitating environment—includes appropriate environmental elements and learning interaction (70, p. 141)

Learning interactions—those interactions which may be described by the postulates of operant conditioning, such as contact or intermittent reinforcement (70, p. 141)

Integrative learning—moving through the types of learning, including tentative trial behavior, active experimentation and retreat into marginal awareness (70, p. 142)

Role learning—superficial acquisition of a behavioral pattern and conscious effort on the part of the individual to utilize the pattern (70, p. 142)

Expected environment—refers to the probable environment in which the patient will live after termination of treatment (70, p. 143)

Social roles—patterns of interaction between two or more persons in which the behavior of one is defined in terms of the behavior of the others (68, p. 52)

State of function—there is evidence of integrated learning of those adaptive subskills which are needed for successful participation in the expected environment (70, p. 143)

State of dysfunction—there is evidence of a lack of integrated learning of the adaptive subskills (70, p. 143)

Meaningful activity—refers to goal-directed action; it is hypothesized that such action enhances integration of sensory stimuli (70, p. 150)

Purposeful activity—is characterized by active response to stimuli, the arousal of interest and a feeling on the part of the individual that he is doing something which is important and significant to the self (70, p. 156)

EXPECTED RESULTS

1. Learn required adaptive skills (70, p. 133)
2. Satisfy inherent needs and the needs of others (70, p. 134)

ASSESSMENT

1. Process/procedures—not specified.
2. Assessment area
   a. Perceptual motor
      1. Ayres Space Test—Ayres
      2. Southern California Motor Accuracy Test—Ayres
      3. Southern California Figure Ground Visual Perception Test—Ayres
      4. Southern California Perceptual-Motor Dysfunction Tests—Ayres
      5. Developmental Test of Visual Perception—Marianne Frostig
      6. Winter Haven Perceptual Copy Forms Test—Winter Haven Lions Club
      7. Developmental Test of Visual Motor Integration—Keith Beery
      8. Illinois Test of Psycholinguistic Ability—Samuel Kirk
   b. Cognitive—none listed
   c. Drive-object—none listed
   d. Dyadic interaction—observation
   e. Group interaction—observation
   f. Self-identity—observation
   g. Sexual identity—observation

INTERVENTION STRATEGIES (70)

1. Media and modalities
   a. Perceptual motor—swinging, spinning, twirling, rolling, pressure, rubbing, brushing, water activities, discriminating objects and shapes, auditory sounds, creeping, crawling, clapping, bicycling, jumping
   b. Cognitive—manipulating objects, play games
   c. Drive object—nurturing relationship, gross motion, resistive activity

    d. Dyadic interaction—therapist as self
    e. Group interaction—none specifically needed, depends on group activity
    f. Self-identity—nurturing relationship activities with established standards and choices
    g. Sexual identity—interaction situation with one or both sexes, discussion

2. Methods (70)
    a. Use of growth-facilitating environments which are responsible for the normal developmental process.
    b. Use sequentially ordered stages of development
    c. Perceptual motor
        1. Integration of primitive postural reflexes through increased vestibular stimulation and opposite reflex patterns
        2. Development of balance reactions through alterations of vestibular stimulation and variations of balancing situations
        3. Balance tactile discrimination and protective touch through increased stimulation to both systems
        4. Form perception development through manual manipulation of objects and increase of distinctive characteristics
        5. Auditory awareness through inhibition of body sounds and increased attention to environmental sounds

3. Equipment (70)
    a. Perceptual motor—scooter board, incline plane, barrel, large beach ball, t-stool, stilts, balance beam, cloth, brush, carpet, objects and shapes, blackboard, weights
    b. Cognitive—toys, tools and games
    c. Drive object—resistive materials, clay, wood
    d. Dyadic interaction—none specifically needed
    e. Group interaction—tools, materials, toys
    f. Self-identity—none specifically needed
    g. Sexual-identity—none specifically needed

4. Precautions (70)
    a. Perceptual motor
        1. Vestibular stimulation—watch for pallor, increased heart or respiratory rate or strong negative reaction
        2. Tactile stimulation is not used if hypertonicity is present

SUMMARY

Recapitulation of ontogenesis is an example of a developmental frame of reference based on the integration of ideas from Ayres, Azima, Fidler and Sechehaye. The basic assumption is that an individual is able to interact effectively and with satisfaction to the self and others through learning those adaptive skills which are characteristic of a mature well adjusted individual. Adaptive skills, it is assumed, develop in an interdependent stage-specific and hierarchical manner through learning processes in various growth-facilitating environments (Fig. 13.2). A person is considered to be in a state of dysfunction when, in one or more adaptive skills, the individual has not attained a level, relatively typical for chronological age and/or the individual has not attained the level needed for effective and satisfying interaction in the environment (Fig. 13.3). One major concern of treatment is to assist the individual in progressing sequentially through the stages of development which were not attempted or never completely mastered (Fig. 13.4). Each individual is assessed in the seven adaptive skills to determine the level of performance attained which can be charted on the Adaptive Skill Development Chart (Table 13.9, Fig. 13.5). As a second concern, information is sought relative to

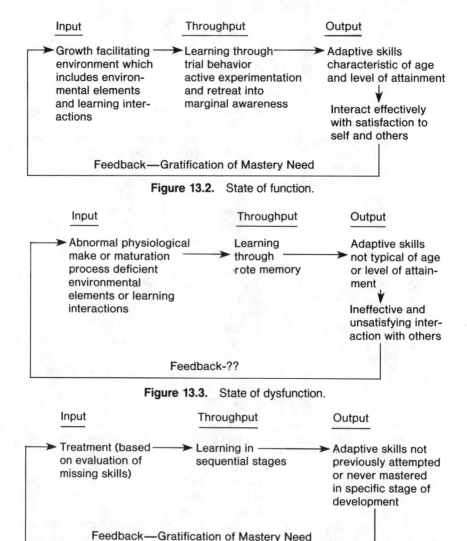

Figure 13.2. State of function.

Figure 13.3. State of dysfunction.

Figure 13.4. Occupational therapy process model for deficient skills.

Table 13.9
Adaptive Skill Development Chart[a]

Perceptual-Motor Skill
The ability to receive, integrate and organize sensory stimuli in a manner which allows for the planning of purposeful movement.
1. The ability to integrate primitive postural reflexes, to react appropriately to vestibular stimuli, to maintain a balance between the tactiile subsystems, to perceive form and to be aware of auditory stimuli.
2. The ability to control extraocular musculature, to integrate the two sides of the body and to focus on auditory stimuli.
3. The ability to perceive visual and auditory figure ground, to be aware of body parts and their relationships, and to plan gross motor movements.
4. The ability to perceive space, to plan fine motor movements and to discriminate auditory stimuli.
5. The ability to discriminate between right and left and to remember auditory stimuli.
6. The ability to use abstract concepts, to scan, integrate and synthesize auditory stimuli and to give auditory feedback

Cognitive Skill
The ability to perceive, represent and organize objects, events and their relationships in a manner which is considered appropriate by one's cultural group.
1. The ability to use inherent behavioral patterns for environmental interaction.
2. The ability to interrelate visual, manual, auditory and oral responses.
3. The ability to attend to the environmental consequence of actions with interest, to represent objects in an exoceptual manner, to experience objects, to act on the bases of egocentric causality, and to seriate events in which the self is involved.
4. The ability to establish a goal and intentionally carry out means, to recognize the independent existence of objects, to interpret signs, to imitate new behavior, to apprehend the influence of space, and to perceive other objects as partially causal.
5. The ability to use trial and error problems solving, to use tools, to perceive variability in spatial positions, to seriate events in which the self is not involved, and to perceive the causality of other objects.
6. The ability to represent objects in an image manner, to make believe, to infer a cause given its effect, to act on the basis of combined spatial relations, to attribute omnipotence to others, and to perceive objects as permanent in time and place.
7. The ability to represent objects in an endoceptual manner, to differentiate between thought and action, and to recognize the need for causal sources.
8. The ability to represent objects in a denotative manner, to perceive the viewpoint of others, and to decenter.
9. The ability to represent objects in a connotative manner, to use formal logic, and to work in the realm of the hypothetical.

Drive-Object Skill
The ability to control drives and select objects in such a manner as to ensure adequate need satisfaction.
1. The ability to form a discontinuous, libidinal object relationship.
2. The ability to form a continuous, part, libidinal object relationship
3. The ability to invest aggressive drive in an external object.

Table 13.9—*Continued*

4. The ability to transfer libidinal drive to objects other than the primary object.
5. The ability to invest libidinal energy in appropriate abstract objects and to control aggressive drive.
6. The ability to engage in total diffuse libidinal object relationships.

Dyadic Interaction Skill
The ability to participate in a variety of dyadic relationships.
1. The ability to enter into association relationships.
2. The ability to interact in an authority relationship
3. The ability to interact in a chum relationship.
4. The ability to enter into a peer, authority relationship.
5. The ability to enter into an intimate relationship.
6. The ability to engage in a nurturing relationship.

Group Interaction Skill
The ability to be a productive member of a variety of primary groups.
1. The ability to participate in a parallel group.
2. The ability to participate in a project group.
3. The ability to participate in an egocentric-cooperative group.
4. The ability to participate in a cooperative group.
5. The ability to participate in a mature group.

Self-Identity Skill
The ability to perceive the self as an autonomous, holistic, and acceptable object which has permanence and continuity over time.
1. The ability to perceive the self as a worthy object.
2. The ability to perceive the assets and limitations of the self.
3. The ability to perceive the self as self-directed.
4. The ability to perceive the self as a productive, contributing member of a social system.
5. The ability to perceive the self.
6. The ability to perceive the aging process of the self in a rational manner.

Sexual-Identity Skill
The ability to perceive one's sexual nature as good and to participate in a heterosexual relationship which is oriented to the mutual satisfaction of sexual needs.
1. The ability to accept and act upon the basis of one's pregenital sexual nature.
2. The ability to accept sexual maturation as a positive growth experience.
3. The ability to give and receive sexual gratification.
4. The ability to enter into a sustained heterosexual relationship.
5. The ability to accept physiological and psychological changes which occur at the time of the climacteric.

[a] Reprinted from A. C. Mosey (63), pp. 134–136, with permission from Charles B. Slack.

the environment in which the person lives or expects to return. Intervention is directed toward the learning of those subskills needed to fulfill the social roles in the expected environment. Thus, learning takes place through patient-therapist nonhuman environment interactions (Fig. 13.6). In both concerns, interactions in the intervention process are synthesized so that they simulate the specific growth-facilitating envi-

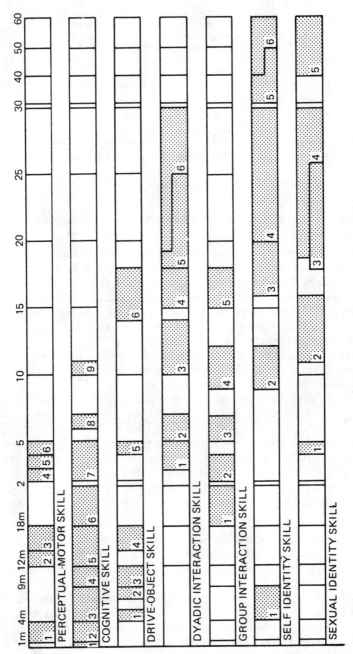

Figure 13.5. Adaptive skills developmental chart. (Reproduced from A. C. Mosey (63), p. 137, with permission from Charles B. Slack.)

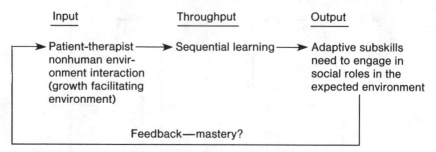

Figure 13.6. Occupational therapy process model for expected environment.

ronment believed to be responsible for the learning of adaptive skills in the normal developmental process.

Analysis and Critique of the Recapitulation of Ontogenesis Model
FRAME OF REFERENCE

The model of recapitulation of ontogenesis is based on a wide variety of philosophical concepts which are difficult to integrate at best. In some cases, the philosophies cannot really be integrated. An example is the use of reward and reinforcement from the mechanistic model (behaviorism) in a model drawn primarily from the organismic metamodel. This problem of mixing concepts from the two metamodels is less evident in the 1970 version of recapitulation of ontogenesis than in the 1968 version. However, the problem should stand as a word to the wise for model builders to be sure the philosophy is consistent before mixing theories and models from various sources together.

A second problem of mixing is that a model or theory used within the frame of reference may be changed by the original model builder or theorist. Such is the case with Dr. Ayres' work. Perceptual motor development is now known as sensory integration; the skills have been regrouped and the assessment instruments have been combined and expanded into one comprehensive assessment tool. Thus, the section on perceptual motor skills needed updating. The problem of revision for updating can occur whenever living people's models or theories are used.

CLARITY

The concept of adaptive skills appears to be useful in explaining the outcome of development and intervention. However, in the 1970 version of recapitulation of ontogenesis, there is no mention of a final outcome. In the 1968 version, the final outcome is adaptation which is defined as "the process of obtaining need gratification for the self concomitant with meeting environmental demands" (69, p. 126). Similar statements appear in the 1970 version but are not related to adaptation as an individual process. The lack of a final outcome reduces the clarity of the model.

Another problem relates to the rationale for the selection of the adaptive skills. Again, the 1970 version provides no clues. In the 1968 version, the explanation is to give some order and structure to the complex process of human development and mature functioning (68, p. 42). Still the reader lacks a clear focus as to how the adaptive skills relate to one another. According to the chart (Fig. 13.5), the first adaptive skills to appear are perceptual motor and cognitive followed by drive object and self-identity. Group skills appear at 18 months, while dyadic skills begin at age 3. Finally, sexual identity begins at 4 years. This development profile suggests that some adaptive skills are more primary than others because those skills begin early. The perceptual motor and cognitive skills could be considered primary to development. It is interesting to note that dyadic skills are not considered primary in view of research on infant-mother bonding. Such bonding would seem to be a critical adaptive skill which would alter the developmental sequence of the adaptive skills. Altering the point of dyadic development, however, would provide a better rationale for selection of the adaptive skills based on developmental psychology. Development in the literature frequently centers around the acquisition of physical and sensory motor, cognitive and language and psychological and social skills. Self-identity and sexual identity are considered to be dependent on the primary skills. Following such a rationale, a model of adaptive skills could be illustrated as shown in Figure 13.7.

The proposed model of adaptation through adaptive skill acquisition provides an integrative rationale for skill development. Furthermore, the model provides support for an interactive rationale between and among the skill areas. The interactive effect in turn supports the rationale for an interdependent relationship of the skill and subskills. In other words, development of adaptive skills is viewed as an integrative, interactive and interdependent process in which each adaptive skill and subskill contributes to the total developmental process. Failure of development in any adaptive skill area will have an effect on the total development and ultimate adaptive potential of the individual.

The most serious limitation in the model appears to be the drive object skill. The concept of drive in psychology is associated with tension-reducing behavior, such as eating to avoid hunger. Mastery, on the other hand, is viewed as a tension-seeking need. Thus, tension-seeking behavior is an active process, whereas tension-reducing behavior is a reactive process. To be consistent with the organismic meta model motivation should be based on a tension-seeking active process. The term "need" is most often associated with the tension while "satisfaction" is associated with meeting the need. Thus, the skill that is labeled "drive-object" would be better named "need satisfaction" skill.

UNIQUENESS

The concept of adaptive skills does provide a basic foundation for occupational therapy as a unique profession. When adaptive skills are viewed as developing through the interaction of the individual and an

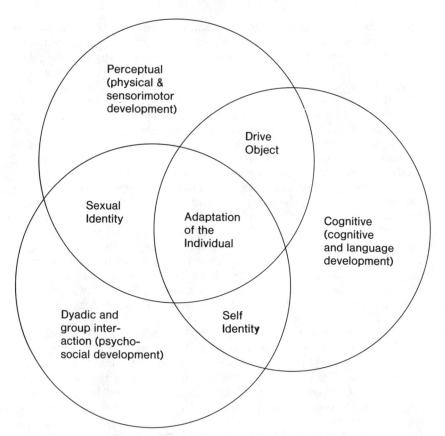

Figure 13.7. Model of adaptation through adaptive skills acquisition.

activity process, the rationale for practice is also supported. In the 1968 version, the use and rationale for activity was explored. Activity was analyzed in terms of objects and interactions which were called activity elements (68, p. 61). Activity elements were viewed as representational of environmental elements which include the objects and interactions needed to support normal development. The representation could be based on similarity or symbolism. Thus, activity used in occupational therapy was considered to represent by similarity or symbolism the normally occurring environmental elements. When learning interactions were combined with either environmental elements or activity elements, learning could occur which developed the components and subskills of adaptive skills (Figs. 13.8 and 13.9). Unfortunately, the activity element was not included in the 1970 version, and thus the rationale for occupational therapy practice through intervention has no support for the use of activity as a medium of change when the normal environment has

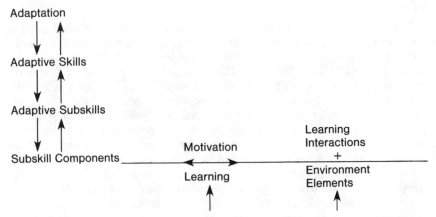

Figure 13.8. Sequence of acquisition of adaptive skills through normal development.

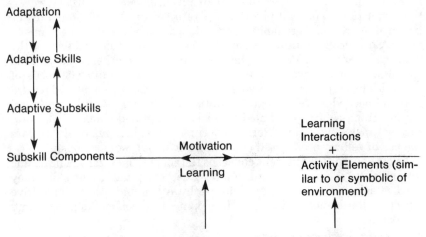

Figure 13.9. Sequence of acquisition of adaptive skills through therapy.

been insufficient or failed. The lack of rationale for activity is a serious deficiency in the 1970 version of recapitulation of ontogenesis.

RESEARCH GUIDE

The model of recapitulation of ontogenesis could be used as research guide to verify or expand the adaptive skill areas, the sequence of subskill development and the characteristics of growth-facilitating environments. In addition, there is a need for evaluation tools in addition to observation in several adaptive skill areas. Furthermore, based on the 1968 rationale for activity, research on activity elements as similar to or symbolic of environmental elements could be explored.

SPECIALIZATION

The 1968 version of recapitulation of ontogenesis states that model may serve as a guide for action in the psychosocial, cognitive and perceptual motor areas. No mention is made in the 1970 version as to areas of specialization. However, the emphasis on psychosocial develop-ment suggests that emphasis on mental functioning has been stressed. Also, there is an emphasis on learning as the major source of development rather than a mix of maturation and learning. Physical motor or sensory motor development is much more difficult to explain as a purely learned behavior. There appears to be some prewired circuits which initiate the contacts with the external environment where learning situations exist. Thus, the model appears to have some limitations as a basis for physical development and physical dysfunction which may have been intention-ally introduced by Mosey when the model was proposed.

ELABORATION AND REFINEMENT

Recapitulation of ontogenesis as a model could be elaborated by paying more attention to the development of physical motor skills. However, the major needs appear to be those of refinement. As mentioned in the frame of reference, there remain concepts which are based on mechanistic views. Specifically, reinforcement and reward are considered part of the learning interaction. Perhaps the concepts of affirmation or consensual validation would serve as well, while maintaining an internal locus of control. The major concern is whether external reinforcement and reward is really needed to develop and maintain a behavior. Maria Montessori did not think so. She used media which could provide their own reward through task completion. Perhaps occupational therapy should explore the use of self rewards or self confirming behavior more seriously.

Another area of refinement concerns the subskill hierarchy. The dyadic relationships seems to begin too late. The perceptual motor skills may need revision in light of later findings by Ayres and others. The drive object skills do not reflect the development of self actualization and competence.

EXPLANATORY USEFULNESS

The concept of adaptive skills provides a useful explanation of how development occurs through learning in a growth-facilitating environment. Unfortunately, the lack of concept of activity element in the 1970 edition reduces the model's explanatory usefulness of the occupational therapy process.

COMMONALITY

The concept of developmental sequence is familiar to other disciplines as a basis for explaining normal behavior. The categories of adaptive skills may seem arbitrary, unless a rationale as proposed in Figure 13.7 is adopted. Learning theory as a means of skill building is familiar also to others. Thus, the model of recapitulation of ontogenesis is fairly recognizable to others.

PRACTICE MODEL

The 1970 model of recapitulation of ontogenesis provides a basis for developmental sequence in a practice theory. However, the 1968 version provides a much better basis for the use of activity in practice. Those who wish to develop practice models based on recapitulation of ontogenesis should be advised to read both versions.

SUMMARY

The recapitulation of ontogenesis model is summarized in Table 13.10.

Activity Therapy—Mosey

FRAME OF REFERENCE

The activity therapy model is based on concepts of therapeutic community or milieu therapy and group dynamics. Activity therapy is based on the belief that many mental health problems are the result of failure to learn to function in the community. Central to the intervention process is the concept of learning by doing.

The therapeutic community concept is based on the work of Maxwell Jones. Milieu therapy is borrowed from Cumming and Cumming and from Robert Hyde. Group dynamics concepts are organized from the works of such leaders as George Homans, Walter Lifton and Theodore Mills. Teaching and learning concepts are borrowed from education psychologists, such as James Bruner, but also from behaviorists, such as Watson and Skinner.

ASSUMPTIONS (71)

1. Psychosocial dysfunction is learned maladaptive behavior in which the individual has developed patterns of behavior that are ineffective in coping with the demands of daily life (p. 5).
2. Psychosocial dysfunction involves the lack of the following (pp. 2–3).
   a. Ability to plan and carry out a task,
   b. Capacity to interact comfortably in a group,
   c. Ability to identify and satisfy needs,

Table 13.10
Recapitulation of Ontogenesis Critique Summary

Criteria	Very Good 1	Moderately Good 2	3	4	Very Poor 5
Frame of reference	X				
Clarity			X		
Uniqueness	X				
Research guide	X				
Specialization	X				
Elaboration/refinement	X				
Explanation	X				
Commonality	X				
Practice model	X				

    d. Ability to express emotions in an acceptable manner,

    e. More or less accurate perception of the self, the human and nonhuman environment, and one's relationship to the environment,

    f. Value system that allows the individual to satisfy personal needs without infringing on the rights of others,

    g. Skill to carry out required activities of daily living,

    h. Ability to work at a relatively satisfying job,

    i. Enjoyment of avocational pursuits and recreational activities,

    j. Ability to interact comfortably in family and friendship relationships.

3. A person does not need to know what past events caused the individual to be in a state of psychosocial dysfunction before change is possible (p. 5).

4. Faulty patterns of (maladaptive) behavior can be unlearned and replaced by other, more effective patterns (p. 5).

5. Growth can be facilitated through action (p. 6).

6. The dynamics of group interaction can be used to foster change (p. 5).

7. The emphasis of treatment should be on the here and now, not on the past (p. 2).

8. The therapist is concerned with where the person is right now and the nature of present life (p. 5).

9. Treatment is directed toward the development of knowledge, skills, and values that the person will need in the future (p. 5).

10. There are two interdependent aspects to activity therapy:

    a. Greater understanding of self

    b. Development of skills (p. 2)

CONCEPTS (71)

Mental illness—psychosocial dysfunction; the inability to meet one's needs in a manner that is satisfying to oneself and not detrimental to the need satisfaction of others (p. 1)

Activity therapy—a method of helping people who are unable to cope with the stresses of daily life to learn to live in and be a part of their community (p. 1)

Treatment—a planned, collaborative interaction between the therapist, the patient, and the nonhuman environment directed toward the development of skills for community living (p. 3)

Planned and collaborative interaction—the idea that the therapist and patient have clearly identified what changes they hope to bring about and what each of them is going to do to attain these previously set goals (p. 4)

Basic skills—those tasks and group interactions which permit a person to function in the community and to satisfy needs (p. 7)

Nonhuman environment—refers to all aspects of the external environment that are not human (p. 4)

Needs—are inherent as opposed to learned or acquired (p. 12)

a. *Physiological needs*—needs that must be satisfied to maintain life, such as air, food, shelter, an optimal amount of sensory stimuli and motor activity and the release of sexually induced tension (p. 12)

b. *Safety needs*—needs that are satisfied through interacting in an environment that is experienced as relatively free of harmful situations (p. 12)

c. *Love and belonging needs*—needs that are satisfied when an individual is accepted by others as being a unique and very special person (p. 12)

d. *Mastery needs*—need to master refers to the desire to explore, understand and to some extent control oneself, other people and the nonhuman environment (p. 13)

e. *Esteem needs*—need to motivate an individual to engage in an activity in order to receive recognition from others (p. 13)

f. *Self actualization*—need to be oneself, to do something that is of particular importance to oneself (p. 13)

Occupational areas

a. *Activities of daily living*—refers to all those *other* things a person must be able to do in order to engage successfully in work, recreation and intimacy (p. 18)

b. *Work*—a person's major occupation and what an individual does to make money (p. 18)

c. *Work habits*—certain basic knowledge and skills involved in the ability to work (p. 19)

d. *Recreation*—those things a person does for fun or relaxation and the involvement in community activities (p. 19)

Types of groups

a. *Parallel group*—individuals work and play in the presence of others, but there is minimal sharing of tasks or mutual stimulation (p. 9)

b. *Project group*—members are involved in short-term tasks that require some sharing or interaction, but there is little interaction other than that necessary to perform the task (p. 9)

c. *Egocentric cooperative group*—members decide on relatively long-term activities and carry them through to completion. Individuals meet each other's esteem needs but not love and safety needs (p. 9)

d. *Cooperative group*—made up of members who have common interests, concerns and values but do not necessarily need an activity as a focal point (p. 9)

e. *Mature group*—made up of people with different backgrounds, interests and ideas who can take a variety of roles as needed to provide a good balance between task accomplishment and satisfaction of group member needs (p. 9)

Terms used in group dynamics

  a. *Group*—an aggregate of people who share a common purpose which can be attained only by group members interacting and working together (p. 45)

  b. *Dynamics and process*—refers to the various facets of small groups that are in a continuous state of change (p. 46)

  c. *Task roles*—those roles that are usually needed for a group to select, plan and carry out a group task (p. 46)

  d. *Social emotional roles*—those roles which are concerned with the function of the group as a group and with satisfying members' needs (p. 47)

  e. *Decision making*—the process of arriving at an agreed upon solution to a problem (p. 50)

  f. *Communication*—the process of giving and receiving information by means of gestures, words and tone of voice (p. 54)

  g. *Group goals*—the future state toward which majority of the group's efforts are directed (p. 56)

  h. *Group cohesiveness*—refers to the degree of closeness group members feel toward each other and the value they place on the group (p. 58)

  i. *Group norms*—value system of a group (p. 60)

  j. *Socialization*—learning about and learning to act in accordance with the normal of the group (p. 63)

  k. *Sanction*—the term used to identify the process whereby a group tries to get one of its members to act within the limits of the group's norms (p. 63)

Terms used in describing relationships

  a. *Intimacy*—the area of human experience that involves a close, sustained relationship with other individuals (p. 20)

  b. *Casual friendship*—the ability to experience pleasure in being with other people (p. 21)

  c. *Chum relationships*—intense relationship of preadolescents in which the individuals want to be together as often as possible (p. 21)

  d. *Love relationships*—mutually satisfying need which is sustained over a long period of time (p. 21)

  e. *Nurturing relationship*—one partner helps the other to grow toward his unique potential (p. 22)

Terms related to self

  a. *Cognitive system*—refers to what a person knows and thinks about himself, other people and the world around him, including factual knowledge, beliefs and ideas (p. 10)

b. *Private self*—aspects of the person which are located within the individual, such as the cognitive system, needs, emotions and values (p. 10)

c. *Public self*—aspects of the person which are more directly related to the interactions with others, such as activities of daily living, work, recreation, and intimacy (p. 17)

d. *Emotions*—inherent responses to need satisfaction and deprivation (p. 14)

e. *Values*—degree of worth ascribed to a person, thing, activity or idea (p. 16)

Terms related to teaching-learning process

a. *Reinforcer*—any event that increases the frequency of a particular act (p. 34)

b. *Differential reinforcement*—process whereby a person is given reinforcement for one kind of behavior and not given reinforcement for another type of behavior (p. 34)

c. *Shaping*—a process whereby successive approximations of the desired behavior are reinforced (p. 34)

d. *Feedback*—the information one receives about the way one's behavior affects other people or things (p. 36)

e. *Generalization*—the ability to apply what was learned in one situation to another appropriate situation (p. 38)

f. *Discrimination*—the ability to determine what is appropriate behavior for one situation as opposed to another situation (p. 38)

g. *Token economy*—way of structuring the treatment setting in which persons are given tokens for appropriate behavior that can be exchanged for foods, events, passes and the like (p. 35)

EXPECTED RESULTS (71)

1. Develop skills for community living (p. 105).
2. Able to perform single task skills.
3. Able to perform at a normal rate.
4. Able to use tools and materials appropriately.
5. Able to satisfy needs by doing tasks.
6. Able to sustain an interest in doing a task until completed.
7. Able to follow instructions, written and oral.
8. Able to perform at an acceptable level of neatness.
9. Able to attend appropriately to detail.
10. Able to solve problems that arise in performing a task.
11. Able to organize a task in a logical manner.
12. Able to function in group situations.
13. Able to participate in a parallel group.
14. Able to participate in a project group.
15. Able to participate in an egocentric cooperative group.

16. Able to participate in a cooperative group
17. Able to participate in a mature group—optional
18. Able to perform activities of daily living needed for living in the expected environment.
19. Able to perform in a work setting (work groups, sheltered workshop, hospital job, community job).
20. Able to participate in homemaking tasks.
21. If a parent, able to function as a parent.
22. If a student, able to function as a student.
23. Able to participate in recreation.
24. Able to form casual relationships.
25. Able to form chum relationships.
26. Able to form love relationships.
27. Able to form nurturing relationships.
28. Able to correctly assess self abilities and limitations according to reality and feedback from others.
29. Able to correctly assess and satisfy physiological, safety, love and belonging, mastery, esteem and self actualization needs.
30. Able to express emotions correctly.
31. Able to identify values and change those values which are detrimental to the person.

ASSESSMENT TECHNIQUES (71)

1. Data collection
   a. Observation—noting a patient's usual patterns of behavior (p. 87)
   b. Structured observation—involves setting up a specific situation and asking the patient to participate in the situation (p. 87)
   c. Interview—one to one discussion with the patient (p. 87)
   d. Questionnaire—a written list of questions the patient is asked to answer as completely as possible (p. 87)
   e. Interview schedule—used to help the therapist obtain the desired information (p. 87)
2. Instruments
   a. Survey of Task skills (pp. 89–91) (Table 13.11).
   b. Group—Interaction Skills Survey (p. 92) (Table 13.12)
   c. Activities of Daily Living (p. 94) (Table 13.13)
   d. Work Survey (p. 98) (Table 13.14)
   e. Child Care Survey (p. 96) (Table 13.15)
   f. Recreation Survey (p. 99) (Table 13.16)
   g. Activity Configuration (p. 102) (Table 13.17)

INTERVENTION STRATEGIES (71)

1. Media and modalities—some are listed in the assessment instruments
2. Techniques
   Activity groups—the composition depends upon the situation or purpose of the group. The process of the group is composed of five steps:

Table 13.11
Survey of Task Skills[a]

Behavior	Comments	Present	Future
Coordination			
Bizarre behavior			
Hyperactivity			
Hypoactivity			
Reliability			
Engagement			
Concentration			
Directions			
Activity neatness			
Attention to detail			
Problem solving			
Organization of task			

Key for Survey of Task Skills

Coordination
    1 = Moves in a clumsy manner, has difficulty manipulating tools and materials
    4 = Is able to engage in activities that require both fine and gross movements

Bizarre behavior
    1 = Stereotyped activities (rocking, playing with hands, repetitive statements), appears to be talking to self, preoccupation with own thoughts, etc.
    4 = Absence of above

Hyperactivity
    1 = Accelerated in speech and/or action
    4 = Speaks and acts at normal pace

Hypoactivity
    1 = Retarded in speech and/or action
    4 = Speaks and acts at normal pace

Reliability
    1 = Cannot be depended on to carry out a given activity; inappropriate use of tools and materials
    4 = Can be depended on to perform in an acceptable manner

Engagement
    1 = Does not engage in activity
    4 = Readily engages in activity without encouragement

Concentration
    1 = Readily loses interest in a given task
    4 = Works at a given task with sustained interest and attention

Directions
    1 = Unable to carry out simple demonstrated, oral and/or written directions
    4 = Readily carries out relatively complex demonstrated, oral, and written directions

Activity neatness
    1 = Performs activities in a sloppy, careless manner
    4 = Performs activities in a neat, orderly manner

Attention to detail
    1 = Overly concise to the point that it interferes with performance
    4 = Attends to detail according to the demands of the given activity

Table 13.11—*Continued*

Problem solving
   1 = Activity behavior is disrupted when confronted with problems that arise in the context of an activity; no attempt is made to solve them
   4 = Identifies and solves problems which arise in the performance of an activity; uses resources in an appropriate manner
Organization of task
   1 = Unable to organize an activity effectively even when tools, materials, and directions are available
   4 = Organizes a task in a logical and efficient manner

[a] Adapted from J. W. Fidler and G. S. Fidler (59). Reprinted from A. C. Mosey (71), pp. 89–91, with permission from Raven Press.

Table 13.12
Group-Interaction Skills Survey[a]

Type of Group	
Parallel group	

Parallel group
   Engages in some activity, but acts as if this is an individual task as opposed to a group activity
   Aware of others in the group
   Some verbal or nonverbal interaction with others
   Appears to be relatively comfortable in this situation
Project group
   Occasionally engages in the group activity, moving in and out according to his own whim
   Seeks some assistance from others
   Gives some assistance when directly asked to do so
Egocentric-cooperative group
   Aware of group's goal relative to the task
   Aware of group norms
   Acts as if he belongs in the group
   Willing to participate
   Meets esteem needs of others
   Able to get others to meet his esteem needs
   Recognizes rights of others
   Not overly competitive
Cooperative group
   Makes own wishes, desires, and needs known
   Participates in group activity but seems concerned primarily with his own needs and needs of others
   Able to meet needs other than esteem needs
   Tends to be most responsive to group members who are similar to him in some way
Mature group
   Responsive to all group members
   Takes a variety of task roles
   Takes a variety of social-emotional roles
   Able to share leadership
   Promotes a good balance between task accomplishment and satisfaction of group members' needs

[a] Reprinted from A. C. Mosey (71), p. 92, with permission from Raven Press.

Table 13.13
Activities of Daily Living Survey[a]

Activity	Present	Future
Adequate hygiene		
Hair combed, appropriately styled		
Dress appropriate for age, current fashion, and occasion		
Clothes cleaned and ironed		
Plan nutritious diet		
Cook		
Shop for food		
Know what change to expect from clerk		
Plan a budget		
Change a bed		
Sweep and dust		
Wash and dry dishes		
Household tasks (hang curtains, change light bulb and fuse, take and appliance to be fixed, etc.)		
Shop for clothes		
Wash clothes		
Iron clothes		
Sew on a button		
Fix a ripped seam		
Make a hem		
Find a number in the telephone book		
Get a number from the telephone operator		
Make a telephone call to request information		
Make a telephone call to leave a message		
Take a telephone message		
Write a personal letter		
Write a business letter		
Fill out various forms		
Travel on a bus, subway, and train		
Read a timetable		
Buy and return a ticket		
Follow a road, subway, and bus route map		
Drive a car		

[a] Reprinted from A. C. Mosey (71), p. 94, with permission from Raven Press.

    a. What is going on here? (encounter or confrontation)
    b. Exploration
    c. What needs to be changed?
    d. Learning
    e. Follow-up
  3. Approaches
    a. A good teacher begins where the learning is and moves at a rate that is comfortable (p. 28).
    b. A good teacher takes into consideration the learner's inherent capacities, age, sex, interests, assets and limitations, and cultural group membership (p. 29).

Table 13.14
Work Survey[a]

Activities	
Alters behavior appropriately on the basis of constructive criticism	
Follows written, oral, and demonstrated directions	
Sustains attention to work tasks	
Organizes tasks relative to priority	
Performs tasks in a normal amount of time	
Works at increased speed when required	
Returns to work when interrupted	
Carries on appropriate conversation when working	
Interrupts work tasks and carries on appropriate conversation	
Completes forms	
Plans work period so that required amount of work is accomplished	
Comes to work on time	
Stays at work for required period of time	
Appears able to work a normal work day	
Evokes a pleasant response from others	
Follows the norms of the work setting	
Gives assistance willingly	
Takes direction from a work supervisor	
Requests only an appropriate amount of need satisfaction from the work supervisor	

[a] Reprinted from A. C. Mosey (71), p. 98, with permission from Raven Press.

Table 13.15
Child Care Survey[a]

Activity	Present	Future
Demonstrates affection		
Cares for physical needs (food, clothes, etc.)		
Plays with a child		
Plans activities for a child		
Disciplines a child in a consistent manner		
Secures periodic physical, dental, and eye examinations		
Maintains a safe home		
Secures adequate baby-sitting facilities		
Shows concern about child's education		
Maintains adequate balance between freedom and control		
Communicates in a forthright manner (does not give double messages)		
Gives child appropriate responsibilities		
Aware of child's needs		

[a] Reprinted from A. C. Mosey (71), p. 96, with permission from Raven Press.

Table 13.16
Recreation Survey[a]

Activity	Present	Future
Swimming		
Table games (poker, chess, bridge)		
Photography		
Drama groups		
Discussion groups		
Choral groups		
Woodworking		
Reading		
Playing musical instrument		
Listening to music		
Social dancing		
Pool		
Sewing		
Bicycling		
Movies		
Going to parties		
Union activities		
Bowling		
Lectures		
Attending classes to learn how to do something		
Gardening		
Shopping		
Church organizations		
Poetry		
Going out to a restaurant		
Political organization		
Modern dancing		
Sketching		
Painting		
Gymnastics		
Boxing		
Wrestling		
Cooking		
Baseball		
Basketball		
Football		
Tennis		
Golf		
Skiing		
Sculpture		
Electronics		
Knitting		
Calesthenics		
Watching TV		
Casual conversation		
Fixing things		
PTA		
Volunteer work		
Community action groups		

[a] Adapted from J. Matsutsuyu (38). Reprinted from A. C. Mosey (71), p. 99, with permission from Raven Press.

Table 13.17
Activity Configuration[a]

Part 1

Time	Mon.	Tues.	Wed.	Thurs.	Fri.	Sat.	Sun.
6–7							
7–8							
8–9							
9–10							
10–11							
11–12							
12–1							
1–2							
2–3							
3–4							
4–5							
5–6							
6–7							
7–8							
8–9							
9–10							
10–11							

Part 2

A. What needs does the activity satisfy? What needs are not satisfied during this activity or not satisfied because of engaging in the activity?

B. I have to do this activity. I want to do this activity. Or both?

C. I want to do this activity and I think this is good. I want to do this activity and I think this is not good. Others make me do this and I am glad they do. Or others make me do this and I wish they did not.

D. I do this activity very well. I do this activity well enough. Or I do not do this activity well enough.

E. I feel joy, liking, love, fear or anxiety, dislike, hatred, anger, depression, guilt, or some other emotion while engaging in this activity. Before and after engaging in this activity, I feel _____ and _____ .

[a] Reprinted from A. C. Mosey (71), p. 102, with permission from Raven Press.

   c. The learner should be an active participant in the learning process (p. 33).

   d. The consequence of an action is important (p. 34).

   e. Opportunity for trial and error imitation enhances learning (p. 36).

   f. Frequent repetition or practice facilitates learning (p. 36).

   g. Learning goals set by the learner are more likely to be attained than goals set by someone else (p. 37).

   h. Practice in different situations encourages generalization and discrimination.

   i. The learner should understand what is to be learned and the reasons for learning (p. 39).

j. Planned movement from simplified wholes to more complex wholes enhances learning (p. 39).
k. Inventive solutions to problems should be encouraged as well as more usual or typical solutions (p. 41).
l. There are individual differences in the ways anxiety affects learning (p. 42).

SUMMARY

Activity therapy is the use of immediate, action-oriented interactions to help people who have been designed as "mentally ill" to learn to live in and be part of their community. It is a method of helping people who are unable to cope with the stress of daily life. Activities are used to provide familiar life situations in which participants are assisted in identifying faulty patterns of behavior and the ideas, feelings and values that support these faulty patterns and are helped to develop more effective ways to acting.

Analysis and Critique of the Activities Therapy Model

FRAME OF REFERENCE

The activity therapy model is based primarily on the organismic view. The focus is on the present, and the emphasis is on learning skills and values for future use. Cause and effect are not emphasized. However, some concepts from behaviorism are included, such as shaping, taken economy, and reinforcers. Mosey continues to attempt to integrate concepts from the organismic and mechanistic viewpoints into one model. The "invasion" or infusion of mechanistic based concepts into an organismic based model must be carefully monitored and explained if the model is to remain true to organismic philosophy that the locus of control should be maintained within the individual and not within the environment, such as a management program.

CLARITY

The problem of how the mechanistically based concepts will be used is not clearly spelled out. Reinforcers can be selected by the therapist to promote behavior which the environment via the psychiatric service determines would be good for the person to learn, or reinforcers can be selected by the person to promote behavior which the person agrees needs to be learned. The difference is the degree of control which the individual maintains.

A second problem is concerned with programming for children. Although the final outcomes are given in the assumption, no subtasks or developmental sequence is provided. In the preface, Mosey (71, p. vi) suggests that the focus for children should be learning by doing, but no details are given to guide the transition. Likewise, no details are provided for modifying the program for older adults. For example, what emphasis should be placed on work satisfaction for a retired individual?

A third problem is the assumption that all psychosocial problems are the result of faulty learning patterns which are maladaptive. There seems to be very little concern for the possibility that some learning may never have occurred at all or that some learning may be nonadaptive. Learning which never occurred may not be under the individual's control. Lack of opportunity due to sociocultural factors should not be classified as maladaptive or faulty learning. There is also a difference in intervention strategy. Lack of learning is corrected by beginning the learning sequence. Faulty learning usually requires unlearning while relearning as simultaneous occurrences. Nonadaptive learning is simply ineffective. The solution does not fit the problem. A hammer cannot be used to tighten the nut on a bolt. Nonadaptive learning usually requires that effective solutions and problems be put together. The missing skills are linkages rather than basis skill development.

Finally, Mosey in the Preface (71, p. V) suggests that activities therapy is a relatively new term in the psychiatric nomenclature. Actually, the term activity therapy has been around for many years, and the frame of reference has been fairly consistent. In the occupational therapy literature the term has been used since at least 1952 (72). Thomas, a registered occupational therapist, describes a program at Chestnut Lodge in which occupational therapy activities are compared to a laboratory and the clinic as a safe place to try various experiments in interacting with people and with activity. Other articles appeared in 1955 (73), 1958 (74), 1965 (75), and 1968 (76). Socialization, productive accomplishment, increased responsibility for making decisions and preparation for life beyond the institution are common themes.

UNIQUENESS

The activities therapy model does not spell out what is unique about occupational therapy or why occupational therapists should be the primary change agents in intervention programs. In fact, the activity therapies model has been written as if any mental health worker could plan and implement an intervention program. The Preface includes reference to "people who simply have the desire and ability to work with psychiatric patients" (71, p. V). Either the profession of occupational therapy is so altruistic that time can be spent on building models for other professional groups, or the profession still has not clearly identified the uniqueness of occupational therapy and thus avoids the issue.

RESEARCH GUIDE

A review of articles in the *American Journal of Occupational Therapy* shows that the activities therapy model as outlined by Mosey has not been used as a basis for research. The general model of activity therapy has been used as a basis for exploring attitudes about an activity program (77). Staff and patients were surveyed as to their opinions about the role of the activity program in the total intervention program. There was substantial agreement between the staff and patients. The major problems appeared to be that both staff and patients were not entirely clear as to the role an activity program could play in helping patients to better recognize problems and to assist patients' skill development in maintaining a job.

The lack of research on Mosey's activities therapy model should not be interpreted as a lack of interest. Hemphill (78) surveyed 241 clinicians to determine what psychiatric evaluations were being used most frequently. All of Mosey's assessment instruments except the Child Care Survey were among the top 10 of 24 evaluations listed. The same six forms also were among the top 10 assessment instruments taught by occupational therapy faculty. Likewise, clinical supervisors demonstrate proficiency in the same instruments. Thus, there appears to be a fairly wide use of the assessments. Whether the program of activities therapy is implemented, however, is difficult to ascertain.

SPECIALIZATION

The discussion of the use of the assessment instruments under research suggests that the activities model as proposed by Mosey may have produced some specialization. However, the impact has not been measured to date. There is definitely a use of the general activity therapy model; the actual use could be assessed by examining the number of articles in the *American Journal of Occupational Therapy* which reference activity therapy programs within a therapeutic community, milieu, or rehabilitation approach to intervention in psychosocial problems.

ELABORATION/REFINEMENT

As stated under the section on clarity, there is a need to elaborate the activities therapy model to include children. An initial start on adapting activities therapy for children may be explored by reading the article by Cermack *et al.* (79). The authors suggest methods for structuring the group and the environment, selecting activities, establishing goals and determining the therapist's role in controlling behavior.

Elaboration is needed also to clarify the norm referenced group for determining basic skills and needs. The goal of providing individuals with the knowledge, skills and clues to meet their needs is laudable, but how are the needs determined? Are the individuals consulted? Is there some master plan for various social economic groups? Is there no plan?

Finally, there should be some refinement within each need category so that progress and attainment can be evaluated. At present, the assessment of progress is dependent on opinion rather than fact.

EXPLANATION

The activities therapy model does provide some explanation of the occupational therapy process. The model is built around the activities which people need to be able to do and usually are doing with some frequency as independent functioning individuals. Such attention to doing and frequency of doing are basic to occupational therapy's definition and process.

The problem appears to be that the activities therapy model does not provide an explanation of the unique role of occupational therapy within the model. The teaching-learning of knowledge, skills and values is not unique to occupational therapy nor are occupational therapists necessarily the most skilled professionals in the teaching-learning process. Therefore, the question arises as to why occupational therapists should be included in an activities therapy program at all. What contribution do occupational therapists make that could not be done as well or better by others?

COMMONALITY

As a common focus, the activities therapy model appears to be fairly successful. The assumption of faulty learning patterns provides a common base for several professional groups. Nurses can instruct in better health procedures, dietitians can teach better nutrition habits, social workers can encourage better family relationships, teachers can provide remedial instruction and occupational therapists can improve occupational skills and performance. Thus, the teaching-learning process offers a unifying strategy. The problem may be in sorting out who does what. Then the failure to identify the unique role of occupational therapy may cause problems because occupational therapists have knowledge and skills to support and reinforce the teaching-learning process of all other professional groups, especially those which are involved in activities, such as music, art, recreation, dance, poetry, drama, etc.

PRACTICE MODEL

At this time, there are no articles in *The American Journal of Occupational Therapy* or *Occupational Therapy Journal of Research* which indicate that practice models have evolved specifically from the activities therapy model presented by Mosey. However, such a statement does not preclude existence of such models but simply means that publication has not occurred. The potential for models or theories related to activity configuration and activities of daily living would seem to be especially good. A summary of the activity therapy model is presented in Table 13.18.

Occupational Therapy Process Model

FRAME OF REFERENCE

Sandra Watanabe (80) has based the frame of reference for the occupational therapy process model primarily on Lewin's concept of life space but the concept is enlarged beyond the totality of forces operating at a given time to include a continuity and specificity of time, space, resources and relationships. However, Arsenion's theory of TEMPO is used also. TEMPO stands for "doing the right things at the right time with the right energy (and expectancy) in the right mode, in the right place and with the right objects" (81). Arsenion recognizes the sociocultural demands on the individual in terms of the flow, pace and timing in the life cycles, as well as the pressure to conform, keep up and get along.

Table 13.18
Activity Therapy Model Critique Summary

Criteria	Very Good 1	Moderately Good			Very Poor 5
		2	3	4	
Frame of reference		x			
Clarity			x		
Uniqueness				x	
Research guide			x		
Specialization		x			
Elaboration/refinement		x			
Explanation			x		
Commonality		x			
Practice model		x			

In addition, White's concepts of competence, mastery, and intrinsic maturation are used to explain the need and ability to recognize options in society. Glasser's concept of responsibility is used as described namely "the ability to fulfill one's needs and to do so in a way that does not deprive others of the ability to fulfill their needs..." (80, p. 441). Allport's concept of proprium is used to describe how a person achieves an integrated personality which can choose and meet the life tasks which make up the individual's place in the society and world. Finally, May's description of the phenomenological method is used as a base for the treatment approach.

ASSUMPTIONS (80)

1. Assumptions about man
   a. Each person has a unique pattern of potential for growth and change (p. 442).
   b. There is an inherent balance in man's productivity—the balance between personal satisfaction and meaning, and social viability and acceptability (p. 442).
2. Assumptions about the life space
   a. The development of life space is based on learning through experience about the spatial and temporal extensions of one's private world (p. 439).
   b. Life space is a fundamental life dimension which is intrinsically related to the other dimensions of life, including energy and time (p. 439).
   c. Life space deals with both the continuity and specific aspects of time, space, human and natural resources and relationships (p. 440).
   d. Some people never develop or expand their life space sufficiently to provide substance and consistency to their self concept or meet the demands of daily life (p. 439).
   e. When a life space is restricted there develops little mastery over one's environment and control over one's life situation (p. 439).

3. Assumptions about mastery
   a. Man has an innate need to manipulate and explore, to stimulate the self by doing and thinking with no other goal than the development of mastery and achievement of success (p. 440).
   b. The development of mastery is motivated by man's need to control what happens to him and around him (p. 440).
   c. The development of mastery in an orderly fashion is necessary for keeping in step with one's reference group (p. 440).
   d. The nature of one's mastery can be noted in the (a) extent and use of life space, (b) mechanisms used in coping with life situations and (c) ease in handling and integrating new experiences (p. 440).
   e. If a person's degree of mastery is insufficient or the attempted mastery inappropriate, he will not be able to handle the stress of daily life (p. 440).
   f. Inability to handle stress increases vulnerability to intrapsychic and interpersonal disorganization and ineffective use of life space (p. 440).
4. Assumptions about responsibility
   a. Responsibility is important to provide the life space with consensual meaning and mastery with performance criteria (p. 441).
   b. Individuals are expected to take the responsibility for choosing and meeting their life tasks at appropriate times in their lives (p. 442).
5. Assumptions about life tasks
   a. For each individual, life tasks differ from functional activities in that he chooses to make a particular investment in a life task and get satisfaction from it while he performs his functions in an uncommitted minimally gratifying manner (p. 442).
   b. An individual's expectations about his personal life tasks and his specific choices of the options are based upon such factors as his inherent (biological) capabilities, his subculture's values, his own perception of the general culture, his socioeconomic position, his family experience, his emotional status, the extent of his life space and his level of mastery and responsibility (p. 442).
   c. The categories from which one's specific life tasks are chosen are developmentally and traditionally associated with specific age groups (p. 442).
   d. Life tasks involve an appropriate commitment to one's own choices, decisions and actions (p. 442).
6. Assumptions about occupational therapy
   a. Occupational therapists are concerned with the extent of the person's life space and how the individual utilizes it (p. 440).
   b. Occupational therapists are concerned with a person's development of the mastery needed to handle daily stresses (p. 441).
   c. Occupational therapy provides opportunity for evoking and fostering responsibility (p. 441).

d. Occupational therapists are involved with persons in active experiences where reality and the possibility of responsibility are essential (p. 441).

e. Issues of decision making, problem solving and responsibility should not be left to chance, or taken over by the therapist, but be the function of therapy (p. 441).

f. Because of its action orientation, occupational therapy has the potential to consciously and concretely put before the person options concerning for what, to what, or to whom the individual understands the self to be responsible (p. 441).

g. Occupational therapy uses self-chosen graded activity and ADL instead of impersonal exercises (p. 442).

h. Occupational therapy process connotes our concern with the evolutionary aspects of the life tasks and the use of objects and activities in the process of becoming (p. 442).

i. The focus on becoming marks an occupational therapist's active orientation to life tasks (p. 442).

CONCEPTS (80)

Life space—The physical, perceptual, cognitive, psychological and socio-cultural realms of an individual (p. 439)

Mastery—ability and skill in recognizing and comprehending the options that society offers and make choices appropriately using one's human and nonhuman environment to meet one's own needs and abilities (p. 440)

Responsibility—the accountability of an individual for his own choices, decisions and actions (p. 441)

Life tasks—the personal and social undertakings from which an individual derives satisfaction and to which he feels a commitment, such as activities of daily living, vocation, socialization, education, creative and avocational interests, family living, and child bearing and rearing (p. 442)

Functional activities, functions—activities performed in an uncommitted, minimally gratifying manner (p. 442)

Functioning—the mechanical, routine follow-through on the aspects of daily life which are seen as necessary to do (p. 442)

Competence motivation—man actively seeks experience which challenges his ability to manipulate his environment (p. 440)

TEMPO—doing the right things at the right Time, with the right Energy and expectancy, in the right Mode, in the right Place, with the right Objects (p. 440)

Anxiety—the state of human being in the struggle against that which would destroy his being (p. 443)

Proprium—the aspects of personality which form the integrated unity that constitutes the individual's uniqueness and sense of individuality (82, p. 81)

Properties of proprium (p. 442)

1. *Bodily sense* (coenthesis)
2. *Self-identity* (temporal, social and spatial awareness)
3. *Ego enhancement* (self-seeking)
4. *Ego extention* (objects of importance)
5. *Rational agent* (in touch with reality)
6. *Self-image* (phenomenal self)
7. *Propriate striving* ("ego-involved" motivation)
8. *The knower* (cognizing self)

▸*Phenomenological approach*—a conscious, lived participation in the patient's world and the acceptance of and respect for things as they are experienced (p. 442)

EXPECTED RESULTS

•1. Expand the life space of neighborhood community, state, country, and world.
2. Expand the life space of personal history and social relationships, and interaction with institutions.
3. Increase mastery of self and environment.
4. Increase sense of responsibility for making decisions.
5. Increase ability and skill to accomplish life tasks in the developmental sequence.

ASSESSMENT INSTRUMENTS

The article mentions a comprehensive interview being done in the home, but no details are included.

INTERVENTION STRATEGIES

1. Media and modalities
   a. Patients own life objects—house, street, store, transportation, library
   b. Natural groups—families, neighbors, community, caregivers
   c. Prevocation exploration and training
   d. Self chosen graded activity
2. Methods, techniques—approaches
   a. Problem identification solving technique
   b. Confrontation
   c. Role playing
   d. Collaborative planning session
   e. Discussion
3. Equipment—that which is in the environment
4. Prerequisite skills and precautions—not specified

SUMMARY

• The occupational therapy process model was created to meet the need of the community mental health therapist who does not have the typical institution and clinic for support. The model served further to identify the role of the occupational therapist as opposed to the other community mental health workers. Intervention was conducted in the person's home and community and made use of the person's own life situations and activities as opposed to the clinical setting.

Four major basic concepts are used in the model to explore a person's relationship to the environment and to examine what might go wrong within the relationship. The concepts are life space, mastery, responsibility and life tasks. Occupational therapy is considered to have a role in facilitating the development and use of each concept. Life space can be facilitated through the active process of doing. Mastery can be enhanced by graded activity directed to problem solving and skill building. Responsiblility is developed through the use of reality-oriented experiences which are mutually planned between the therapist and the person. Life tasks are influenced by utilization of a phenomenological approach which involves active participation in the person's world. Evaluation and intervention are based on the acceptance of and respect for events as the person experiences them.

Analysis and Critique of the Occupational Therapy Process Model
FRAME OF REFERENCE

• The occupational therapy process model clearly is based on the organismic view in which self-control, self-mastery and sense of responsibility are stressed. Developmental process is used also, although the stages and sequences are not provided. As frames of references are organized, the occupational therapy process model has an unusually broad and varied input. No less than 12 major writers of theory and six lesser known writers are referenced as providing portions of the total frame of reference. Such diversity can create problems of integrating concepts into a unified system.

CLARITY

Figure 13.10 is an attempt to outline the concepts mentioned in the occupational therapy process model. An analysis of the model suggests that the major difficulty is in the throughput process. Are all those mechanisms necessary? Is there some way to combine needs, motivations, value perceptions, emotions, learning and development into few categories or at least into a more organized system which ties the mechanisms to some specific output? The model looks more like a laundry list than an integrated approach.

The same problem occurs when the model of dysfunction is illustrated as in Figure 13.11. Connections between throughput and output are not clearly stated. Furthermore, several mechanisms listed under the model of function do not appear in the model of dysfunction, but the rationale is not clear for either inclusion or exclusion.

Part of the difficulty of the model is the result of trying to combine so many different theories and model builder's ideas into one practice model. The concepts and assumptions need to be carefully selected and even

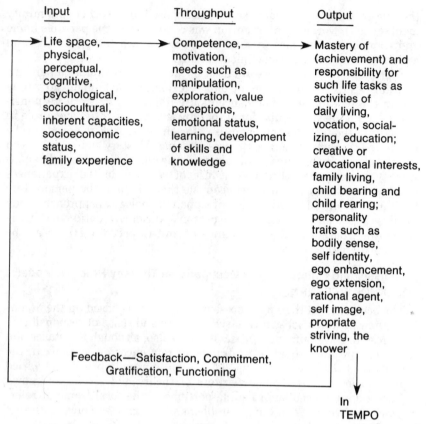

Figure 13.10. Occupational therapy process model of function.

more carefully integrated into the practice model so that the organization of input, throughput and output is comprehensible and has some face validity.

The model does somewhat better at suggesting how the occupational therapy process can be organized to provide intervention for persons who have dysfunction in life tasks. The sequence of assessment, selection of media and methods and expected results is reasonably clear (Fig. 13.12). The difficulty is that details of assessment and use of media and methods is incomplete.

UNIQUENESS

The uniqueness of the occupational therapy process model is the attempt to organize a number of concepts which have a basic appeal to the beliefs and values which underlie occupational therapy. Mastery of the skills needed for life tasks and the sense of responsibility to perform the skill in the appropriate life space are assumptions and concepts consistent with the goals of functional independence and adaptation.

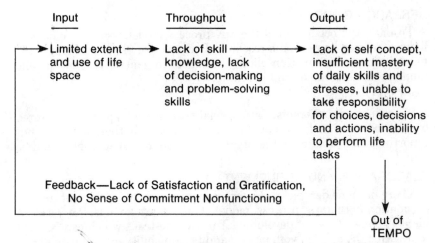

Figure 13.11.   Occupational therapy process model of dysfunction.

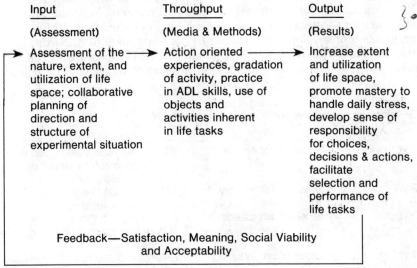

Figure 13.12.   Organization of occupational therapy intervention within the occupational therapy process model.

The problem is that such assumptions and concepts are not unique to occupational therapy and do not adequately define or describe the uniqueness of occupational therapy as an intervention approach. Rather mastery and responsibility are central concepts to many models developed from the organismic view. Somewhere the concept of occupation and the assumptions that occupations should be individually organized or balanced must be identified in any model which claims to represent occupational therapy and practice.

RESEARCH GUIDE

To date, the occupational therapy process model does not appear to have generated any specific research. Perhaps one major problem is the need for more information about the model in general and specifically more about assessment and planning.

SPECIALIZATION

If occupational therapists are specializing in the approach suggested by the occupational therapy process model, such therapists are not reporting their practice in the literature. No published accounts could be found.

ELABORATION AND REFINEMENT

There is considerable need for elaboration and refinement in the occupational therapy process model. One major area is the need to identify some stages of development in the life tasks which can be used to describe the concepts of mastery and responsibility more fully and can be used as the basis for evaluation. A number of scales outlining the sequence of basic activities of daily living could be adapted or refined. Maurer's analysis of vocational development could be included. Watanabe mentions Allport's stages of proprium but does not outline the progression of development. Table 13.19 is a summary of Allport's eight stages. These could be used to evaluate the person's sense of self. In addition, Havighurst's developmental tasks could be adapted to look at

Table 13.19
Development of the Proprium according to Allport

Age	Stage	Description
1 yr	Sense of bodily "me"	Infants learn that their bodies exist because of the sensation which is experienced
2 yr	Sense of self-identity	The realization that there is self continuity over time
3 yr	Sense of self esteem	Feeling of pride that emerges from learning to do things by oneself
4 yr	Sense of self extension	Extension of self to include external objects which are "mine"
4–6 yr	Emergence of self-image	Development of a conscience which can compare "good me" and "bad me"
6–12 yr	Emergence of self as a rational coper	Thinking becomes a means of problem solving
12 through adolescence	Emergence of propriate striving	Long-term goals are created which give organization and meaning to one's future life
Adulthood	Emergence of self as a knower	Synthesis of the previous stages

[a] Adapted from G. W. Allport: *Patterns and Growth in Personality*. New York, Holt, Rinehart and Winston, 1961, pp. 110–138.

Table 13.20
Developmental Tasks according to Havighust[a, b]

Infancy and early childhood
MS	1. Learning to walk
MS	2. Learning to take solid foods
MS	3. Learning to talk
MS	4. Learning to control the elimination of body wastes
C	5. Learning sex differences and sexual modesty
C	6. Forming concepts and learning language to describe social and physical reality
C	7. Getting ready to read
S	8. Learning to distinguish right and wrong and beginning to develop a conscience

Middle childhood
MS	1. Learning physical skills necessary for ordinary games
S	2. Building wholesome attitudes toward oneself as a growing organism
S	3. Learning to get along with age-mates
S	4. Learning an appropriate masculine or feminine social role
C	5. Developing fundamental skills in reading, writing and calculating
C	6. Developing concepts necessary for everyday living
S	7. Developing conscience, morality, and a scale of values
SM	8. Achieving personal independence
S	9. Developing attitudes toward social groups and institutions

Adolescence
S	1. Achieving new and more mature relations with age-mates of both sexes
S	2. Achieving a masculine or feminine social role
I	3. Accepting one's physique and using the body effectively
I	4. Achieving emotional independence of parents and other adults
S	5. Preparing for marriage and family life
P	6. Preparing for an economic career
S	7. Acquiring a set of values and an ethical system as a guide to behavior; developing an ideology
S	8. Desiring and achieving socially responsible behavior

Early adulthood
S	1. Selecting a mate
S	2. Learning to live with a marriage partner
P	3. Starting a family
P	4. Rearing children
P	5. Managing a home
P	6. Getting started in an occupation
S	7. Taking a civic responsibility
S	8. Finding a congenial social group

Middle age
P	1. Assisting teen-age children to become responsible and happy adults
S	2. Achieving adult social and civic responsibility
P	3. Reaching and maintaining satisfactory performance in one's occupational career
L	4. Developing adult leisure-time activities
S	5. Relating oneself to one's spouse as a person
I	6. To accept and adjust to the physiological changes of middle age
S	7. Adjusting to aging parents

Table 13.20—*Continued*

Later maturity		
I	1.	Adjusting to decreasing physical strength and health
P	2.	Adjusting to retirement and reduced income
S	3.	Adjusting to death of spouse
S	4.	Establishing an explicit affiliation with one's age group
S	5.	Adopting and adapting social roles in a flexible way
SM	6.	Establishing satisfactory physical living arrangements

^a Adapted from R. J. Havighurst: *Developmental Tasks and Education*, 3rd ed. New York, McKay, 1972.

^b Code: occupational areas: SM, self maintenance; P, productivity; L, leisure. Performance areas: MS, motor sensory; C, cognitive; I, intrapersonal; S, interpersonal (social).

occupational and performance areas (Table 13.20). The outline is too sketchy but could be expanded by integrating other theorists ideas.

EXPLANATORY USEFULNESS

The occupational therapy process model is consistent with the organismic, humanistic and developmental concepts of occupational therapy. It does focus on facilitatory rather than directive relationships of the therapist and person receiving service. Furthermore, the model is based on concepts available for community work where assistance is possible, but some degree of independence is assumed for the recipient of service. Otherwise, hospitalization would be required.

The major drawback of the model is the failure to identify a unique feature or aspect of occupational therapy. Nothing in the model speaks on how the occupational therapist's knowledge skills are superior to others in accomplishing the teaching-learning of life tasks. The only hint of a unique role is the emphasis on learning by doing which is useful but could be articulated by many good teachers.

COMMONALITY

The occupational therapy process model does provide a common focus for mental health workers interested in the humanistic or developmental approaches to dealing with mental health problems. Responsibility and mastery are familiar terms. Likewise the learning by doing method is familiar to teachers and educators. Thus, the model is successful in communicating some common themes which others can understand and accept or reject. Also, the model is clearly not based on psychoanalytic concepts except for reference to the work "ego." For a core of mental health workers trying to develop approaches not based on traditional psychiatry the model offers a truly different perspective.

PRACTICE MODEL

Although some specific practice submodels or theories may exist, there is no identifiable literature available. Certainly, the possibility exists for submodels on theories to develop especially along age or diagnostic

Table 13.21
Occupational Therapy Process Model Critique Summary

Criteria	Very Good 1	Moderately Good		Very Poor 5
		2	3	4	5
Frame of reference	x				
Clarity		x			
Uniqueness				x	
Research guide			x		
Specialization			x		
Elaboration/refinement			x		
Explanatory usefulness				x	
Commonality			x		
Practice model			x		

classifications. There is room for much creative thinking and development.

SUMMARY

A summary of the model is provided in Table 13.21. The strongest point is the frame of reference. Weaknesses are the uniqueness and explanatory usefulness. If these were overcome, the model could show considerable improvement in the other criteria.

References

1. Thayer AS: Work cure. *J Am Med Assoc* 51:1485–1487, 1908.
2. Barrus C: *Nursing the Insane.* New York, Macmillan, 1908, p. 210.
3. Van Nuys JD: The value of occupation in the treatment of the insane. *Kansas State Charit Institut* 6:7–11, 1911.
4. Schwab SI: Therapeutic value of work in hysteria and neurasthenia. *Interstate Med J* 9:248–255, 1902.
5. Atwood CE: The favorable influence of occupation in certain nervous disorders. *NY Med J* 86:1101–1103, 1907.
6. Sawyer CW: Occupation for mental cases during institutional care. *Mod Hosp* 5:85–87, 1915.
7. Haviland CF: Occupations for the insane and their therapeutic value; what is now done and what, if anything further should be done. *NY State Hosp Bull* 5:13–26, 1912.
8. Ricksher C: Occupation in the treatment of the insane. *Ill Med J* 23:380–385, 1913.
9. Cohn E: The systematic occupation and entertainment of the insane in public institutions. *J Am Med Assoc* 50:1249–1251, 1908.
10. Fields GE: The effect of occupation upon the individual. *Am J In* 68:103–109, 1911.
11. Wade JP: Occupation of the insane. *Md Psychiatr Q* 1:10–11, 1911.
12. Herring AP: Diversional occupation of the insane. *Proc Am Med Psychol Assoc* 19:245–248, 1912.
13. Moyer TJ: Occupation in the treatment of the insane. *J Am Med Assoc* 48:1664–1666, 1907.
14. Frost HP: Occupation of patients in state hospitals for insane. *Mod Hosp* 5:151–155, 1915.
15. Evans BD, Mikels FM: The therapeutic and economic value of diversional occupation. *Proc Am Med Psychol Assoc* 22:311–322, 1915.
16. Barton GE: Occupational therapy. *Trained Nurse Hosp Rev* 54:138–140, 1915.

17. Tracy SE: The place of invalid occupation in the general hospital. *Mod Hosp* 2:386–387, 1914.

18. Dunton WR: *Prescribing Occupational Therapy.* Springfield, Ill, Charles C Thomas, 1928.

19. Atwater MM: Suggestion for a classification of occupations in occupational therapy. *Arch Occup Ther* 1:389–394, 1922.

20. Tracy SE: *Studies in Invalid Occupations: A Manual for Nurses and Attendants.* Boston, Whitcomb and Barrows, 1910. Reprinted by Arno Press, New York, 1980.

21. Tracy SE: Getting started in occupational therapy. *Trained Nurse Hosp Rev* 67:397–399, 1921.

22. Tracy SE: Some profitable occupations for invalids. *Am J Nurs* 8:172–177, 1907–08.

23. Tracy SE: The development of occupational therapy in the Grace Hospital, Detroit, Mich. *Trained Nurse Hosp Rev* 66:401–403, 1921.

24. Tracy SE: Invalid occupation in the curriculum of the training school. *Mod Hosp* 3:56–57, 1914.

25. Tracy SE: The place of invalid occupation in the general hospital. *Mod Hosp* 2:386–87, 1914.

26. Tracy SE: Power versus money in occupation therapy. *Trained Nurse Hosp Rev* 66:120–122, 1921.

27. Tracy SE: Twenty-five suggested mental tests derived from invalid occupations. *Maryland Psychiatr Q* 8:15–18, 1918.

28. Dunton WR: A nurse's occupation course. *Proc Am Medico-Psychol Assoc* 19:269–278, 1912.

29. Dunton WR: *Occupation Therapy.* Philadelphia, Saunders, 1915.

30. Dunton WF: Occupation as a therapeutic measure. *Med Rec* 83:388–389, 1913.

31. Dunton WR: Occupational therapy. In Barr G: *Modern Medical Therapy in General Practice, Vol. I.* Baltimore, Williams & Wilkins, 1940.

32. Dunton WR: *Prescribing Occupational Therapy.* Springfield, Ill, Charles C Thomas, 1928.

33. Dunton WR: The principles of occupational therapy. *Public Health Nurse* 10:316–321, 1918.

34. Dunton WR: Occupational therapy. In Mack HE, Pemberton R, Coulter JS: *Principles and Practices of Physical Therapy,* Vol. I. Hagerstown, Md, Prior, 1935.

35. Dunton WR: Occupational therapy. *Occup Ther Rehabil* 10:113–121, 1931.

36. Dunton WR: Should there be a recreation schedule? *Proc Am Medico-Psychol Assoc* 22:337–342, 1915.

37. Dunton WR: The importance of interest in occupational therapy. *Occup Ther Rehabil* 30:384–386, 1951.

38. Matsutsuya JS: The interest check list. *Am J Occup Ther* 23:323–328, 1969.

39. Wittkower ED, La Tendresse JD: Rehabilitation of chronic schizophrenics by a method of occupational therapy. *Br J Med Psychol* 28:42–47, 1955.

40. Wittkower ED, Azima H: Dynamic aspects and occupational therapy. *Arch Neurol Psychiatry* 79:706–710, 1958.

41. Azima H, Wittkower ED, LaTendresse J: Object relations therapy in schizophrenic states. *Am J Psychiatry* 115:60–62, 1958.

42. Azima H, Azima FJ: Projective group therapy. *Int J Group Psychother* 9:176–183, 1959.

43. Azima H, Azima FJ: Outline of dynamic theory of occupational therapy. *Am J Occup Ther* 13:215–221, 1959.

44. Azima H, Wittkower ED: Gratification of basic needs in treatment of schizophrenics. *Psychiatry* 19:121–129, 1956.

45. Azima H: Dynamic occupational therapy. *Dis Nerv Syst Monogr Suppl* 22:138–142, 1961.

46. English HB, English AC: *A Comprehensive Dictionary of Psychological and Psychoanalytical Terms.* New York, McKay, 1958, p. 541.

47. Shoemyen CW: Occupational therapy orientation and evaluation. *Am J Occup Ther* 24:276–279, 1970.

48. Shoemyen CW: The Shoemyen battery. In Hemphill RJ: *The Evaluative Process in*

Psychiatric Occupational Therapy. Thorofare, NJ, Charles B. Slack, 1982, pp. 63–83.

49. Goodman M: Basic instructions for administering Goodman battery. In *Evaluation Procedures in Occupational Therapy.* Illinois Committee on Practice, Illinois Occupational Therapy Association, 1969.

50. Evaskus MG: The Goodman battery. In Hemphill BJ: *The Evaluative Process in Psychiatric Occupational Therapy.* Thorofare, NJ, Charles B. Slack, 1982, pp. 85–125.

51. Gillette NP: Standardizing observation techniques through available occupational therapy media. In *Proceedings of the Special Programs of the Psychiatric Subcommittee.* New York, American Occupational Therapy Association, 1964, pp. 3–6.

52. Owens C: Developing an evaluation test battery. *Patterns for Progress in Psychiatric Occupational Therapy.* New York, American Occupational Therapy Association, 1965, pp. 7–13.

53. Owen C: *Activity Battery Manual.* San Jose, Calif, Sparton Book Store, 1967.

54. Hemphill BJ: *Training Manual for the B.H. Battery.* Thorofare, NJ, Charles B. Slack, 1982.

55. Hemphill BJ: The B.H. battery. In Hemphill BJ: *The Evaluation Process in Psychiatric Occupational Therapy.* Thorofare, NJ, Charles B. Slack, 1982. pp. 127–138.

56. O'Kane CP: *The Development of a Projective Technique for Use in Psychiatric Occupational Therapy.* Buffalo, State University of New York, 1968.

57. Capra F: *The Turning Point.* New York, Simon and Schuster, 1982.

58. West W: *Changing Concepts and Practices in Psychiatric Occupational Therapy.* New York, American Occupational Therapy Association, 1959.

59. Fidler JW, Fidler GS: *A Communication Process in Psychiatry: Occupational Therapy.* New York, Macmillan, 1963.

60. Fox JVD, Jirgal D: Therapeutic properties of activities as examined by the clinical council of the Wisconsin schools of occupational therapy. *Am J Occup Ther* 21:29–33, 1967.

61. Fidler JW, Fidler GS: *Introduction to Psychiatric Occupational Therapy.* New York, Macmillan, 1954.

62. West WL (ed): *Changing Concepts in Psychiatric Occupational Therapy.* New York, American Occupational Therapy Association, 1959.

63. Mosey AC: *Three Frames of Reference for Mental Health.* Thorofare, NJ, Charles B. Slack, 1970.

64. Weinroth LA: Dynamic occupational therapy. *Am J Occup Ther* 9:243–245, 1955.

65. Gratke BE, Lux PA: Psychiatric occupational therapy in a milieu setting. *Am J Occup Ther* 14:13–16, 1960.

66. German SA: Group approach to rehabilitation: occupational therapy in a psychiatric setting. *Am J Occup Ther* 18:209–214, 1964.

67. Hansen PJ: Evolution of a rehabilitation program in family living. *Am J Occup Ther* 20:193–195, 1966.

68. Mosey AC: *Occupational Therapy: Theory and Practice.* Boston, Pothier, 1968.

69. Mosey AC: Recapitulation of ontogenesis: a theory for the practice of occupational therapy. *Am J Occup Ther* 22:426–432, 1966.

70. Mosey AC: *Three Frames of Reference for Mental Health.* Thorofare, NJ, Charles B. Slack, 1970.

71. Mosey AC: *Activities Therapy.* New York, Raven Press, 1973.

72. Thomas LR: Activity therapy in a psychiatric hospital. *Am J Occup Ther* 6:115–117, 1952.

73. Bobis BR, Harrison AM, Traubil L: Activity group therapy. *Am J Occup Ther* 9:19–21, 50, 1955.

74. Springfield FB, Tullis LH: An intensive activity program for chronic neuropsychiatric patients. *Am J Occup Ther* 12:247–249, 1958.

75. Shannon PD, Snortum JR: An activity group's role in intensive psychotherapy. *Am J Occup Ther* 19:344–347, 1965.

76. Howe MC: An occupational therapy activity group. *Am J Occup Ther* 22, 176–179, 1968.

77. Barton GM, Scheer N: A measurement of attitudes about an activity program. *Am J*

Occup Ther 29:284–287, 1975.
78. Hemphill, BJ: Mental health evaluations used in occupational therapy. *Am J Occup Ther* 34:721–726, 1980.
79. Cermack SA, Stein F, Abelson C: Hyperactive children and an activity group therapy model. *Am J Occup Ther* 26:311–315, 1973.
80. Watanabe S: Four concepts basic to the occupational therapy process. *Am J Occup Ther* 22:439–445, 1968.
81. Arsenian J: Life cycle factors in mental illness. *Mental Hyg* 52:19–26, 1968.
82. Chaplin JP: *Dictionary of Psychology.* New York, Dell, 1975 (new revised ed).

CHAPTER 14

Parameter Models

Parameter models describe types of service delivery patterns used to provide occupational therapy service. Such models delineate the characteristics or attributes of different methods of organizing practice.

COMPREHENSIVE OCCUPATIONAL THERAPY MODEL
Frame of Reference

The model was developed by a special task force of the Council on Standards in 1972 and defined by another task force in the same year (1, 2). It was designed as a position or statement paper of the American Occupational Therapy Association. Generally, the ideas appear to be based on the biopsychosocial model of health and drawn from the World Health Organization's concept of health. The model is directed toward stating the place of occupational therapy services in a comprehensive health care model in which the treatment- or pathology-oriented concept is enlarged to include a broader range of services. This model also was used in the 1973 Essentials of Accreditation for an Occupational Therapy Education Program.

Assumptions

VIEW OF HEALTH (1)

Good health may be dependent upon the opportunity each individual has to seek and receive those services which achieve the following.

a. Control his environment in the interest of health
b. Prevent barriers to health
c. Provide medical care for acute illness and traumatic injury
d. Provide restoration
e. Serve to identify and maintain health

VIEW OF OCCUPATIONAL THERAPY (1)

1. Activities are primary agents for learning and development and an essential source of satisfaction (to the individual).
2. Task occupation is an integral part of human development.
3. Activities are "doing," and such focus upon productivity and participation teaches a sense of self as a contributing participant rather than recipient.
4. The end product inherent in a task or an activity provides concrete evidence of the ability to be productive and to have an influence on one's environment.
5. When activities match or are related to the developmental needs and interests of individuals, these activities provide an intrinsic gratification which promotes and sustains health and evokes a strong investment in the restorative process.

6. Occupational therapy is designed to help individuals whose abilities to cope with tasks of living are threatened or impaired by developmental deficits, the aging process, poverty and cultural differences, physical injury or illness, or psychological and social disability.

7. Occupational therapy seeks to have an impact upon those forces that influence man's health and affect his ability to perform the tasks necessary for promotion or maintenance of his sense of well-being.

Concepts (1)

Occupational therapy—the art and science of directing man's participation in selected tasks to restore, reinforce and enhance performance, facilitate learning of those skills and functions essential for adaptation and productivity, diminish or correct pathology, and to promote and maintain health.

Occupation—refers to man's goal-directed use of time, energy, interest and attention.

Health—an individual state of biological, social and emotional well-being whereby an individual is capable and able to perform those tasks or activities which are important or necessary to him to promote and maintain a sense of well-being.

Prevention and health maintenance program—purpose is to foster normal development, sustain and protect existing functions and abilities, present disability, and/or support levels of restoration or change.

Remedial program—focuses on the reduction of pathology or specific disability, provides task and activity experience which may diminish the particular impairment, restore or develop the individual's capacity to function.

Daily life tasks and vocational adjustment programs—concerned with work adaptation and work role adjustment, and where the tasks chosen are those which will promote and teach independent functioning, develop and enhance the ability to work and/or fulfill age-specific life tasks and roles.

Process of service delivery

1. Evaluate the individual client or patient's performance capacities and deficits.
2. Select tasks or activity experiences appropriate to the defined needs and goals.
3. Facilitate and influence client or patient participation and investment.
4. Evaluate response, assess and measure change and development.
5. Validate assessments, share findings and make appropriate recommendations.

Adaptation, adaptive skills, Productivity, Performance capacity—not defined

EXPECTED RESULTS
1. Development of adaptive skills and performance capacity.
2. Reduction of factors which serve as barriers or impediments to the individual's ability to function.
3. Augment those factors which promote, influence or enhance performance.

Assessment Instruments
None are listed or discussed.

Intervention Strategies
See Table 14.1

Summary
The comprehensive model of occupational therapy services and programs is divided into three major categories. These categories are:

1. Prevention and health maintenance
2. Remedial
3. Daily life tasks and vocational adjustment.

The categories are based on a comprehensive health care plan which defines health in relation to biopsychosocial factors, the capacity to perform activities and the forces of heredity and environment (Table 14.1).

Each of the three program categories stresses a different aspect of health. Prevention and health maintenance are designed to address the concepts of promoting normal development and preventing the loss of functions. Remedial programs are designed to reduce the effects of pathology and restore function. Daily life tasks and vocational adjustment programs are organized to promote and develop skills, roles and life tasks.

The programs are seen as mutually interdependent and overlapping. Each is accomplished through the process of evaluation, goal setting, participation, measurement of change, sharing findings and making recommendations.

PREVENTION MODEL OF OCCUPATIONAL THERAPY—WEIMER
Frame of Reference
The prevention model of occupational therapy is based on the assumptions of preventive medicine which is concerned with the quality of life as well as the quantity (3). Preventative medicine also is interested in the possibilities of limiting health problems and the stresses arising from them.

Assumptions about Health (3)
1. Everyone has health.
2. Health is a continuum which is meaningful when related to wellness and illness.

Table 14.1
Outline of Occupational Therapy Service in the Comprehensive Model[a]

Prevention and Health Maintenance	Remedial	Daily Life Tasks and Vocational Adjustment
Purposes	Purposes	Purpose
1. Foster normal development	1. Reduce pathology or specific disability	1. Increase work adaptation
2. Sustain and protect existing functions, skills, capacities and strengths	2. Diminish particular impairment	2. Improve work role adjustment
3. Prevent disability and/or support levels of restoration or change.	3. Restore or develop individual capacity to function	Methods
Methods	Methods	Choose tasks which:
Provide activity experiences which:	Select tasks or activities which:	a. Promote and teach independent functioning
a. Enable the individual to use productivity, existing skills, capacities and strengths	a. Provide specific exercise and motor learning	b. Develop and enhance ability to work and/or fulfill age-specific life tasks and roles
b. Provide personal gratification	b. Offer sensory stimuli	c. Identify and examine roles and skills essential for individual's adaptation
c. Meet basic human needs	c. Promote muscle strength	d. Assess and nurture level of work capacities, attitudes and self care skills
d. Provide opportunities to pursue and develop interests	d. Alter disorders in thinking and feeling	e. Identify needed learning and sequence
e. Explore potential	e. Teach or enhance interpersonal skills	f. Provide graded task experiences to teach necessary skills and attitudes.
f. Develop capacities	f. Offer need gratification	
g. Learn resources within self and environment	g. Correct faulty self concepts and identity	
	h. Develop attitudes and skills basic to pursuit of independent functioning	

[a] Adapted from ref. 1.

3. Health is dynamic, not static; thus disability may coexist with ability, disease with freedom from disease.
4. Health behavior is characteristic of a man and man's mores.
5. Health includes a state of well-being, a quality of life and a dimension of purpose or worth.
6. Health may be influenced by intrusions of elements, personal habits and life-style and by social value judgments.

Assumptions About Occupational Therapy (3)

1. Occupational therapy is an art and science with an identifiable body of knowledge to support it.
2. Occupational therapy is a viable discipline that paces with the times and responds to the demands of practitioners and consumers.
3. Occupational therapy is medically, socially oriented and has a long history of identification with liberal arts and medicine.
4. Occupational therapy is premised on the concept of man's need for self-occupying tasks which influence the state of his health.
5. Occupational therapy holds a constellation of thought relevant to man's need for productivity and creativity.
6. Occupational therapy is wellness-oriented and focuses on the residuals and compensation to lessen the impact of disease or disability and the enrichment of remaining ability.
7. Occupational therapy is based on humanistic philosophy and is directed to the quality and dignity of living.
8. Occupational therapy should be identified by the person as relevant to home and job.
9. Occupational therapy attempts to normalize the person's environment by using familiar media and building upon the interaction of person and milieu.
10. Occupational therapy fosters the role of self-involvement in shaping the status of one's health, overcoming illness and disability, and holding health gains.
11. Occupational therapy has a responsibility for health of those persons who are treated directly.
12. Occupational therapy is the specialty concerned with the influence and impact of hand-mind productivity upon health.

Concepts (3)

Health—is an equilibrium state which can be manipulated by the individual, society and the elements.

Preventive health—a continuum which begins with the promotion of wellness and carries through easement in terminal illness.

Service functions continuum

a. *Promotion*—is consumer education through attempts to bring certain conditions that affect health to awareness of individuals.
b. *Protection*—is concerned with high risk factors known to be related to disability or injury.

   c. *Identification*—is concerned with early screening and evaluation procedures for the purposes of identifying defects or problems that may lead to disability or of identifying existing disabilities.

   d. *Correction*—is the remediation or treatment of identifiable pathology that interferes with man's ability to function.

   e. *Accommodation*—is designed to help an individual with impairments adjust to disability.

Balance of health—is analyzed by evaluating body systems, body structure, tangible and intangible health supports.

Continuum of health—medically oriented

   a. *Wellness*—no signs of illness

   b. *Latent illness*—state of apparent wellness but possessive of predisposing factors and suggestive of future illness

   c. *Subclinical illness*—refers to patient-known and patient-unrecognized illness

   d. *Clinical illness*—covers acute and chronic, reversible, irreversible and degenerative pathologies

   e. *Transience or terminal*—focuses on the tenuous transition from life to death

Continuum of health—life-style oriented

   a. *Optimum*—not defined

   b. *Acceptable*—not defined

   c. *Marginal*—not defined

   d. Deficient—not defined

   e. *Destructive*—refers to the failure to support customary life-style.

   f. *Intolerable*—designates that degree of illness incompatible with life.

Expected Results (3)

1. Health can be promoted.
2. Health can be protected.
3. Health and illness can be identified.
4. Health problems and illness can be corrected.
5. Health problems and illness can be accommodated.

Assessment Instruments

These are not discussed but mentioned in Identification.

Intervention Strategies

See Table 14.2.

Summary

The primary thrust of the prevention model is to focus on the range of services which occupational therapy can provide and to view the range of services as a continuum of health services based on preventive health

Table 14.2
Outline of Occupational Therapy Service in the Prevention Model[a]

Promotion	Protection	Identification	Correction	Accommodation
Purpose Promote health	Purpose Protect health	Purpose Identify health (problems)	Purpose Correct health (problems)	Purpose Accommodate health problems
Methods Health education Eradication of taboos and cultural habits Training in hygiene activities conducive of good health Consumer education Career development education	Methods Accident prevention in homes and cars Hazards of sports Playground plan for handicapped	Methods Multiphasic screening Consultant evaluations Physical examination Diagnostic workups	Methods Treatment Rehabilitation Mastery of activities	Methods Change environments Alter customs Interpret medical facts Counsel families Reduce architectual barriers

[a] Adapted from R. B. Wiemer (3).

concepts. The services themselves concern not only the individual but also are related to factors that exist within the physical and social environments which may impact on health and the ability to perform everyday activities.

Five service programs are described. These are promotion, protection, identification, correction and accommodation. Promotion and protection are designed to keep health problems from occurring. Identification programs should assist in pinpointing potential or real problems. Correction and accommodation programs provide services to correct or solve problems which have already occurred (Table 14.2).

ANALYSIS AND CRITIQUE OF THE PARAMETER MODELS
Frame of Reference

The frame of reference for occupational therapy programs needs to be consistent with the organismic philosophy and the assumption that occupational performance is evidence of and synonomous with health and wellness. By definition, then, to the occupational therapist health and wellness is the ability to perform occupations to the degree or level of performance that meets individual and social demands.

Both of the models in this section define health as a state of being in relation to environmental conditions rather than defining health as a state of active process in relation to actions, activity and doing. In other words, the models look at action as an outcome of health rather than viewing health as an outcome of action. One again, the philosophic view is important. The medical model views health as a result of actions taken by the physician. The occupational model views health as an outcome of actions taken.

Clarity

The two models present some overlap and some differences. The concepts of remediation and correction appear to be referring to rehabilitation or restoration of function. Prevention and health maintenance in the comprehensive model and protection in the prevention model appear to be similar. Also, there appear to be similarities between the daily life tasks and vocational adjustment in the comprehensive model and the promotion model in the prevention model. On the other hand, there do not appear to be correlations for the categories of identification and accommodation in the prevention model (Table 14.3).

The category of identification seems out of place with the other four in the prevention model. Identification is an assessment process only and does not involve intervention. Assessment which does not require intervention by occupational therapy is always a possibility. Therefore, a separate category appears unncessary. On the other hand, the category of accommodation appears to be a useful one because it stresses the need to adapt the environment to the person in situations where individual adaptation alone is not sufficient. The concept of adapting the environment to the individual is missing from the comprehensive model.

Table 14.3
Comparison of Similarities and Differences between the Two Program Models

Comprehensive	Prevention
Remedial	Correction
Prevention and health maintenance	Protection
Daily life tasks and vocational adjustment	Promotion
None	Identification
None	Accommodation

Table 14.4
Revision of Purposes to an Occupational Outcome

Comprehensive model
1. Prevent loss of ability and maintain ability to perform occupations and tasks.
2. Remediate (restore) ability to perform occupations and tasks.
3. Develop and promote ability to perform occupations and tasks.

Prevention model
1. Promote ability to perform occupations and tasks.
2. Protect ability to perform occupations and tasks.
3. Identify problems in the ability to perform occupations and tasks.
4. Correct (individual) problems in the ability to perform occupations and tasks.
5. Accommodate the individual by changing the environment to reduce problems in the ability to perform occupations and tasks.

Both models propose the outcomes or purposes in terms of health rather than occupation as discussed in the section on Frame of Reference. Actually, most of the categories can be maintained while changing the emphasis to occupations rather than health (Table 14.4).

Uniqueness

The two models do not present occupational therapy as a unique service because neither focuses on the unique aspect of occupational therapy which is occupation. As Table 14.4 shows, such a focus is possible and would improve both models. Also, neither model stresses the adaptive function of occupations in performing tasks within the occupational areas.

Research Guide

Very little research has been done in relation to the effectiveness of different types of delivery of occupational therapy services. The major studies on efficacy have been concerned with the total effects of rehabilitation and not with occupational therapy service by itself. Efficacy studies of occupational therapy could serve a useful function in substantiating the purpose and role of occupational therapy in working with various types of problems.

Specialization

The area of remedial or corrective programs has been the most common area of specialization in service delivery profiles. Next most common would be those programs which develop or promote health and function. Third would be the prevention, maintenance and protection programs. Identification programs only, which offer no intervention, are less common. Accommodation programs are most common as extensions of the remedial or corrective programs.

Elaboration and Refinement

Elaboration would appear to be helpful in explaining the relationship of health and occupation and in describing services in relationship to occupational and task performance. Refinement could be achieved by being more specific regarding the occupational problem the individual is assumed to have in performing occupations and tasks and by stating the working assumption upon which assessment and intervention are based. The entering level and working assumption could be followed by examples of expected results, examples of methods and techniques used in program

---

Table 14.5
Service Programs of Occupational Therapy: Preventative (Protection) Model

1. Entering level— individual(s) is currently performing occupations and tasks in the normal community environment to relative personal satisfaction.
2. Working assumption—loss of functional ability/skill (disability) in occupational performance can be prevented by active intervention of therapists to inform citizens of potential dangers to health.
3. Examples of expected results (outcomes)
   a. Prevent developmental regression, physical and psychosocial
   b. Prevent biogenic disorders
   c. Prevent psychogenic disorders
   d. Prevent sociogenic disorders
4. Examples of methods and techniques used in program planning and implementation
   a. Scheduling and performing activities of daily living
   b. Instruction in efficient home management
   c. Recommending change of work situation or job change
   d. Instruction in planning for retirement activities
   e. Instruction in the development and use of adapted equipment
   f. Programmed activities designed to prevent loss of physical and sensory functions, such as range of motion, coordination, muscle strength, physical tolerance, cognitive-perceptual motor capacity
   g. Instruction in work simplification and energy conservation
   h. Information and instruction on the availability and use of adapted devices
   i. Instruction in the elimination of architectual barriers and hazardous furniture and equipment
   j. Planned activities to make constructive use of leisure time
5. Outcomes accomplished through:
   a. Individual or group lecture, discussion and demonstration
   b. Development of illustrated booklets, tapes and films
   c. Consultation to community organizations concerned with the health and general welfare of its citizens

Table 14.6
Service Programs: Developmental/Abilities Model (Promotion)

1. Entering level—Individual has not learned or developed occupational skills and abilities appropriate to the age level or life task. Program includes individuals throughout the life-span.
2. Working assumption—disability can be understood in terms of a deviation in a profile of skills from normal performance.
3. Examples of expected results (outcomes)
   a. Increase motor and sensory functions to appropriate age level or life task
   b. Increase psychosocial (behavioral) skills to appropriate age or life task
   c. Increase abilities to perform activities of daily living
   d. Increase ability to perform life tasks—play, work, leisure
4. Examples of methods used in program planning and implementation
   a. Instruction in and opportunity to perform skills and activities within the individual developmental level
   b. Instruction in performing ADLs
   c. Programmed activities designed to develop concept of self, interpersonal relationships, group interaction skills
5. Outcomes accomplished through
   a. Explanation and demonstration
   b. Normal developmental sequencing
   c. Repeated practice and feedback
   d. Behavior modification
   e. Simulation—role playing
   f. Task analysis

planning and implementation and examples of media or modalities used to accomplish the outcomes (Tables 14.5 to 14.8). Such an outline approach permits a more thorough presentation of program factors and permits comparison of the programs to each other.

Explanatory Usefulness

Both of the models fail to describe the real essence of occupational therapy service which limits their usefulness as a means of explaining occupational therapy to other professionals or consumers. The most useful explanation would be to describe how the performance of occupation can be organized into different delivery patterns to meet different personal or community needs and problems. Of the two models, the preventive model is somewhat better organized and complete except that identification should not be a separate category.

Commonality

The organization of services into major categories is a common means of pulling together information in various fields and should be understood. Specifying outcomes and means of achieving those results also is common and should facilitate understanding by other disciplines. The major concern is to specify how occupational therapy combines infor-

Table 14.7
Service Programs: Remediation/Restoration (Correction)

1. Entering level—individual has lost occupational skills and abilities due to illness or trauma but can be expected to regain at least some skills and relearn some activities through specialized treatment and training.
2. Working assumption—disability can be understood by varying the conditions, task performance.
3. Examples of expected results (outcomes)
   a. Increase independence in performing activities of daily living
   b. Increase motor and sensory functions
   c. Improve home management skills
   d. Improve work proficiency and task performance
   e. Control energy expenditure
   f. Improve job-related skills
   g. Improve psychosocial performance
   h. Prevent deformity
   i. Prevent extension of disease or trauma pathology
4. Examples of methods and techniques used in program planning and implementation
   a. Increase physical and sensory functioning in such areas as range of motion, muscle strengthening, coordination, physical tolerance, sensory discriminative and integrative function through planned activities
   b. Instruction in performing ADLs
   c. Instruction in selected aspects of home management
   d. Instruction in specific work-related skills
   e. Instruction in and development of recreational activities
   f. Instruction in behavior/psychosocial skills
5. Outcomes accomplished through
   a. Individual or group-planned specific activities
   b. Environmental control—structured or nonstructured
   c. Development of home program

mation and skills into a unique service orientation. The unique combination is the role and function of occupation in producing and maintaining health.

Practice Models

Program models should present a very useful format for the development and further refinement of practice models and theory. The major concern is to better articulate the program models so that the service functions are defined and described clearly. Both the philosophy and the assumptions need to be understood and accepted as well.

Summary

A summary of the parameter models is provided in Table 14.9. The models do support specialization and practice, but both are weak in explaining the uniqueness of occupational therapy as a profession.

Table 14.8
Service Programs: Environmental Adjustment/Prosthetic Model (Accommodation)

1. Entering level—individual change and recovery have achieved a level of occupational performance that can be expected in the immediate or long-range period. Further improvement in function can be expected if the external environment is changed to reduce barriers to performance.
2. Working assumption—devices and environments can be developed and applied which will extend, enlarge and facilitate the occupational performance (physical and mental) of the handicapped person
3. Examples of expected results (outcomes)
   a. Further improve physical and sensory functions
   b. Further improve psychosocial/behavior functions
   c. Further increase ability to perform ADLs
   d. Further increase ability to perform work/play activities
4. Examples of methods and techniques used in program planning and implementation
   a. Modification and instruction in use of equipment
   b. Construction and instruction in use of splints
   c. Elimination of architectual barriers
   d. Reconstruction of physical surroundings
   e. Instruction in use of prosthetic devices
5. Outcomes accomplished by
   a. Task analysis
   b. Explanation and demonstration
   c. Repeated practice
   d. Consultation

Table 14.9
Parameter Models Summary Critique

Criteria Statements	Very Good 1	Moderately Good			Very Poor
		2	3	4	
Frame of reference			X		
Clarity			X		
Uniqueness				X	
Research guide			?		
Specialization		X			
Elaboration/refinement		X			
Explanatory usefulness			X		
Commonality		X			
Practice model		X			

References

1. Occupational therapy: Its definition and function. *Am J Occup Ther* 26:204–205, 1972.
2. Report of the task force on social issues, Part VII. *Am J Occup Ther* 26:350–351, 1972.
3. Wiemer RB: Some concepts of prevention as an aspect of community health. *Am J Occup Ther* 26:1–9, 1972.

CHAPTER 15

Toward Better Models of Occupational Therapy

REEXAMINATION OF PHILOSOPHY ISSUES

There are a number of philosophical issues which models of practice in occupational therapy ultimately must resolve. The issues are much broader than occupational therapy practice but do influence the outcome of therapy. As stated in Chapter 2, a model should be inherently logical. That is, aspects of the model should fit together and follow from one aspect to the next. Philosophical issues may form the base for the continuity. The first section of this chapter concerns issues relevant to building a basic model while the second section discusses issues related to building practice models. Some of the issues have been previously mentioned in Chapter 5 but are presented in this chapter in more detail as to the impact on occupational therapy.

Heredity vs. Environment

One of the oldest issues is the relative influence of heredity vs. environment in determining human development and behavior. This issue also has been called nature vs. nurture, nativism vs. cultural relativism, genetics vs. social controls or maturatism vs. learning. The central question concerns how much of a person's development and behavior is governed by controls which are inborn and how much is governed by external environmental influences. Those who favor the inborn or hereditary influences have included the preformationists and the predeterminists. The preformationists believe that all of the person's developmental and behavioral characteristics exist completely formed within a person at birth. As the child grows, the characteristics unfold on a prearranged schedule, regardless of the environmental situations. Predeterminists also believe that heredity is the primary determinant but believe that the physical and social environment does have some effect.

On the other side are the environmentalists who believe that environmental experience is the critical determinant in development and behavior. Environmentalists believe that a person is born with a blank notebook (tabula rasa) or a void which is filled in as the person experiences events. Thus, a good environment is critical to provide the guidance and experiences which will foster the best developmental and behavioral characteristics.

In recent years there has been a swing away from the question of how much heredity or environment is responsible for developmental and behavioral characteristics. Rather the question has become, in what manner do heredity and environment interact? The question permits a look at both sides together rather than favoring an either/or situation. The interactionist approach suggests that heredity determines the range of potential and the environment determines the extent to which the range will be achieved. Also, the interactionist approach permits one to accept that heredity may be more important at certain times in an individual's life, such as in puberty, while environment may be more important at other times, such as in adulthood. Furthermore, heredity may be more important in the development of certain characteristics, such as height, while environment may be more influential in the development of emotional controls. In some cases, the contribution of heredity and environment may be about even.

The interactionist approach seems much more fruitful for model building and research in occupational therapy. If heredity were all important, there would be little for therapists to do except to watch the unfolding of genetic and maturation influences. On the other hand, if environment was all important, therapists should be able to help people overcome almost any problem or handicap. All that would be needed is the proper environmental influences. The actual potential for therapy seems to be somewhere in between. The question is: Where is the in between position?

For therapists, the real importance of heredity and environment seems to focus on nervous system functioning. Reilly (1) has suggested that adaptation or change in the nervous system occurs in three ways: evolution, development and learning. These mechanisms work through the process of instincts, needs and values. Based on Reilly's analysis, there is actually a continuum rather than a polar model of change. It seems possible that the nervous system has organized itself to accommodate such functions into three interrelated subsystems seen in the brain (2). The archi-system is the oldest and seems to contain the stereotyped reactions and reflexes associated with instincts. The paleo-system could control the patterns of motions associated with development which are centrally programmed but require some environmental support to develop properly. Finally, the neo-system is the newest. It responds to environmental situations and can change or modify the acquisition of skilled movements to meet a variety of personal and social values. Table 15.1 illustrates the organization and change potential of the nervous system.

Table 15.1
Change Potential in the Nervous System and Effect on Behavior

Nervous System Organization	Mechanism of Change	Process for Change	Outcome of Change in the Nervous System
1. Archi (very old)	1. Evolutionary (genetic)	1. Instinct (inherited)	1. Reflexes/reactions (stereotyped change)
2. Paleo (intermediate)	2. Development (maturation)	2. Needs (interactive)	2. Patterns of motion (some modifications of pattern possible)
3. Neo (new)	3. Learning	3. Values (environmentally controlled)	3. Skilled movement, dexterity, coordination (very plastic, flexible, changeable)

Use of the model of change as a base for models of practice provides a rationale for why some behaviors and skills can be changed or modified by therapy intervention while others cannot. Behaviors which originate in the archisystem are not easily changed, whereas those originating in the neosystem have potential for change. Perhaps the methods for promoting change should be separated for the three levels as well. Different organizations within the nervous system may respond best to different methods of encouraging whatever change potential may be available.

In summary, there are three questions a model builder who accepts the interactionist approach should consider: (a) How wide are the boundaries set by heredity, maturation and learning for various aspects of development and behavior? (b) What environmental forces influence the way these aspects will manifest themselves in the person's development and behavior? (c) How will this interaction of inherited potential and environmental forces operate at different stages of a person's life?

Direction and Progression of Change

Another issue which arises frequently in model building concerns the nature of change. This issue is not whether change occurs but how it occurs. Although the issue has been described in many ways, there seem to be five major formats which can be illustrated and described (Fig. 15.1). The first format illustrates change and development as a continuous process which progresses toward a final outcome at a constant and predictable rate. This view may be called the "onward and upward" approach. Once change has begun, it continues uninterrupted although perhaps imperceptibly to the end point. Nothing basically interferes with the course or pathway. This approach is reminiscent of the hereditarian viewpoint.

The second view is similar to the first except that some downward or regressive movement occurs at various intervals. In other words, change may fall back slightly in one area because another aspect of development is commanding more attention or perhaps because of minor environmental changes such as illness or temporary trauma. This view is labeled "slide up and down."

A third view that development and behavior change perceptibly at various points should be recognized as a separate stage with a separate name. Progress thus is marked by specific changes on an upward trend. This view is called the "step by step approach."

A fourth view is a modification of the third. Again the principal difference is the recognition that development and behavior may regress as well as progress. Regression does not last too long and ultimately helps to satisfy the gain. This approach may be called the "step up and step down" approach.

Finally, there is the spiral approach which suggests that development and behavior will progress and fall back and then progress again. Moving forward and backward is expected and desirable to promote integration of previous learning with new experience.

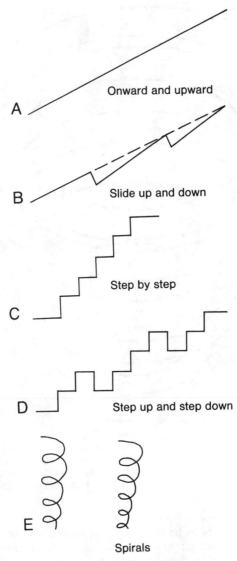

Figure 15.1.   Models of direction and continuity of change.

Views one and three seem to have little value for occupational therapy models. They tend to suggest that human performance will march onward in one way or another regardless of what therapists do or do not do. Views two and four offer some advantage to model building because there is a recognition that not everything goes smoothly all the time. Some backward movement might be stopped or reversed earlier if therapy and a helpful environment were available. The best view for occupational

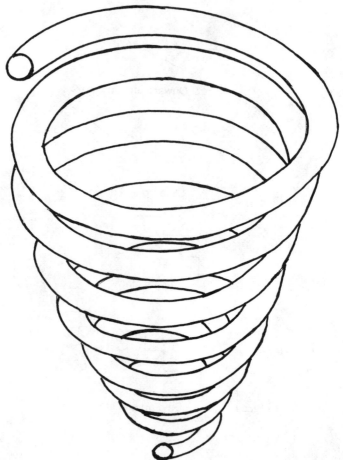

Figure 15.2. Direction and progression of change model. (Adapted from Willard H. Spackman CS: *Occupational Therapy*, 4th ed. Philadelphia, Lippincott, 1971, p. 404.)

therapy models appears to be the spiral approach. The falling back and regrouping of development and behavior as part of the forward and upward progression offers several entrance points for therapy programs. Therapy can be aimed at reducing the total decline and fall, at facilitating the recovery and at maximizing the forward thrust. For an example of how such a model might be used, see Figure 15.2.

Evil vs. Good

A third issue is the continuing concern among various social institutions as to whether humans are basically evil or basically good. The view that humans are basically bad and sinful has had support from religion, science and history. Christian doctrine has taught that the whole human race was corrupted when Eve succumbed to eating the apple and what is more, humans continue to be unable to resist temptation or live a good life without divine intervention.

Darwin's theory of evolution also lends support to the evil philosophy. He suggested that the world is a battleground for a constant struggle for survival wherein only the strongest live. This concept of survival of the fittest helped reinforce the idea that humans are essentially cruel, selfish and aggressive.

History itself is replete with stories of man's inhumanity to man. In recent times is the example of the German extermination camps where many people were killed because they did not fit the picture of the Aryan race. The daily newspapers frequently have stories of persons killed over a single argument in a local bar, or infants physically abused because they did not "obey" a parent's command to stop crying. Thus the pattern of perceiving humans as competitive, hostile and aggressive again is reinforced.

On the other hand, people can be cooperative, loving and kind hearted. Several scientists have reported groups of people in primitive tribes who, as a rule, are helpful and gentle to their neighbors and rarely become hostile or aggressive. The early settlers in this country are known to have helped new neighbors build a house or participate in barnraisings. The daily newspaper is also a source of good deeds as when people willingly donate clothing and household goods to a family whose home is burned down. Such contrasts suggest that humans are neither basically evil nor good but rather have the potential to develop in either direction. The key is the type of educational training that is received in a specific culture.

Models of occupational therapy should include reference to evil or good because the techniques of practice will be influenced by the decision. If humans are basically selfish and predatory then therapists must try to protect the ill and handicapped and insist that society adopt a strong system of discipline and control so the strong cannot take advantage of the weak. If, however, the model is based on the philosophy that humans essentially are good, then therapists can foster friendly constructive behavior by encouraging spontaneity, openness and self direction.

It seems that if the stated outcome of occupational therapy process is to return to or maintain in society an independent, functioning individual then models of occupational therapy should adopt a positive view of human beings. The view that people basically want to be good permits the occupational therapist to work with the family, friends and community to seek cooperative and understanding relationships with people who have been ill and disabled.

Normal vs. Abnormal

The philosophical issue of normality vs. abnormality also includes the related issues of desirable vs. undesirable or healthy vs. unhealthy. As a term the word "normal" has several descriptions. These include natural, typical, average, well adjusted, or getting along nicely. When normal is used to mean natural it usually implies that nature is to take its course and humans are to do nothing to prevent or alter the course. The problem of implying that normal is natural is that the meaning may be interpreted as good or bad. If normal is considered desirable or healthy then the attribute being considered is good. If normal is considered undesirable or unhealthy then the attribute is bad. For example, the puritans considered that children were naturally bad and lazy and must be taught not to follow their natural tendencies but to learn to be good, hard working citizens. On the other hand, Rousseau, an 18th century philosopher, felt that children were naturally good and would develop wisdom and virtue of their own accord if given a suitable environment. Thus, the term normal can be misleading when used to mean natural.

If the term "normal" is meant to convey typical or average, there are other pitfalls. Typical or average means what is most common under the prevailing conditions. However, again the prevailing conditions may not represent the desired or healthy state. If a group of recent graduates is surveyed and found to have the reading comprehension level of a sixth grader, that may not be the desired outcome of a high school level education. In the same vein, if a survey is done which finds that the average child has four colds each winter, that may not be the preferred state of health.

Other misinterpretations of the term normal occur when it is used to mean well adjusted or getting along nicely. In this case normal means that the person fits into a pattern of behavior in which the individual looks and acts like most peers. The problem is that the peers may be doing things that society does not consider desirable or healthy. For example, an adolescent may be considered well adjusted and may fit in with his peers if the individual smokes and pops pills at teenage gatherings. Cigarettes and drugs, however, may not be considered desirable by parents and certainly can be unhealthy. Thus the term "normal" must be used with care in models of occupational therapy. Therapists should be aware of what is meant when the term is used.

Need vs. Drive

Most models assume that there is some moving force which causes humans to seek certain things. Such an energy force is generally called motivation. Reilly (3), for example, assumes that occupation is such a moving force. She assumes that occupation is a primary motivating force in the development of health. There are two basic forms of motivation stated in the literature. These are called need and drive. Although the two terms may in reality be synonymous, a distinction in the literature has been made. Drive "implies output of pent up energy searching for a place in which to invest or expend itself" while need "implies intake, a void seeking to be filled." Behavioral theorists seem to use drive, whereas humanistic theorists prefer need (4).

The best description of either term has been made by Maslow (5) who prefers to use need. He distinguishes two types: deficiency needs and growth or self actualization needs. Deficiency needs which threaten survival and self maintenance can be recognized by five objective and two subjective criteria. These are (a) its absence breeds illness, (b) its presence prevents illness, (c) its restoration cures illness, (d) it is preferred over other satisfactions in most free choice situations, (e) it is generally inactive or absent in a healthy person, (f) there is a conscious or unconscious yearning or desire, and (g) there is a lack or deficiency with the individual. The overriding characteristic of all deficiency needs is the continuous endeavor of the body to preserve the steady state and maintain equilibrium.

On the other hand, growth or self actualization needs go beyond the steady state and strives for expression and improvement of the self. The focus is on potential, talent, and capacity. There appears to be four general directions of such growth: (a) toward development and use of potential in constructive and creative ways, (b) toward enrichment of life experiences, (c) toward increased relatedness with others and "human enterprises" and (d) toward "becoming a person" and answering the questions of who am I and what am I doing here? (5).

Maslow (6) also has suggested that needs can be placed in a hierarchy ranging from basic physiologic needs at the bottom to self actualization at the top. Physiologic needs include air, food, drink and rest. The second group involves safety needs such as those for security and stability. A third group involves belongingness, love needs and rootedness. The fourth level involves esteem needs such as self-respect and self-worth. Finally, at the top is self actualization which includes what a person is and what a person has become.

The role of occupation in relation to these needs has not been well explained. Reilly has proposed that occupation does indeed fulfill some of the deficiency needs stated by Maslow but what about the role of occupation in self actualization? Although intuitively there is an acknowledged role, models of occupational therapy do not seem to speak to the issue. Perhaps more important is the role of occupation in fulfilling more than one level in the hierarchy at one time. Occupational therapists are aware of the concepts of work efficiency. What about *occupational efficiency*? Could occupations be explored to determine which ones will fulfill the most needs of an individual with the fewest number of occupations? While healthy people may be able to pursue many occupations, a person with health problems or handicapping conditions may need to select occupations in a more efficient manner to meet needs without undo expenditure of energy.

Needs vs. Values

Needs tend to focus the individual's behavior toward a goal or direction which will increase or reduce a level of tension within the individual. Values, on the other hand, focus behavior by establishing a set of standards or norms which are considered by society to have worth. Needs organize individual behavior directly, while values organize group behavior and thus contribute indirectly to the organization of individual behavior. Furthermore, behavior based on values can complement behavior based on needs. For example, a person might be hungry, but there are many kinds of food which can be consumed in a number of eateries or food serving places. Values provide the parameters of what food is available where. The individual must be aware of the values concerning food as well as the physiologic need for food.

Another example is occupational choice. A person has the need for action and occupation, but there are many ways to be active and many occupations which may be done. Values suggest those occupations which society agrees to support and the level of support society chooses to award a specific occupation. Thus, society values a carpenter and a lawyer but awards the lawyer more value by increasing the level, status and power.

Occupational therapists traditionally have not articulated much concern about values in general and a person's ability to discern or respond to values. However, the increasing interest in community-based practice and various subcultural groups should increase the concern for value development and clarification. Institutional values tend to be rigid and easily identifiable. Social values, on the other hand, have more latitude and variability. In the community a person must respond to those values which operate in that community if the person is to "fit in" and be accepted as a community member. Hall (7) has suggested that values are developed in four phases which form a hierarchy. The first phase is concerned with self-preservation and self-delight. The second involves self-worth and self competence. The third includes self independence and self as a being, and finally the fourth centers on harmony and synergy. Each phase can be differeniated by age, maturity of mental and emotional processes and skills. Table 15.2 lists the ages and stages. However, Hall cautions that not many people obtain phase IV, and some do not achieve phase III. That is, such persons do not obtain self independence and a sense of self as someone with skills to construct and create. However, persons who have not obtained phase III can be helped through occupational therapy which specializes in learning to do and to become independent. The contribution of occupational therapy to phase IV is not as clear-cut but may be feasible through further analysis.

Table 15.3 shows the changing focus in the mental processes through

Table 15.2
Ages and Values[a]

Age	Phase	Values
0–6	I	a. Self-preservation—security, survival
		b. Self-delight—pleasure, wonder
7–16	II	a. Self worth—belonging
		b. Self competence—work
17–39	III	a. Self independence—equity, rights
		b. Being self—construct, creation
40+	IV	a. Harmony—with self and others
		b. Synergy with self and of world

[a] Adapted from B. P. Hall (7).

Table 15.3
Mental Process and Values

Level	Phases of Consciousness
I. Ego (dominant) and the world	World as mystery (physical)
II. "Theory"	World as problem (social)
III. "I"	World as project and invention (conscience act)
IV. "We"	World as mystery cared for (interdependent)

a Adapted from B. P. Hall (7).

the four phases. Initially, the focus of values is concerned with the self as the center of the world and with physically related values such as security and pleasure. In the second phase, the focus shifts to dealing with others and the values of society. The third phase focuses on the self as a creator and inventor whose values reflect a conscious concern for the rights of the individual. Finally, the fourth phase focuses on togetherness and the values of interdependence.

Hall suggests that a person must complete all of one phase before the next phase is begun. If any value in the first phase reappears as a need, the person returns to the phase until the value is met. Thus, the upper phases are only possible when the values and needs of lower phases have been met. Since values are learned, however, the person must know what values to have and what skills are necessary to achieve the values. In a complex society which changes there may be many people whose value system is incomplete and nonfunctional. When the values are related to occupational performance, occupational therapists are the professionals who should have the skills to help develop, refine and clarify.

Values also can be explored in terms of sources. Coleman (8) suggests that there are four major sources: culture, science, religion and the individual. Culture includes five basic concerns: (a) Is human nature basically good, bad or neutral? (b) Are humans basically pawns or do they have some degree of free will? (c) Should humans live for the present or for the future? (d) What activity is of most value? (e) What is the dominant or desired relationship among group members? Science provides truthful dependable information and facts about the biological, physical and social science areas of the human and nonhuman environment. Its contribution is to provide reliable criteria for making decisions about choices in value orientation. Religion also is concerned with truth but as that truth has been passed on to generations through the reevaluations of a greater power such as God, Buddha and Mohammed. Many of the values are illustrated through the rituals, dogma and trappings which served previous generations but may not serve present day problems. Finally, life experience provides a source of values based on past success or failure, satisfaction or dissatisfaction in dealing with different situations. In addition to individual experience, a person can draw upon the experience of others, such as friends or leaders. Further information may be obtained by reading history or observing current events.

By being aware of the sources of values, occupational therapy may learn the sources of influence on the people receiving services and know the effects of values derived from each source. In particular values drawn from religion may be difficult to modify, since such values are not based on knowledge but on faith. For example, family planning might be an effective means of increasing the mental and physical health of a young mother with several children but will not be successful if the woman does not accept any of the currently known methods for limiting family size.

Occupational therapists need to consider the possibility of assessing value orientations more closely. Values can govern a large segment of behavior and provide a focus or direction for behavior change. Values can provide the basis for good development and goal-directed behavior.

Irrationality vs. Rationality

The irrational viewpoint of humans has been supported by two major psychological models and by the swiftly changing times. Psychoanalytic theory has upheld irrationality by its stress of the unconscious as a motivating source of behavior. Since the behavior is the result of forces from the id or possibly the superego, there is little chance to monitor the behavior against a rational or real world. Behaviorists support the irrational view by suggesting that humans are passive and *malleable*. Thinking is shaped by the environment rather than by internal processes.

Modern events tend to support the irrational point of view simply by rapid occurrence. By definition rational thinking requires time and reflection. Frequently decisions have to be made rapidly without much benefit of reflection; thus the hasty decision making may appear irrational. Furthermore, there is a variety of cultural, emotional and motivational forces which can lead to irrational behavior and decisions.

In spite of evidence to the contrary, there continues to be a belief in reason and common sense. Indeed it seems possible that rationality is important to survival. Obviously rational behavior is helpful in exploring and making sense of the physical and social surroundings. Rationality is useful, particularly in solving complex problems. The rational view of man seems to be a useful philosophy for models of occupational therapy to adopt. People faced with chronic conditions and handicaps have many problems which are complex and convoluted. Accepting the client as a rational person who needs help in learning to solve the problems but is basically capable of doing so is consistent with the concept of promoting independent living.

Determined vs. Free

Determinism has two forms. One deals with fate and the other with the law of cause and effect. Fate is a cultural religious concept which states that everyone in the final analysis is programmed by culture or religion to perform certain actions in their life and sometimes in death also. A person cannot escape the inevitability of actions which may include a preselection for salvation or damnation. The concept of fate is similar to predeterminism except that the originating source is culture or religion rather than heredity or biology.

The other form of determinism comes from the scientific assumption that the universe is an orderly place where all events occur in response to the natural law of cause and effect. Thus, all human activity is also lawful and follows a cause and effect relationship. If the cause of an action or behavior appears to be unknown, the problem is that not enough is known about the individual's past experiences. There is a cause. The cause is simply not clear in the present circumstances. However, the cause has to be tied in some way to the concept of conditioning through the use of rewards and punishments. All behavior thus exists because of a series of rewards and punishments an individual received from the environment. Therefore, although a person may think that the choice of rewards can be freely selected, such freedom is an illusion because the choices are really determined by past conditioning.

The concept of freedom has been best described by the existentialistic approach. Freedom involves the choice of deciding what sort of person to become and the courage to pursue the established goal. Freedom includes a sense of valuing the self as important and the willingness to accept the responsibility for maintaining self-determination. As a concept, freedom is very familiar. Democracy is founded on freedom. Freedom of speech and freedom of vote are taken for granted. However, freedom is difficult for many people to fully accept. The requirements for decision making and responsibility are more effort than the concept of freedom might imply. Thus, the concept of freedom is not always used in models of practice in its most complex sense. Rather a middle ground between freedom and determinism may be suggested.

The middle ground approach views freedom as an emerging process. As such the process of freedom provides the potential for planning ahead. A person is not completely bound by past experiences, but the experiences do provide a fund of knowledge upon which to consider building a future or to consider rejecting as not useful.

The concept of freedom along with its traveling companions, choice and responsibility, has an important place in models of occupational therapy practice. Freedom of choice provides a potentially wide range of change possibilities. A person who feels that choices can be made, and that choices of forward or backward movement are under some degree of self-control, has a sense of being active and of being in partial control of destiny rather than a total victim in it. Freedom can include the choice of being part of a team which develops the management plan rather than being a spectator. Freedom can be the responsibility to actively participate in the management program once it is established and to make recommendations for further involvement in their own programs. Freedom is one of the key concepts of this involvement.

Responsibility vs. Irresponsibility

Responsibility implies that the person is capable of, and can be held accountable for, monitoring individual actions, whereas irresponsibility implies that the person is incapable of making the necessary judgments to monitor actions unless specifically conditioned by the environment.

These two issues raise several points of concern which ultimately affect the outcomes or goals of treatment. First, if the individual is viewed as basically responsible for personal action, then the individual must be an integral part of any intervention strategy from the planning stage to the implementation stage. The role of the therapist is that of an advisor and a facilitator but not an authoritarian leader. Furthermore, the results of intervention are in large measure the responsibility of the client because the client knows the plan and what is required. Failure to follow through can be viewed as the client not maintaining responsibility. Failure in therapy cannot be solely the therapist's fault because the arrangements were an agreement or plan developed in cooperation with the client. Only if the therapist fails to provide the services promised is the therapist contributing to a failure to meet the objectives and goals.

On the other hand, if the individual is viewed as basically irresponsible the burden of results falls on the therapist. The therapist is responsible for developing the intervention plan, although the client may concur. The therapist is responsible for conducting the intervention program, although the client may comply by coming at the scheduled time. If results are not obtained, the therapist should alter the plan or program, or both. Failure to achieve results is primarily a reflection on the therapist who did not control sufficiently the antecedent or consequent events.

Occupational therapists have felt in general that clients should be involved in planning and be responsible for carrying out as much of the program as possible. Thus, occupational therapy subscribes to the idea that the individual is at least in part responsible for the intervention process. However, the degree of responsibility varies according to the therapist's analysis of the client's age, condition and level of understanding as well as the value the therapist places on client responsibility.

REEXAMINATIONS OF ASSUMPTIONS

There are two underlying assumptions about how occupational therapy works which are in conflict with each other. One assumption is that occupation works because it diverts a person's attention away from problems and replaces the attention with healthy thoughts and activities toward which the person can strive. The other assumption states that occupation works because it directs attention toward the problem and encourages the person to learn ways of overcoming or solving the problems. As problems are overcome or solved, the person's state of health improves.

Originally, the founders suggested that the value of occupation was its power to turn the person's attention away from disability (9). Therapists using the diversional approach tried to (a) make occupation interesting, (b) use normal and familiar occupations, and (c) keep the person as unaware of abnormality as possible. Others, however, suggested that disability is uppermost in the person's mind (10). Thus, occupations should address the disability directly and provide the consumer with a means of decreasing the effects of disability while increasing ability. In the direct application approach the consumer learns to measure improvement by increased skill, longer work periods and better functional capacity of body and mind.

Recent theories on the nature of occupational therapy suggest that therapy does not so much divert, disengage or distract the mind and body as it directs, focuses, channels or engages the mind and body toward healthful, or at least more adaptive, tasks of living (11). Although an ill person may be capable only of keeping the mind alert and oriented to reality, the convalescent person is capable of actively doing tasks and skills which will contribute to recovery of function and reduce the impact of dysfunction or disability. Concentration on the directional focus of occupational therapy should make the description of occupational therapy services more understandable to consumers and payers who find it difficult to believe that diversion is a worthy goal in helping a person become a functioning individual capable of performing in all occupational areas.

Occupational therapy has plenty of ways to change the direction of thinking processes without resorting to simple diversion. Besides, if the intervention is successful, an individual should have sufficient problem-solving skills to find simple diversions through resources in the community.

A second problem has been the failure of occupational therapists to understand the importance of following through to the completion of occupational performance. Occupational therapy is more than the teaching of individual, specific skills. It also is the integration and combination of skills into sequences and patterns of occupations (activities) to facilitate the total functioning of an individual in the environment. Helping a person learn individual skills such as eating with a fork is not enough. The person needs to integrate self-feeding with meal time and meal time as a self maintenance activity in the total day of activity. Part of the reason some clients do not carry out activities at home which were learned in the clinic seems to relate to the failure to build a total occupational pattern which fits newly learned or relearned skills together in a gestalt or whole pattern. Clients have difficulty adjusting the changes in skill level or performance time into the schedule. Family members are used to doing the job for the client or do not wait until the client is finished. Thus, the total pattern of occupational performance is disrupted.

Perhaps there is a failure to understand the sequential or chaining phenomena involving a number of different occupations and not just a piecemeal approach to occupational performance. Effective behavior is more than a collection of skills. The skills must be organized into habits or routines based on a sequence of performances which lead to a total production.

A third problem is to clarify the role of occupation in health and wellness. Occupational therapy has never clearly stated why occupation is effective in developing, regaining and maintaining health. In short, there is a need to specify health in relation to occupation. The most direct assumption appears to be that health can be defined as the capacity/ability to perform those occupations necessary to adapt to and cope with personal needs and values, and social demands and expectations of everyday life. Such an assumption suggests that a critical determinant of health is occupational performance. If a person can perform the occupational tasks or arrange for their performance that person has health or wellness. When a person cannot perform or arrange for the performance of occupations then health is impaired. The body functions through the demand for performance. When no performance is required or is restricted, the body quickly loses its functional capacity. Immobilization is one example as is inactivity. Doing facilitates body function; not doing hinders body function. Thus, health, performance and doing are positively related, while lack of health, nonperformance and not doing are likewise related.

REEXAMINATION OF CONCEPTS
Vocation vs. Occupation

One concept which needs to be reexamined in occupational therapy is that of vocation vs. occupation. Basically vocational selection and application is product-oriented. The product or end result is the focus of attention. On the other hand, occupational performance is process-oriented. The doing or performing is the central focus. Such a focus does not negate the importance of an outcome but rather controls the product through the process as opposed to permitting the product to dictate the process. Inherent in the assumption of process vs. product is a philosophical issue. When process is the central focus, the individual maintains control and interest in the occupation as a means of doing and performing. The product is an affirmation of having done or performed. The value, however, is not in the product but in the doing.

When the focus is on the product the emphasis shifts from person to external environment. The environment controls the value of the product. An individual is valued only if the product meets the environmental criteria. Likewise, the individual's vocation is valued only if the vocational product is satisfactory to external criteria. Thus, the process is externally controlled or determined also. Individual workmanship is only valued if the product meets specifications.

Occupational therapy was founded on the importance of occupational performance and not on vocational production. The emphasis is on helping an individual to learn to control one's own performance and thus the product achieved. The emphasis is not on production control which required the individual to conform to external criteria for performance.

Purposeful Behavior vs. Purposeful Activity

The previous discussion of process vs. product may contribute to clarifying the concepts of purposeful behavior and purposeful activity. A purposeful behavior is part of a process which leads to a useful or satisfying occupational performance. Likewise, a purposeful activity is part of a process. Behavior and activity are two sides of the same coin. Purposeful behavior leads to purposeful activity and purposeful activity facilitates purposeful behavior. Both are inherent in the process of the occupational performance of an individual who is able to adapt to the environment or adapt the environment to personal needs and satisfaction.

Purposeful behavior and purposeful activity can be combined into the term "purposeful doing" (Fig. 15.3). Purposeful doing thus involves an individual who is controlling more than half of a situation in which the

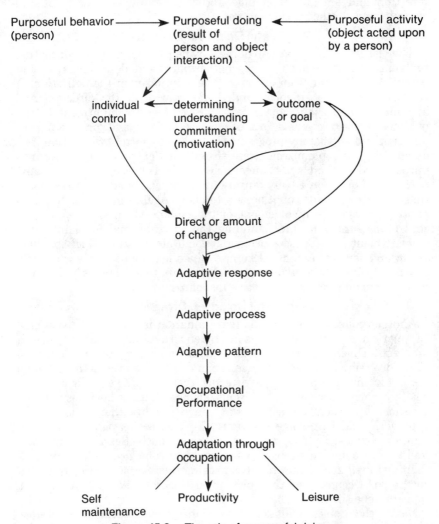

Figure 15.3. The role of purposeful doing.

purposeful doing is occurring. The control has a direction and amount of change within the specified outcome or goal which the individual understands and is motivated (wants, needs) to achieve. The direction and outcome lead to an adaptive response which is part of an adaptive process which in turn is part of an adaptive pattern. The adaptive pattern or sequence is functional in performing the occupations and life tasks of the individual. Occupational performance leads to adaptation with the environment through the use of occupations in self maintenance, productivity and leisure. Purposeful doing, therefore, is the result of person-object interaction which the individual controls through determining the direction and amount of change and through understanding of and committment to the outcome or goal.

Purposeful Doing vs. Exercise

The discussion of purposeful doing may help clarify another conceptual problem. This problem concerns whether purposeful doing (behavior and activity) is different from exercise. The solution is in the definition. If the term "exercise" involves individual control of the direction and amount of change and an understanding of and commitment to the outcome then exercise is a form of purposeful doing and can be a part of an occupational therapy program. However, if control or direction, understanding and committment are absent then exercise is not a form of purposeful doing and is not a medium or method of occupational therapy.

A related question is why purposeful doing elicits adaptive responses that exercise alone does not appear to elicit. Again the answer seems to relate to the active involvement of the person which is necessary for controlling direction, understanding the situation and in maintaining committment (11). These aspects may facilitate learning which is inherent in an adaptive response. Exercise which is done passively with little control of direction, understanding and commitment probably does not produce much learning of adaptive responses.

Purposeful Doing vs. Diversion

Another concept which needs reexamination is the term "diversion." In American society, diversion is not taken as a serious solution to health problems. Diversion seems to be equated with play or frivolousness. Thus, diversion is something anyone can do (play) and something people spent too much time doing (frittering their time away). In contrast, health problems are viewed as serious business. Serious business requires a serious approach; namely work. The possibility that a nonserious approach could help solve a serious situation seems paradoxical. The solution obviously is too simple to be taken seriously. Besides, if diversion could solve a health problem why would anyone need education and training to tell people how to do something that everyone already knows how to do? Occupational therapists must clarify to the public that what appears to be simple is in fact complex.

Next is the problem of dosage. Diversion appears to depend on interest and attention. No interest and no attention equals no diversion. Consequently, the more interest and attention, the more diversion. Therefore, interest level must be determined before diversion can be applied. Frequently, the determination of interest was either overlooked or incomplete. Thus, activities were not selected with the greatest potential for maintaining interest and attention. There is a large area for research in learning how to develop and maintain interest and attention in people who have health needs.

A third problem relates to how diversion was applied. Diversion can be thought of in two ways. One is to turn the attention away from the immediate situation of pain, confinement or healing process to anything else regardless of value to the client. The second is to turn the attention in another direction that is of value to the client and which can be done within the immediate situation. If time is used to achieve a constructive purpose, such as continued learning of a subject or skill or learning a new subject or skill, there would seem to be more value. Unfortunately, many diversional activities seemed to have lacked a direction or purpose. Perhaps better assessment is needed to determine value.

Good Definitions vs. Poor Definitions

A third concept which needs reevaluation is the definition of occupational therapy itself. Throughout the recent history of occupational therapy, the profession has been plagued with definitions that really do not do the field justice. For example, occupational therapy should not be defined as the use of *any* activity, as appears in early definitions of the field (13). *Any* activity includes those which are not goal-directed or purposeful. For example, turning a paper clip upside down endlessly on the desk is an activity. Swinging the crossed leg at the knee is an activity. Neither are goal-directed purposeful occupations. At best they may be diversional activities.

Instead, occupational therapy should be defined as the use of *selected* occupations or activities which are purposeful, meaningful and goal-directed as delineated by the client. Without the focus on value of occupation and on a goal-directed purpose, occupational therapy becomes a high class form of babysitting or entertainment. Selection is a key defining word because it implies that a rationale was used to "pick" the occupation as opposed to the random approach implied by the word "any." Occupational therapists select and choose, with the client's cooperation, those occupations which will best meet the client's needs, best fit the client's interests and best maintain or gain attention.

Balance vs. Imbalance

Another concept which needs clarification and reexamination is that of balance. The term "balance" or equilibrium appears in occupational therapy literature with some frequency. The problem is that the word is used in several ways. There appears to be at least six different usages. These are (a) balance as a response to gravitation force in space, (b) balance as a physiologic process, (c) balance as a time organizer (d) balance as an emotional stabilizer, (e) balance as a goal for harmonious proportion and (f) balance as social organizer of power and influence.

As a response to gravity balance is concerned with stability and mobility. Stability involves maintaining (static) balance or equilibrium in order to hold a particular posture or position in space such as sitting or standing. Dynamic balance is concerned with maintaining balance while moving (mobility) through space such as for walking, running or dancing. Occupational therapists are concerned with helping people achieve and maintain balance against gravity in and through space. Examples include activities to encourage protective and equilibrium reactions and activities to promote or decrease responses to linear and angular acceleration.

Balance as a physiological process is basically a synonym for "homeostasis." The word was first used by Cannon (14) to describe the mechanisms used by the body to correct deviations from the state of dynamic equilibrium. Through a series of sensors and feedback loops, the body is able to monitor and correct chemical changes and make corrective actions to maintain health and prevent illness. When the mechanism of homeostasis fails, then the person is much more likely to succumb to disease and dysfunction. Although many of the homeostatic mechanisms operate below the level of consciousness, there are certain conscious acts which can facilitate homeostasis, such as sufficient rest, proper activity, and good nutrition. Occupational therapists can help the person learn to recognize the value of determining the quantity and quality of selected tasks which facilitate homeostatic balance.

Balance as a time organizer is one of the more identifiable uses of the term. Meyer (15) speaks of the need to balance the amount of time spent in sleep, rest, work and play. Kielhofner (16) has suggested that the use of time is learned and is an important means of adapting to the environment. The balance of time can be viewed in terms of daily occupational activities or over a life-span of activities. Daily balances can be determined by an activity schedule of time and a record of what was done during that time. Life-span analysis could be assessed by time spent in certain occupational areas over the years (Fig. 15.4).

Balance as an emotional stabilizer makes some use of the concepts of homeostasis and time organization. The emphasis is on maintaining a sense of emotional integrity by controlling factors which seem to influence emotions. For each person certain amounts of physiologic needs such as sleep, security and food seem to promote emotional stability. Likewise, certain amounts of activity and occupational performance seem to facilitate emotional stability. Deficiencies and excesses of physiologic or time amounts seems to adversely affect emotional stability. The early proponents of occupational therapy expressed concern for the effects of too little activity as the work of the devil (17) and too much activity as a cause of "neuresthenia" (18).

Balance as a goal for harmonious proportion seems to be a part of the

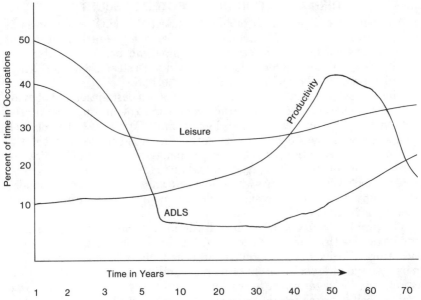

Figure 15.4. Model of time spent in occupational performance in a life-span.

self actualizing process. Whereas the concept of balance as emotional stability is an example of Maslow's (19) "basic or deficiency need." The concept of harmonious proportion is an example of "being" needed or valued. The person is motivated by inner growth to seek a balance of unity or wholeness. Through attainment of such balance a person can acheive a high level of psychological health. Occupational therapists can attempt to help the person clarify and seek such harmonious proportion and balance.

Balance as a social organizer of power and influence recognizes the interacting effect between persons in terms of dependence and independence. The term "maximum level of independence" seems to be used to acknowledge the proper balance between total helplessness and total self-sufficiency (20). As independence is achieved in self maintenance tasks the individual can direct energy to productivity and leisure. Through productivity many people achieve recognition of social value and may gain influence. Occupational therapists are used to help people learn, relearn or maintain self maintenance skills.

Throughout the different ideas on balance seems to be a similar theme that the ability to organize and perform certain occupations and tasks in the right amount and sequence is facilitatory to health and promotes adaptation. The common denominator is purposeful doing which facilitates organization and promotes the performance of sensorimotor, physiologic, temporal, emotional, motivational and social balance.

REEXAMINATION OF EXPECTED RESULTS

Another set of concerns is related to expected results or outcomes of intervention. Results or outcomes have been explained in terms of competence, mastery, achievement, functional independence, autonomy and adaptation. Related terms have included self-esteem, self-confidence, satisfaction of needs, self actualization and others.

The central problem with all of these terms is a description of behavior or performance criteria which permits a person to determine whether the outcome really has been fulfilled. For example, White (21) has defined competence as the "means to be sufficient or adequate to meet the demands of a situation or task." What behaviors or performances are sufficient or adequate for a given individual? How will such behaviors be determined? Who will judge when the performance meets the demands? How many situations or tasks should a person be able to meet before therapy is terminated?

The problem is to operationalize the definition into a procedure which can be used with a variety of clients with individualized needs and unique situations. Various theorists have suggested different approaches. The most general approaches seem to be roles and developmental tasks. Role competence is determined by listing the roles the person has acquired and the behaviors which the person performs to fulfill those roles. When the person can perform the behaviors which comprise the roles, the individual can be discharged. Competence in development tasks is determined by analyzing what tasks the person should be performing or wants to perform and then evaluating the person's ability to perform those tasks. When the person can perform all the tasks within the developmental profile of tasks the individual is ready for discharge.

A third approach is to analyze the occupations a person needs or wants to perform in terms of self maintenance, productivity and leisure. Considerations include age, performance level, social situation, cultural expectations and individual preferences. When a list of performances is determined, the person is evaluated to assess which occupations need further skill acquisition. When performance meets individual and social expectations, the person is discharged.

Although each approach offers some guidance in determining outcome criteria, precision is still lacking. Occupational therapists must work on becoming more skilled in determining and applying outcome criteria which are measurable and explainable to others.

REEXAMINATION OF ASSESSMENTS

One of the major problems in assessment is to provide a comprehensive assessment profile. Therapists traditionally have developed instruments within their area of interest or within a given framework of practice. Some instruments developed within a narrow framework are of value in collecting specific information about a client's performance skills. However, the total value of limited scales is diminished when a complete assessment of all five performance areas and three occupational areas is not accomplished. At least some general knowledge in motor, sensory, cognitive intrapersonal and interpersonal performance areas should be gathered to determine if the performance is within normal limits of development, self-satisfaction and social expectation. Likewise, the occupational areas of self maintenance, productivity and leisure should be assessed. Even if the length of stay is short, such assessment should facilitate discharge planning and referral to other professionals or community resources.

A related problem in assessment is the style in which the data are acquired. According to the book of sample forms (22), most occupational therapy forms are of the checklist type. Either the therapist or the client checks off a response such as "yes" or "no," "sometimes" or "never," etc. Checklist forms can be helpful to the therapist if the form lists all possible items which need to be considered. If the therapist follows the checklist, all information needed for intervention planning should be obtained. However, when checklists are used with clients, the format may inhibit rather than augment responses. A checklist suggests the nature of expected responses rather than promoting a free exchange of information. The checklist also suggests a termination point. When the last item is checked off the task is done. An example is Matsutsuyu's Interest Check List (23). When the form is completed, the task is finished. However, the client may not have exhausted personal interests. While the form may be representative of many people's interest, the purpose in using the form is to determine an individual's interests. Unless a reasonably good effort is made to be comprehensive, the checklist may reduce the amount of information rather than increase the data base.

An alternative is an open ended form which might ask the questions which the individual items illustrate. Table 15.4 is an example of such format. The open format does have limitations if administered alone. Some people are unable to think of answers unless choices are available. For such persons, a checklist may be useful, but an interview approach might be useful also. The advantage remains that the open format reduces

Table 15.4
Open Question Interest Form

1. What activities which require manual (hand) skills do you enjoy?
2. What physical sports do you enjoy?
3. What social recreation activities do you enjoy?
4. What daily activities do you enjoy doing?
5. What cultural events or educational activities do you enjoy?
6. Please indicate whether each of the items you listed is a strong interest (s) or casual interest (c).
7. Please provide a summary of interests, hobbies, and pastimes from childhood to the present
8. Please indicate which of the activities in your history you liked best (b) and which you like least (l).
9. Are there interests which you have never done or pursued? If so, please list.

the built-in bias of a checklist form since beliefs and values can vary within socially acceptable boundaries.

Therapists need to become more aware of the problems in collecting data when personal preferences and social values are being assessed. If the belief in self-control is to be maintained, then the form should provide maximum opportunity for client response with a minimum of therapist direction and bias.

REEXAMINATION OF INTERVENTION

The central problem in intervention is to explain why or how occupational activities work to produce changes in performance. There appear to be four major situations or tasks which occupational activities can address. Thus, there are four rationales for providing such change. These rationales are to compensate, substitute, reinforce or duplicate situations and tasks which a person needs to perform for self-satisfaction or social requirement. Compensation occurs when a situation or task is employed to develop skills and performance in an area which should have been learned earlier in life but was not. An example is learning to measure with a ruler. Such a task is usually learned as a young grade school child. Thus, when an adult cannot use a ruler for measuring and must be taught the skill, then learning is compensating for an earlier situation which was missed.

Substitution or replacement is used when the previous situation or task is unsuitable in the present circumstances and does not promote continuing skill development. The concept according to Hall (24) is to put something new and better in place of the old, such as a new interest, a new belief in self or a new skill. An example is to substitute occupational performance for hallucinations. Performance develops skills and may lead to improved self concept. Hallucinations may "protect" the self concept but do not contribute to socially acceptable behavior. Improved skill performance may provide a means of demonstrating more socially acceptable behavior.

Reinforcement occurs when occupations are used to augment the situation or skills which previously were being developed but now are incompletely or inadequately developed to meet current demands. For example, a person may have learned to shop for groceries at the best price and quality. However, after a recent divorce, the person now must learn to buy furniture and arrange for housing as well. The basic skill of money management for food must be expanded to meet the needs for purchasing furniture and determining the amount of money required for housing.

Duplication or equivalence is incorporated when a situation or task is used in which the requirements are equal to another situation or task which is inaccessible or impractical in the current situation. For example, a person in a wheelchair may prepare a meal in the occupational therapy kitchen for three fellow patients as though she were cooking for her family of three who are at home some distance away. Duplication permits practice to occur in a simulated and safe environment. Furthermore, the performance can be evaluated and changes made with less risk of the undesirable consequences of failure and the additional injuries which could occur.

To summarize, the four rationales suggest that occupational therapy functions by constructing environments and providing situations or tasks which for a given individual will compensate, substitute, reinforce or duplicate those which are needed to accomplish a specified outcome or goal. The therapist determines which environment and what situations or tasks are needed through assessment and planning. The terminal or final outcome is to enable the individual to live in as normal an environment as possible through the facilitation and promotion of performance skills and level that will satisfy individual needs and meet the demands of society.

REEXAMINATION OF THE FRAME OF REFERENCE FOR PRACTICE

Occupational therapy has evolved into a practice discipline without an identifiable basic science. For example, medicine is based in biologic science; social work in sociology, counseling in psychology and physical therapy in physical science. However, occupational therapy has no single identifiable base. Instead, occupational therapy has tried to use a multiple base approach by combining biology, psychology and sociology into the biopsychosocial (25, 26). The multiple base leads to a variety of models and theories which are barely related to each other and confuse the definition of occupational therapy rather than clarify it.

Llorens (27) has suggested that there should be a field of study called "occupationology" which would study occupation and lead to a scientific knowledge of occupation. Such a study could examine the phylogenesis and ontogenesis of occupation on collective and individual man and on the ability to adapt or adjust to the environment through such occupation.

Some of the literature is available. It is scattered, however, through such fields as cultural anthropology, social psychology, industrial psychology, business organization and biological adaptation. Specific topics include daily routines, occupational roles, vocational choice, sensorimotor development, cognitive skills, educational methods, social awareness, individual interests, concept of self, play activities and values clarification. Questions to be answered are the (a) meaning and role of occupation in human life, (b) evolution of occupations in human existence, (c) transmission of occupation skills and values from one generation to the next, (d) variability of occupational choice in a given society and (e) problems in occupational performance as related to health and wellness.

The knowledge gained through occupationology could be used to explain and provide rationale for the selection of occupational activities and methods used in therapy. Such knowledge also would provide assumptions and concepts on which to base new methods of intervention.

REEXAMINATION OF THEORY IN A PRACTICE DISCIPLINE

A final area of problems are theoretical or research issues which occupational therapy seems to have potential for addressing but which lack both discussion and research findings in the occupational therapy literature. These issues can be posed in terms of a series of questions.

One question is whether the characteristics of occupations or activities can be identified which facilitate the reduction of response to stress levels. Gal and Lazarus (28) have shown that activity can reduce the level of stress hormones in the system. What remains is for occupational therapy to show which activity or activities are more useful in reducing reactions to stress. For example, is activity more effective if it relates directly to the nature of the stress or is it more effective if the activity diverts attention from the stress? Such a study might provide an answer to the question of whether directional, diversional, or both types of activity, are the major purpose of occupational therapy.

Another question relates to the role of occupation/activity in reducing the effects of sensory deprivation. What are the characteristics of an occupation or activity which counter the effects of lower sensory input situations. Could activity be selected, for example, by a person before surgery which would be used after surgery to prevent sensory deprivation and reality disorientation. Types of activity might be passive watching or listening initially but rapidly change to require more involvement of the person as homeostatic mechanisms in the body are stabilized.

A third question concerns the role of occupation or activity in the maintenance of health and well-being. Can patterns or configurations of occupations be analyzed to determine the health status of an individual before clinical signs of illness or general deterioration are apparent? Can preventive maintenance programs of occupation be individualized by each person based on general configurations? Can nursing home personnel be instructed as to how to help residents develop and maintain an occupational program to prevent or retard loss of health through basic aging and deterioration?

A fourth question is a professional one. How can occupational therapists learn to be more responsive to changes in the role of occupation in society over time? Although arts and crafts are not the only occupation, these media provide an example. During the formative years of the profession many arts or crafts could be used to provide a significant portion of a person's income. For example, basket making, sewing and pottery making were legitimate vocations as well as occupations. As technology in industry advanced hand-made articles were devalued, and the unit cost became too expensive to compete with industrial production. Thus, the role of arts and crafts in society changed from positive to impractical. People did not make things; factories did. Hand-made articles were for diversional and recreational purposes; not for productive purposes. However, occupational therapy continued to use the same media as though they had the same productive purpose. Little wonder that patients and administrators saw occupational therapy as an expensive and unnecessary luxury. The value of arts and crafts of course had not disappeared, but it had changed. The skills learned from the art or craft no longer could be applied directly to productive needs but could be applied indirectly if analyzed properly. Arts and crafts can be excellent prevocational learning tasks and remain excellent leisure activities. However, they must be evaluated in terms of today's culture in order to maximize use. Occupational therapists must come to recognize that much of the media of occupational therapy is socially and culturally dependent. For example, toys change in appearance with each new successful children's television program or movie. Analysis, however, will show that the functions remain similar: fantasy, manipulation and exploration. Yesterday's toys though are boring to today's children. Occupational therapists in pediatrics must keep their toys looking up-to-date, although the functions in play do not change. The question is how can such awareness of social and cultural impact be taught to and practiced by occupational therapists so that occupational therapy remains oriented to the changing world?

References

1. Reilly M: *Play as Exploratory Learning.* Beverly Hills, Calif, Sage, 1974, p. 126.
2. Moore JC: *Concepts from the Neurobehavioral Sciences.* Dubuque, Iowa, Kendall/Hunt, 1973, p. 33.
3. Reilly M: Questions and answers. *Am J Occup Ther* 20:66, 1966.
4. Thomas RM: *Comparing Theories of Child Development.* Belmont, Calif, Wadsworth Publishing, 1979, p. 45.
5. Maslow AH: *Toward a Psychology of Being,* Princeton, NJ, Van Nostrand, 1962, pp. 20–23.
6. Maslow AH: *Motivation and Personality,* 2nd ed. New York, Harper & Row, 1970, pp. 39–46.
7. Hall BP: *The Development of Consciousness: A Confluent Theory of Values.* New York, Paulist Press, 1976.
8. Coleman JC: *Psychology and Effective Behavior.* Glenview, Ill, Scott Foresman, 1969.
9. Dunton WR: *Occupation Therapy.* Philadelphia, Saunders, 1915, p. 25.
10. Upham EG: *Ward Occupations in Hospitals.* Federal Board for Vocational Education Bulletin 25. Washington, DC, Government Printing Office, 1918, p. 18.
11. King LJ: Toward a science of adaptive responses. *Am J Occup Ther* 37:432, 1978.
12. White RW: The urge toward competence. *Am J Occup Ther* 25:273, 1971.
13. Pattison HA: The trend of occupational therapy for the tuberculous. *Arch Occup Ther* 1:19, 1922.
14. Cannon WB: *The Wisdom of the Body.* New York, W.W. Norton, 1939.
15. Meyer A: Philosophy of occupation therapy. *Arch Occup Ther* 1:1–11, 1922.
16. Kielhofner G: Temporal adaptation: A conceptual framework. *Am J Occup Ther* 31:235–242, 1977.
17. Sawyer CW: Occupation for mental cases during institutional care. *Mod Hosp* 5:85, 1915.
18. Hall HJ: The systematic use of work as a remedy in neurasthenia and allied conditions. *Boston Med Surg J* 152:29, 1905.
19. Maslow AH: *The Further Reaches of Mankind.* New York, Viking, 1971, pp. 299, 318–319.
20. Pedretti LW: *Occupational Therapy: Practice Skills for Physical Dysfunction.* St. Louis, Mosby, 1981, p. 110.
21. White RW: The urge toward competence. *Am J Occup Ther* 25:273, 1971.
22. *Sample Forms for Occupational Therapy.* Rockville, Md, American Occupational Therapy Association, 1980.

23. Matsutsuyu J: The interest check list. *Am J Occup Ther* 23:323–328, 1969.
24. Hall HJ: *Occupational Therapy—A New Profession.* Concord, Mass, Rumford Press, 1923, pp. 15–21.
25. Reilly M: The educational process. *Am J Occup Ther* 23:302, 1969.
26. Mosey AC: An alternative: The biopsychosocial model. *Am J Occup Ther* 28:137–140, 1974.
27. Llorens LA: A journal of research in occupational therapy: The need, the response. *Occup Ther J Res* 1:4, 1981.
28. Gal R, Lazarus RS: The role of activity in anticipating and confronting stressful situations. *J Hum Stress* 4:4–20, 1975.

A Proposed Model: Adaptation through Occupation

In previous chapters various problems with existing frames of reference and philosophy used in occupational therapy theory have been noted. Among these are:

1. Use of the mechanistic philosophy in which the locus of control is external to the individual.
2. Use of reductionism in which the problem is reduced to the smallest identifiable unit.
3. Use of the biomedical model which focuses on pathology and treatment through drugs and surgery.
4. Borrowing extensively from other applied fields in order to make occupational therapy theory fit into existing philosophies, models or theories of temporary dysfunction.
5. Concentration on acute, short-term problems rather than longer term chronic problems of living.
6. Misinterpretation regarding the purpose of occupational therapy.

What appears to be needed is a frame of reference and philosophy which responds to the essence of occupational therapy as a unique and identifiably separate discipline. Factors to be considered are:

1. What is the unique organizing concept of occupational therapy and how can it be defined?
2. How does this concept operate in the environment naturally to describe a normal health process (frame of reference and assumptions)?
3. What happens when the concept is not operating or operating poorly (assumptions)?
4. What environmental conditions are needed to exist in order to start the concept operating again or improve the output of a poorly operating concept?
5. What environmental conditions hinder the concept from operating?
6. How can the concept be further studied (taxonomy)?

A review of these questions has produced some possible answers which are contained in the model presented. First, the unique organizing concept of occupational therapy is occupation which can be defined as that which engages a person's time, energy and attention. A general frame of reference and assumptions are contained in the following statements:

The role of occupation on human life

1. Occupation is fundamental to human existence and health because it maintains and provides for the life support systems and because it gives meaning to life.

2. Occupation is performed as a holism or gestalt in which the whole is different from the sum of its parts.
3. Occupation is a dynamic process which changes in form and complexity over time and in different spaces.
4. Occupation is influenced, altered and changed by the physical, biological and sociocultural environments in which an individual lives.
5. Occupation can be used to facilitate adaptation to the environment or facilitate the deliberate manipulation of the environment.

Problems in occupations

1. Occupation may become nonadaptive or maladaptive when certain alterations or changes occur in the physical, biological or sociocultural environments.
2. Certain occupations may hinder adaptation to the environment or hinder the deliberate manipulation of the environment.
3. Lack of adaptive occupation affects health adversely.

Environmental facilitation

Optimal learning environments for occupational adaptation are the social institutions in which people play, work and interact together toward common goal(s) of individual members.

Environmental hindrance

Nonoptimal learning environment for occupational adaptation is physical institutions which separate people from a community, some families and other social structures which serve primarily the physical institution, one member or part of a social structure.

Taxonomy

1. Occupation can be divided into three subcategories: self maintenance, productivity and leisure which in turn can be subdivided (Table 16.1).
2. Occupation can be divided into component tasks:
   a. Orientation—includes the three dimensions of space, the individual, family or community and three dimensions of time plus clock, circadian and psychologic.

Table 16.1
Taxonomies in Occupational Therapy: Occupational Areas

Self Maintenance	Productivity	Leisure
Self-care	Work	Recreation
ADL	Play	Avocation
Economic budgeter	Volunteerism	Play
	Student amateurism	
	Prevocation vocation	
	Homemaker	
	Home management	
	Vocation	

    b. Order—includes patterns of forward and backward, sideways, up and down, circular, spiral and fixed or flexible.

    c. Activation—includes the ability to move all or part of the body in certain prescribed ways as well as the thinking or rehearsal of movement in order to do an occupation.

3. Occupations can be divided into five performance areas: motor, sensory, cognitive, intrapersonal and interpersonal, which can be subdivided (Table 16.2).

The answers to the initial questions lead to a second set of questions. These are:

1. What is the nature of human beings?
2. How does the performance of occupations affect human beings?
3. Under what circumstances does occupational dysfunction occur?
4. What is the role of occupation in relation to adaptation, health and wellness or lack of same?
5. What rights do humans have in receiving health care services?
6. What contributions to health care delivery can be made through occupational therapy?
7. How can occupations be used therapeutically?
8. What is occupational therapy?

These eight questions can be answered by examining the assumptions on which occupational therapy is based. Appendix A provides a list of the assumptions related to each question.

The answers to the second set of questions leads to a third set of questions. There are:

1. What is the scope of occupational therapy?
2. What is unique about occupational therapy?
3. What are the major concepts and assumptions?
4. What are the major goals or expected results?
5. Who should receive services?
6. What assessments should be made?
7. What media or modalities can be used?
8. What methods and techniques can be used?
9. What is the total process of therapy intervention?
10. What are the outcomes of occupational therapy service?

SCOPE

Occupational therapy is a means of providing effective problem solving through increasing the variety of possible actions until the best or preferred action(s) is found to decrease, minimize or eliminate the patient/client's problems. In other words, the sequence of therapy is (a) a person has problems which limit the ability to perform certain occupations, (b) the occupational therapist has suggestions for possible solutions to a number of potential problems in performing occupations, (c) therapy occurs when a solution(s) is found which reduces or eliminates the person's problems and which is satisfactory to the person. The

Table 16.2
Taxonomies in Occupational Therapy: Performance Areas

Motor	Sensory	Cognitive	Intrapersonal	Interpersonal
Dexterity	Tactile	Concept formation	Feelings	Dyads
Strength	Kinesthesis	Attention	Emotions	Small group
Coordination	Vestibular	Problem solving	Mood/affect	Large group
Accuracy	Proprioception	Communication verbal	Self concept	Community
Speed	Vibration	Time management	Reality orientation	Country
Tolerance	Temperature		Interests	World
Reflex	Pain		Motivation	Values/beliefs
Reactions	Taste			Roles
Gestures	Smell			
Speech	Vision			
Developmental	Hearing			
milestones	Pressure			
	Sensory			
	Awareness			
	Sensory integration			
	Perceptual motor			

occupational therapist's job is to work with the person to find solutions which can be used to effectively reduce or eliminate the problems in occupational performance which the person is experiencing. Occupational therapy is concerned with a person's use of orientation such as time and space, ability to activate or do and the acquisition of order in terms of sequences and patterns of behavior in relation to the occupations of self maintenance, productivity and leisure which are needed to provide adaptive or coping responses to and with the environment. In other words, occupational therapy is concerned with the activities or routines of daily living that a person does within a given time and space and the meaning of those activities in terms of adaptive behavior for that individual. If a person is able to perform the occupations or activities adequately to meet the physical, biopsychological and sociocultural environmental demands and to the individual's satisfaction in terms of achievement and balance then the person has obtained adaptation through occupations. Adaptation through occupation thus means the organization and management of occupational activities and tasks in a manner that meets the goal of achieving maximum autonomy or functional independence, actualization or satisfaction and accomplishment. This scope is summarized in Figures 16.1 and 16.2 and Table 16.1.

WHAT IS UNIQUE ABOUT OCCUPATIONAL THERAPY?

The uniqueness of occupational therapy lies in the reasons and rationale for what occupational therapists do in society and how they assess and plan to accomplish the objectives and outcomes. The outcomes themselves, the media and modalities in some cases, the methods, techniques and equipment are similar to those used by other professionals. It becomes apparent that occupational therapists must be able to explain the purpose and function of occupational therapy thoroughly in order to avoid confusion. Since much of what can be seen in an occupational therapy program is not unique except for some specialized adapted equipment and splints it is difficult to show what occupational therapy is. Rather the key is in the explanation. The key explanation is the use of occupation to help people develop, restore or maintain a normal routine of occupational activities in self maintenance, productivity and leisure. By occupation is meant those activities and tasks which a person performs as part of a daily living routine and which engage the individual's resources, time and energy.

Basically, it appears that occupational therapy functions to help people relate to occupational activities in six ways:

1. Occupational therapy can help people learn or relearn the performance of occupations necessary to adapt to daily life.
2. Occupational therapy can help people to organize and balance the sequence of activity within their occupational performance.
3. Occupational therapy can help provide suggestions for alternative (adaptive) ways of performing occupations which may facilitate performance for those with disability.

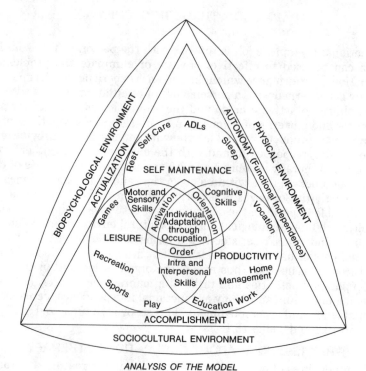

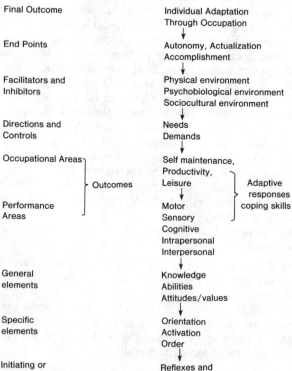

Figure 16.1. Adaptation through occupation model.

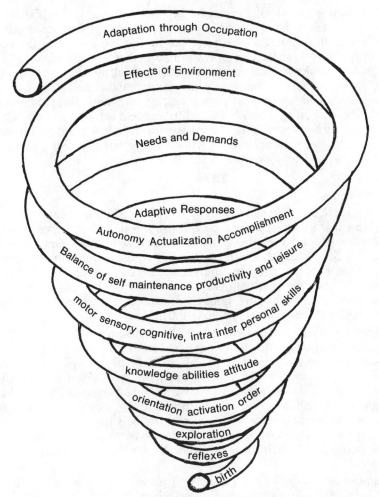

Figure 16.2. Scope of adaptation through occupation model.

4. Occupational therapy can provide the resources for practicing and trying out different ways of performing occupations for those with disabilities.
5. Occupational therapy can help identify the areas of dysfunction in the total performance of occupations.
6. Occupational therapy can provide specialized equipment to assist in the performance of daily occupations for those with disabilities.

WHAT ARE THE MAJOR CONCEPTS AND ASSUMPTIONS?

The basic assumption of occupational therapy intervention is that man, through the use of purposeful, goal-directed occupations/activities can influence positively the achievement of health/adaptive responses and minimize their loss. Purposeful occupation occurs when the senso-rimotor system is doing something which is meaningful to the cognitive, psychological, and social aspects of the individual, and when the occu-pation/activity is successful in meeting a demand in the physical, bio-psychological or sociocultural environment. Healthy adaptive responses involve being able to perform the occupations in self maintenance, productivity and leisure which are necessary to maintain health, prevent disability, and bring satisfaction and to problem solve effectively, which changes may be needed in the future to protect independent functioning.

The following concepts and definitions are used in this chapter to explain the models of practice in this chapter.

CONCEPTS

A. Outcomes

Occupational adaptation and adjustment—occupational adaptation and adjustment is obtained when a person has the skills in the five perform-ance areas which are needed to perform those self maintenance, produc-tive, or leisure occupations to the level of actualization, autonomy, and accomplishment required by individual, social and physical environ-ments. Further, occupational adaptation requires that the total person be involved in the planning, implementation and feedback to the maxi-mum degree the individual is able to participate.

Autonomy—functional independence. The collective skill/ability to per-form, or make arrangements to have performed, all activities which the person needs to participate in the physical, biopsychological and socio-cultural environments. The activities include those of self maintenance, productive and leisure activities which must be performed to fulfill the person's role and function. To be functionally independent does not require that the person do each activity totally without help. The key is management rather than self performance. A person can arrange to have some activities done by others either by trading off or payment for service.

Actualization—satisfaction. The collective feeling and emotional sense of well-being that a person experiences when the individual is able to perform the occupations successfully to meet demands of the environ-ment. Actualization is based on fulfilling a want, need, desire or appetite. Generally, the degree of gratification is determined by the degree to which the person is pleased or satisfied with the result of an occupation. If the person is very pleased with the results of a completed project, generally the degree of actualization will be positive and vice versa. Although there are some observable signs of actualization the primary measure of actualization is subjective. Possible observable signs include smiling, sigh of pleasure, frequent attention to the object or activity, and favorable comments about the object or activity. Subjective measure-ments must be made in relation to choice factors based on values.

Accomplishment—the collective knowledge and recognition that the per-son experiences when the individual knows how the occupations can be performed. Accomplishment pertains to the completion of the requirements such as skills or sequence of skills which are necessary to perform an occupation. The sense of accomplishment is achieved when the person knows that the skills have been acquired through training or practice to such a degree that performance of the task meets individual or social expectations. As a result of the accomplishment, a person is able to execute, carry out or do something that was not performed before the training or practice occurred or had been lost and was relearned. Accomplishment is both an objective and subjective quality. Objectively, accomplishment can be measured by comparing the individual's performance to a standard. Subjectively, accomplishment can be measured only by the individual. The individual can state a feeling or sense of accomplishment in terms of degrees.

B. Environment

Physical environment—the inanimate, nonhuman aspects of the environment which include objects, space, weather and other elements

Biopsychological environment—the individual self or being, including the body and mind which form the human being

Sociocultural environment—the other humans with which the individual relates, including the customs, mores, norms, roles and laws which humans use to organize behavior

C. Occupations—those activities and tasks which engage a person's time, energy and resources

Self maintenance occupations—those activities or tasks which are done routinely to maintain the person's health and well-being in the environment, *i.e.*, dressing, feeding

Productivity occupations—those activities or tasks which are done to enable the person to provide support to the self, family, and society through the production of goods and services to promote health and well-being, *i.e.*, secretary, mechanic, homemaker

Leisure occupations—those activities or tasks done for the enjoyment and renewal that the activity or task brings to the person which may contribute to the promotion of health and well-being, *i.e.*, bowling, collecting antiques

D. Occupational performance areas—includes the ability and skill to perform in each of the performance areas of motor, sensory, cognitive intra- and interpersonal skills. Each individual does not have to perform each and every possible skill which is needed to complete the requirements in each part of the repertoire of occupational areas in self maintenance, productivity and leisure.

Motor skills—the level, quality and/or degree of range of motion, gross muscle strength, muscle tone, endurance, fine motor skills and functional use (1)

Sensory skills—the level, quality and/or degree of acuity, range, perception and integration of the sensory systems

Cognitive skills—the level, quality and/or degree of comprehension, communication, concentration, problem solving, time management, conceptualization, integration of learning, judgment and time-place-person orientation (1)

Intrapersonal skills—the level, quality and/or degree of self-identity, self-concept and coping skills (1)

Interpersonal skills—the level, quality, and/or degree of dyadic and group interaction skills (1)

E. General elements

Knowledge—facts, truths or principles which are learned through experience, study or investigation

Abilities—capacity or power to perform physically and mentally one or more tasks or activities

Attitude/value—manner, disposition, feeling toward a person or thing regarding the relative worth, merit or usefulness

F. Specific elements relative to occupational therapy

Orientation—includes the three dimensions of space, plus the individual, family or community and the three dimensions of time plus clock, circadian and psychologic.

Order—includes patterns of forward and backward, sideways, up and down, circular, spiral and fixed or flexible

Activation—includes the ability to move all or part of the body in certain prescribed ways as well as the thinking or rehearsal of movement in order to do an occupation

G. Types of adaptation

Adaptive behavior—includes knowledge and skill to arrive at a balance of self maintenance, productivity and leisure activities consistent with social norms and self-satisfaction

Maladjustive, maladaptive behavior—that which is unacceptable to the individual, other persons or society or that which does not produce the results intended; the inability of the individual to develop patterns of behavior which make for success in the environment

Nonadaptive behavior—that which does not produce the results intended but is not objectionable to the individual, other persons or society; behavior which fails to bring the individual into harmony with the social or physical environment

H. Occupational terms

Adaptive occupations—those occupations which permit an individual to meet personal needs and live a satisfying life in the community. Adaptive occupations are individually specific because each person has a unique set of occupational skills. Occupational skills are developed to meet individual needs to respond to the environments (biopsychological, social, cultural and physical).

Occupational activities—those which are part of, or concerned with, the performance of an occupation. Thus activities which lead to or facilitate the performance of occupation in self maintenance, productivity or leisure by an individual are occupational activities. Examples of occupational activities are self-care tasks, work habits or leisure skills. Occupational activities must have the added dimension of relevance or purpose to the individual which will lead to a goal-directed outcome. Thus, some activities are inherently not occupational activities because they are never a part of goal-directed occupational performance, while others are not occupational activities to some individuals because the person has no purpose for such activity.

Occupational dysfunction—includes problems of planning for occupations to be done, actually performing the occupations and evaluating the effectiveness (feedback) of such performance. Dysfunction may be observed in the (a) failure to perform an occupation in which the skills are available, (b) inability to perform an occupation because the skills cannot be done, and (c) nonperformance of an occupation because the opportunity has not arisen or has not been taught.

Therapeutic occupations—those occupations or activities which are used as part of an intervention program. To qualify as a therapeutic occupation there must be a purpose or goal toward which the occupation is being directed. Although most occupations can be used for therapeutic purposes, the most common ones are those which fall into the categories of self maintenance, productive or leisure time activities.

Occupational balance—a state in which a person's needs and demands are met through the performance of occupations in all three areas—self maintenance, productivity and leisure. Occupational balance requires an understanding of the person's needs and demands and an analysis of the types of tasks being done, their effectiveness in meeting needs and demands and the amount of time being spent or not spent to perform them. Balance is influenced by individual situations, performances (values) and age. Balance should be a dynamic process which can change as needs and demands change. It may be useful to evaluate balance by using Lewin's force field model.

Occupational standard (norm, criteria)—a minimum level of acceptable performance which is determined both by social and personal values. The standard is composed of a series of subtasks which lead to a final output. Some standards are evaluated by society only as final outcomes, such as most self maintenance tasks. The individual sets the standard of the subtasks. Other standards are evaluated during the subtasks as well as in the final outcome, such as most productive tasks where the employer oversees the total performance. Standards for leisure, on the other hand, may be evaluated totally by the individual, or a combination of both individual and societal evaluation may be used. The level or degree of standard also is subject to age and role criteria. Generally, the level of the standard is increased with age until a maximum is reached. As new roles are assumed the standards are applied. Furthermore, a given standard may be applied in one situation and not in another. For example, the mode of dress changes with the setting or event. Acceptable dress for the beach is not acceptable for the office. The standards are different, although the process of putting on the clothes may be essentially the same for each.

Occupational roles—collections of specific subcategories of occupational areas. Roles depend on age, ability and circumstances. Roles have occupational standards. Generally roles become more complex with age until retirement, at which time roles may be simplified. Roles depend on occupational performance of selected skills in various combinations and patterns.

Meaningful occupations—those occupations which have meaning or significance to the individual in terms of personal needs and environmental demands. The activity may be seen as a part of a goal to be reached or accomplished or the activity may be done deliberately because the person wants to be able to do it. Purposeful activities have a reason or intention for being done as opposed to doing something just to fill up spare time or doing something because it's a challenge to do but has no real usefulness in everyday life, such as wiggling one's ear. Among the possible needs or demands which activities could fulfill are physiologic, security, belonging, societal and self actualizing needs. Such needs or demands form the basis for most goal-directed behavior which a person may wish to set as an objective, with the occupational therapy as part of a management plan. Occupations which are meaningful must be measured primarily by subjective means. Only an individual can state whether an activity is meaningful or valuable and whether it can serve as a direction for goal-oriented behavior. Occupations which are meaningful to one person are not to another. The degree or significance of meaning also can vary. It is possible to create a list of occupations which more often have meaning to a group of persons in a specific society and culture, but an individual may not share all the values of the society. Meaning also is changed with the intention of new technology and fads. Before cars were invented, few people were interested in learning to drive, but today learning to drive is a common goal-directed occupation. Fads influence the perceived purpose of an activity by increasing the social interest. If "everyone" is making objects with macrame then the value of macrame tends to increase as an activity with a purpose.

Purposeful occupations—those occupations which are valued and sanctified by society and culture as completed tasks. Although the person performs the task, the individual may not understand the meaning or significance of the task except to know that the socioculture environment values the outcome that task completion brings about. Purposeful occupations are most common in self maintenance and productivity occupations. They are measured by sociocultural standards based on the values and norms adopted by a group of citizens. Such factors as socioeconomic status, educational level, and aptitude may be considered in establishing or applying criteria.

Goal-directed occupations—those occupations which are used as part of a therapeutically defined program. They may be either meaningful or purposeful occupations, depending on the goal. Generally, leisure occupations should be meaningful and self maintenance and productive occupations should be purposeful in the final analysis.

Challenging occupations—an occupation is challenging if it is stimulating to or arouses interest in the individual so that there is full use of abilities, energy or resources. A challenging occupation increases the attention and motivation of a person, whereas the opposite is true for an unchallenging occupation. Challenge can be affected by internal and external factors. A person who is rested and not in too much pain is more likely to view performing an occupation as a challenge than a person who is fatigued and in pain. Challenge is affected also by competition. Doing an activity with others may make it more challenging than doing it alone. Challenge can be measured best by subjective measures of value to the individual. Some possible objective measures could be the length of time a person performs an activity and the relative attention which is paid.

WHAT ARE THE MAJOR OUTCOMES OR EXPECTED RESULTS?

Occupational therapy involves the use of therapeutic occupations to prevent and diminish the loss of skills and function in occupational performance or to restore and maintain occupational performance. A therapeutic occupation is an activity or task which is selected for the purpose of promoting the motor, sensory, cognitive, intra- or interpersonal performance of an individual.

The ultimate goal of selecting and employing various therapeutic occupations is to facilitate the maximum autonomy, actualization and achievement level of a person in the occupational areas of self maintenance, productivity and leisure to achieve an occupational balance which in turn will permit the adaptation of the individual to, and with, the physical, biopsychological and sociocultural environments. These outcomes can be stated as:

1. The person will be able to perform or have performed those occupations which meet the individual's needs and are acceptable to the person and society.
2. The person will have the necessary performance skills which compose the occupations in the individual's repertoire of self maintenance, productivity and leisure.
3. The person will have a balance of occupations such that actualization, autonomy and achievement are attained to a maximum degree of adaptation.
4. The person will be able to adapt to the environment or cause the environment to adapt to the individual.

5. The person will be able to meet both deficiency needs and growth needs.
6. Where the person is unable to perform the skills independently, assistive devices or equipment or other environmental adjustments may be used.

WHO SHOULD RECEIVE SERVICES?

Any person (a) who has failed to develop occupational skills in any of three areas, (b) who has a temporary or a permanent loss of occupational skills, (c) whose performance of occupational skills will require nonroutine modification or (d) who is at risk for losing occupational skills, is a primary candidate for occupational therapy assessment, analysis and possible intervention. Those who probably are not candidates for occupational therapy services are those (a) who have a transient loss of occupational skills of less than 1 month duration (b) who have minimal loss of occupational skills, (c) whose performance is within normal limits of performance in occupational skills and (d) who is able to maintain occupational skills without special assistance.

Examples of the former are a child with poor play skills, a dancer who becomes quadriplegic, a houseperson whose right side is flaccid after a stroke or a retiree with no plans for retirement. Examples of persons who are unlikely to need occupational therapy are an office worker who has an uncomplicated appendectomy, a construction worker who loses the distal joint of the ring finger on the nondominant hand, a child with controllable diabetes and a person with osteoarthritis who has developed a sound time activity management plan without professional help.

To view occupational therapy from a physical perspective, the need for services arises from problems in performing the routine occupations. Any physical problem where routine occupations are not being performed or are performed with difficulty is a potential candidate for occupational therapy services. The length of the health problem is one general indicator. Chronic conditions tend to interfere with occupational performance. A second indicator is a health problem which affects the neuromuscular skeletal system for more than a few days. A third indicator is a cardiovascular disorder which suddenly alters the vital capacity and energy level. These problems have been summarized in Table 16.2.

Social or psychological problems which may result in occupational dysfunction are those which interfere with regular performance. Depression which is more than temporary in length is an indicator. Syndromes which interfere with reality orientation and time management are also indicators. These problems are summarized in Table 16.3.

WHAT ASSESSMENTS SHOULD BE MADE?

There are two major areas of assessment which need to be completed. One concerns the analysis of occupations and the other relates to the assessment of individuals.

Table 16.3
Occupational Therapy Referral Checklist

If the patient/client indicates or needs any three or more of the items listed below, referral to occupational therapy is probably indicated.

I. Patient has physical problems such as:
_____a. Muscle weakness—especially in one or both of the upper extremities or hands.
_____b. Physical skills are delayed or lost, especially fine motor skills of the forearms and hands.
_____c. Physical tolerance is limited.
_____d. Loss of a limb or any part of a limb, especially of the upper extremities.
_____e. Range of motion limitations, especially of the upper extremities or hands.
_____f. Reflexes are abnormal or delayed in development.
_____g. Sensory function is poorly developed or has been diminished, especially in association with neuromuscular disorders.

II. Patient needs assistance in:
_____a. Adapting equipment for self-care and maintenance.
_____b. Adapting his performance (Example: learning one-handed skills).
_____c. Cognitive learning and memory tasks.
_____d. Developing coordination and dexterity skills.
_____e. Learning homemaking/child care activities.
_____f. Performing perceptual-motor tasks (Example: crossing the street).
_____g. Learning or relearning self-care activities.
_____h. Planning and carrying out common tasks (shopping for groceries, opening a checking account).
_____i. Practicing basic job-training skills (interviewing, following directions).
_____j. Learning work simplification and efficiency methods (energy conservation).

III. Patient needs to develop or increase such psychosocial abilities as:
_____a. Making independent decisions.
_____b. Expressing or sublimating certain defense mechanisms.
_____c. Functioning in group situations.
_____d. Motivating self to action.
_____e. Responding to human and nonhuman objects in the environment.
_____f. Distinguishing reality from nonreality.
_____g. Fulfilling role expectations.
_____h. Exercising self-control.
_____i. Building self concept.
_____j. Practicing social skills.
_____k. Organizing daily activities and short-range goals.

IV. Patient needs to develop and/or practice:
_____a. Avocational interests and skills.
_____b. Verbal and nonverbal communication skills—basic level.
_____c. Leisure time planning.
_____d. Play skills (child).
_____e. Spatial organizaion of self to the environment.
_____f. Organizing a time schedule.

Analysis of Occupations

The process of determining the therapeutic potential or value of an occupation is determined through an activity analysis. An activity analysis is accomplished by examining the properties of a specific activity in relation to the five performance areas. In addition, the sequence or pattern of activities is examined and the usual amount of time and space used are noted. Furthermore, possible variations are explored to simplify or alter the task(s), to decrease energy consumption, to reduce the cognitive demand, to eliminate the need for some equipment or to substitute for other equipment. Variations are to explore and determine alternate ways in which an occupation activity or task may be accomplished if the original or "normal" method cannot be done because of limitation in performance capacity, such as physical disability or reduced cognitive functioning.

Assessment of Individuals

Table 16.4 summarizes the types of data which assessment instruments should collect. The questions are adapted from the eight stages of learning as developed by Gagne (2). There are two basic styles for requesting information from subjects. One specifies and structures the type of responses to be given and the other is open ended to permit the subject to give any answer. The "closed" style usually is easier to record, since the range of responses is known in advance and the behavior to be measured can be defined precisely. Examples include forced choice tests, tests with examples of answers given, or tests which do not include space for all possible answers.

One problem of the closed styled is that the subject must confine the answers to the choices available. If none fits or more than one fits the individual, the subject may (a) select an answer which is not characteristic of the individual (b) confound the data by providing too many answers or (c) fail to answer at all.

Table 16.4
Occupational Dysfunction[a]

Skill development (activation)	Does the person have adequately developed skills? Is the person missing skills or are some skills inadequately developed?
Chained behavior (order)	Is the person able/unable to combine skills into sequences of actions? (motor and verbal)
Information (orientation)	Does the person have adequate/inadequate knowledge of the physical, personal and social environment to make discriminations and generalizations?
Problem solving (adaptation)	Is the person able/unable to use knowledge and skills to collect and organize data, elect a solution and review the consequences?

[a] Adapted from R. M. Gagne (2).

A second problem is that the test itself may provide clues to answers. The subject may select one of the clues because it is easier than thinking of a more characteristic answer, or the subject may feel that the clues are more acceptable answers than those the individual might provide. Another problem is that closed style may not address at all an area of concern to the individual. Thus, important data are not collected.

These problems result in a similar outcome. The individual subject does not provide correct or true answers which reflect the situation as the individual feels or remembers the facts to be. Obviously the problem is more critical in the assessment of cognition, intrapersonal or interpersonal data. Motor and sensory data are less subject to such error but are not immune.

In comparison the open ended style has the advantage of permitting a person to answer in any manner the individual feels or wants to reply. As a result, the information more accurately reflects the facts and truth as the person believes things to be. The problems are that the data must be analyzed more carefully since the subject may answer in a manner which is not easy to interpret or the answer may be incomplete. Also the subject may choose not to answer at all because the person cannot think of an answer or is afraid to reveal personal feeling for fear of what others will think. For an example, a person might not squeeze the dynamometer as hard as possible because strength is associated with returning to the job situation which the individual is not ready to face. By being "weak," the person hopes to buy additional time. Another example is the man who enjoys needlework but will not list needlework on an activity interest survey for fear others will laugh at such an interest.

MEDIA AND METHODS

Tables 16.5 and 16.6 outline the media, methods, equipment, precautions and prerequisite skills which may be used or considered in an intervention program. Appendix B outlines in more detail the types of media and methods used in occupational therapy.

WHAT IS THE TOTAL PROCESS OF THERAPY ASSESSMENT INTERVENTION?

The process of assessment intervention begins with the philosophy or frame of reference regarding human beings, occupations, health and wellness and occupational therapy. In general, the philosophy of occupational therapy is drawn from the organismic view of humans. Based on the philosophical decisions, paradigms and models of organization can be developed to cluster a group of assumptions and concepts selected from philosophy together with some ideas regarding general approaches to intervention.

Philosophical decisions and models of organization provide the framework for practice development directed to achieve some targeted results. The results will be obtained by selecting methods (how to interview) from the models of organization and media (what to use) consistent with

Table 16.5
Intervention Stategies Tools

Media and Modalities		Methods, Approaches and Techniques		
Media or Agent Types	Modalities Agent Groups	Teaching Methods	Therapeutic Approaches	Specialize Techniques
A. Inanimate 1. Creative arts 2. Manual skills 3. Games and sports 4. Education and learning tasks 5. Toys B. 1. Self 2. Dyad 3. Group 4. Animals 5. Plants and nature	1. ADLs or ODLs 2. Work related activities 3. Recreational avocational activities 4. Homemaking activities 5. Functional activities	1. Demonstration and performance 2. Exploration and discovery 3. Explanation and discussion 4. Problem solving and decision making 5. Audiovisual aids 6. Role playing and stimulation 7. Practice and repetition 8. Behavioral management	1. Normal developmental sequencing 2. Normal activity sequencing 3. Task analysis 4. Graded activities 5. Adapted activity 6. Consulting 7. Normal environment 8. Adapted environment 9. One to one 10. Activity group 11. Time scheduling 12. Progressive resistive exercise 13. Relaxation 14. Reality orientation	1. One-handed techniques 2. Work simplification/efficiency and energy conservation 3. Prosthetic orthotic training 4. Joint protection 5. Adapted techniques 6. Adapted equipment and devices 7. Adapted therapy equipment 8. Activity configuration 9. Work tolerance/ physical tolerance 10. Modified learning sequences 11. Sensory integration 12. Sensory motor 13. Splinting 14. Barrier free design

Table 16.6
Intervention Strategies

Equipment (Samples)	Precautions	Prerequisite Skills
Clothes	Fatigue	Postural and equilibrium reactions
Eating devices	Flushing	Initial synergy patterns
Hand tools	Dizziness	Some muscle tone and strength
Needles (knitting, crochet)	Palor	Some range of motion
Leather tools	Seizures	Some coordination
Looms		Awareness and initial attention
Kitchen utensils		Basic memory
Balls		Initial interaction on a one to one
Tables and chairs		
Table games		
Mats		
Pencils and crayons and marking pens		
Puzzles		
Blocks		

the frame of reference. Thus, in the final analysis assessment and intervention processes are influenced by philosophy, paradigm and practice issues and decisions. The specific issues and decisions are drawn from frames of reference, models of organization and expected results. The actual details of assessment and intervention depend on the selection of assumptions and concepts, media and modalities, and method techniques and approaches. The relationship between assessment and intervention to philosophy, paradigms and practice is illustrated in Figure 16.3.

The process of therapy can be outlined in four interlocking repetitive steps as seen in Table 16.7. These four steps are assessment, planning, implementation and reassessment.

WHERE SHOULD OCCUPATIONAL THERAPY FOCUS IN THE FUTURE?

The last question affecting the development of occupational therapy models is to examine where model building goes from this point. There appears to be three major lessons from history which occupational therapists should learn and integrate into model building, analysis and application. These lessons are: (a) society changes, (b) technology changes, and (c) depth and breath of information changes. All three have a profound effect on the theory and practice of occupational therapy.

Society changes its system of values about the role and type of occupational activities that are given a high priority. Occupational therapists must be alert to the changes and reorganize its media and modalities or its explanation of use in response to the changing values. The failure to understand and respond to the change in value from handmade articles to mass produced articles appears to be one major failure

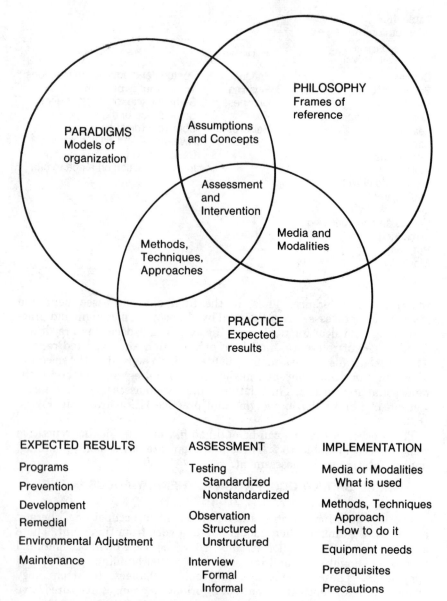

Figure 16.3. Relationship of philosophy paradigms and practice.

EXPECTED RESULTS	ASSESSMENT	IMPLEMENTATION
Programs	Testing	Media or Modalities
Prevention	Standardized	What is used
Development	Nonstandardized	
Remedial	Observation	Methods, Techniques
Environmental Adjustment	Structured	Approach
Maintenance	Unstructured	How to do it
		Equipment needs
	Interview	
	Formal	Prerequisites
	Informal	Precautions

in application of occupational therapy philosophy to practical application. In the search for models for this book, no examples were found of occupational therapists alerting others of the possible need to adjust the use of crafts to those which could include some small scale mass production approaches, with the possible exception of printing. The adherence

Table 16.7
Process Model

	Step 1: Assessment	Step 2: Planning	Step 3: Implementation	Step 4: Reassessment
Questions:	What are the problems and strengths of patients or clients?	What is the priority and objectives/goals of intervention?	How will the intervention be accomplished and who will do it?	What are the results of intervention? How can it be changed?
Information on list:	Obtain information through standardized test, nonstandardized test, interview checklist or survey observation	List of problems and objectives	List of media, or modalities, methods, techniques or approaches, equipment and supplies to be used and therapist, assistant, aide, volunteer, or family member who will carry out the program	Obtain information through repeating assessment techniques or other assessment, measure change against goals, reestablish plan or discharge
Consistency:	Type of testing and information must be based on and consistent with the frame of reference and model of organization	Problems identified and objective selected must be based on and consistent with frame of reference and model of organization	The use of media, techniques, methods, equipment and supplies must be based on and consistent with frame of reference and model of organization	Determination as to when objectives/goals have been reached or how to alter the plan must be based on and consistent with the frame of reference and model of organization

to individually made items which did not fit the current productive patterns of society appears to be a serious miscalculation in model development in the 1930s and 1940s.

Perhaps another example is the failure to understand or apply the differing value of crafts to upper class women therapists and lower class patients. Crafts were valued by upper class women as a means of self-expression and as a means of accomplishing productive occupation. Such crafts could be given as gifts or exchanged for other items. For lower class persons, the need was to direct rehabilitation efforts toward a wage-earning skill. Unless the crafts were carefully selected and explained they probably seemed irrelevant as preparation for return to self maintenance and productive living.

The second major change which influences occupational therapy is technology. Technology made possible mass production which overtook the manual skilled crafts which used to earn many people a living. Suddenly, leather could be sewn by machine and large ceramic factories could mass produce pottery so that each piece was identical. Machine-made products even resulted in a reduction of the value of hand-crafted wood products, such as furniture or toys. Unfortunately, occupational therapists did not modify their values of crafts products to match the changing social values. Part of the problem may be that occupational therapists value the results obtained in improved skill and performance more than the article produced. However, from the client's point of view, the product may be seen as a confirmation of the improved skill and performance. Thus, a meaningful end product confirms the value of the intervention process. Therefore, occupational therapists must be creative in finding media and modalities that are meaningful to the client. For example, why not use the assembly and disassembly of small machines such as an engine or units of machines such as a carburetor? What about small punch presses which make some plastic item like checkers? Could range of motion be increased by using a series of types of joints put together in various patterns? Why not use door locks, nuts and bolts or other hardware items for finger dexterity, eye-hand coordination and following directions?

A third change is the information base. More is known about what kinds of dysfunctions occur and how to correct the problems. In mental health problems of time distortion can be identified and programs begun to clarify use of time and time relationships. In physical dysfunction strengthening coordination and integration programs can be begun based on knowledge of how the skills and performances occur. In part diversional programs are not needed because intervention can be started earlier instead of waiting for "nature to take its course." Thus, the focus of change needs to be identified in occupational therapy models.

Another type of informational change which occurs is modification of theories used in other health areas. For example, the popularity of psychoanalytic approaches to mental health programs seems to be decreasing. Instead stress and learning theories are being advanced. Such theories have different explanations for mental health problems and suggest different methods of intervention which in turn require rethinking about what media or modalities to use. Furthermore, the explanation of use must be changed. Hammering a nail may be an aggressive act, a stress reducer and a structured learning task, depending upon which theory is being used as the frame of reference.

Finally, one aspect of model building should not change. The philosophical base should remain firm. Occupational therapy is centered on the human organism as a totality which is not divisable into a collection of parts. Occupational therapy is designed to focus on maximizing self-control, self responsibility and self-selection which result in self initiated and directed action. When any of these views plus others in the organismic philosophy are violated, occupational therapy is in danger of being derailed (3). The essence of occupational therapy must be maintained and preserved in any model of practice which occupational therapists develop or adopt.

Such a position may not be easy to maintain in the face of the scientific method of research and biomedical models of health. Nevertheless, occupational therapy must seek methods of research which do not require reductionism to elementary particles to provide answers. Occupation is a multifactored force in human activity. The interactive effects of occupation may be more important to health and adaptation than any single occupation or collection of performance skills. Thus, research designs which provide the methodology to examine multiple dimensions are likely to be the most useful approaches to studying occupationology and occupational therapy.

References

1. *Manual on Administration.* Rockville, Md, American Occupational Therapy Association, 1978, pp 73–75.
2. Gagne RM: *Conditions of Learning,* 2nd ed. New York, Holt, Rinehart and Winston, 1970, pp 63–64.
3. Shannon PD: The derailment of occupational therapy. Am J Occup Ther 31:229–234, 1977.

Assumptions Underlying the Theory and Practice of Occupational Therapy

ASSUMPTIONS ABOUT A HUMAN BEING

1. A person is a biopsychosocial being
   a. The life force has structure and function, pattern and organization
   b. There is a sequential process of growth and development from birth to death which is unidirectional
   c. The person exists in a group of meaningful others
2. A person is a unified whole
   a. Behavior is synergistic
   b. The person interacts in the environment as a total being
   c. All behavior is meaningful
3. A person is an open system energy unit
   a. There is a constant interchange of energy between the person and the environment
   b. A person can adapt to many environments
   c. A person dynamically affects the environment and is affected by it
   d. A person can achieve a balance between using and conserving energy in the environment
4. A person has the capacity for thought and sensation
   a. A person is capable of abstraction, imagery and language
   b. A person is capable of perception, feeling and has emotions
5. A person has needs
   a. Each person develops a unique pattern to meet these needs
   b. The needs are met on a priority basis within the pattern
   c. The environment through society influences the patterned behavior of meeting needs
   d. Society attempts to ensure that needs will be met by sanctifying a variety of occupations
6. A person has responsibilities
   a. A person must decide what that person wishes to become and the methods to be used to attain the goals.
   b. A person assumes position/roles in the society each with its set of expectations.
   c. Several positions and roles may be occupied at one time—which compounds the responsibilities.
7. A person has potential
   a. Potentials are in part biologically determined.
   b. Potentials can be hindered or facilitated by the environment.
   c. Every person has the potential for continuous learning.

8. A person is the sum total of individual experience.
   a. Current behavior is the result of past experiences.
   b. Current experiences will influence future behavior.
9. A person has basic rights.
   a. A person has the right to maximum individual potential
   b. A person has the right to have physiological security and belonging needs provided if unable to provide for the self.
10. A person is an active being.
   a. Humans have an inherent need for action.
   b. Humans respond to internal and external sources of motivation to action.
   c. Humans achieve action through multiple systems, including motor, sensory, cognitive, intra- and interpersonal.

ASSUMPTIONS ABOUT OCCUPATIONS

1. Each person must perform some occupations or have the occupations performed for the person to survive, *i.e.*, occupation is a primary need.
2. All occupations may be performed by one person or different persons may perform some occupations.
3. A person adapts or adjusts through the use of various occupations.
4. Through occupations a person may adapt to the environment or adapt the environment to the person.
5. The occupations a person learns and is able to perform determine the degree to which a person is able to adapt.
6. Occupations are composed of abilities, knowledge and attitudes.
7. All occupations are determined by the environment (physical, psychobiological and sociocultural).
8. Some occupations are performed to maintain or change the physical environment.
9. Other occupations are performed to meet the expectations of the sociocultural environment.
10. Still other occupations are performed to maintain or change the biopsychological environment.
11. Occupations permit a person to fulfill individual and group needs.
12. A balance of occupations is facilitory to the maintenance of health and a satisfying life.
13. Autonomy, actualization and accomplishment can be achieved by promoting a balance of occupational performance in the areas of self maintenance, productivity and leisure.
14. Occupations may be divided into three major areas:
   a. Self maintenance—those occupations permit man to maintain individual life support needs (food, shelter, belonging).
   b. Productivity—these occupations assist society to facilitate each person to meet individual needs by the use of collective resources.
   c. Leisure—these occupations permit the individual or group to express the needs for creative outlet and renewal of interest in self maintenance and productive occupations.

15. Occupations involve positions, roles and responsibilities which change over the life-span.
16. Occupational performance is goal-directed and purposeful.

ASSUMPTIONS ABOUT OCCUPATIONAL DYSFUNCTION

1. Occupational dysfunction can occur whenever the skills in occupational performance are inadequate to meet the individuals needs or to provide satisfaction.
2. Occupational dysfunction may occur because a person does not have a sense of purpose or goal-directed plan.
3. Injury, accident, trauma or disease may disrupt a person's sense of goal directedness by changing the individual's self assessment of ability or skill to perform those occupations which are of interest or are valued.
4. Injury, accident, trauma or disease may disrupt a person's sense of goal directedness by decreasing the individual's actual skill in performing those occupations which will provide for needs and bring satisfaction.
5. Occupational dysfunction may occur as a result of failure to develop occupational skills, failure to organize skills into effective occupational performance, failure to maintain skills, loss of skill components, loss of effective organization of skills.
6. Occupational dysfunction may occur as a result of environmental changes in the physical, psychobiological or sociocultural environments.
7. Occupational dysfunction may alter the performance of self maintenance, productivity and leisure occupations.
8. Occupational dysfunction may alter the performance components of motor, sensory, cognitive, intrapersonal or interpersonal skills.
9. Occupational dysfunction will reduce the individual's ability to adapt or adjust through the use of occupations.

ASSUMPTIONS ABOUT HEALTH, WELLNESS AND ILLNESS

1. Health is a dynamic and changing phenomenon
2. The optimal level of wellness varies due to factors such as age, genetic inheritance, social and environmental factors
3. Health is a total condition of a biopsychosocial being—it cannot be divided into physical, mental, or social health
4. Illness may interfere with a person's pattern of meeting needs by:
   a. Reducing the energy level available
   b. Disrupting the events and persons in the pattern
   c. Changing the ability to perform occupations
5. Regaining health requires energy which reduces the available energy for engaging in occupations, fulfilling needs and accepting responsibilities
6. Illness interferes with a person's ability to meet responsibilities by:
   a. Altering potential methods of reaching a goal
   b. Changing the positions/roles a person occupies

c. Reducing the number of occupations which the person can perform

ASSUMPTIONS ABOUT RECEIVING HEALTH CARE SERVICES

1. A person has the right to decide whether to seek and accept health care services within legal limitations.
2. A person has a right to determine the state of health and level of wellness that the person will seek to attain or maintain as long as the decision does not threaten or endanger the health and wellness of other persons.
3. A person has a right to be consulted with regarding the objectives/goals and methods to be used in individual health care plans.

ASSUMPTIONS ABOUT DELIVERING HEALTH CARE THROUGH OCCUPATIONAL THERAPY

1. A person may need assistance at times from occupational therapy to meet individual needs and responsibilities to perform occupations.
2. A person's occupational performance and adaptive behavior can be identified and analyzed to determine assets and liabilities in meeting those needs and responsibilities.
3. A management program can be developed with the person's active involvement which will attain or maintain a person's occupational performance and adaptive behavior.
4. A management program is most useful to the client if it begins at the sequential level of the client's current functioning and maintains the existing level or increases the functional level to progressively higher (advanced) levels.
5. A management program should be oriented toward enabling the client to:
   a. Achieve the highest level of occupational performances and adaptive behavior consistent with the client's goal
   b. Return to a normal living environment in the community if possible
   c. Increase independent adaptive behavior and decrease dependent, maladaptive or nonadaptive behavior
   d. Increase successful occupational performance and decrease nonproductive occupational performance.

ASSUMPTIONS ABOUT THE THERAPEUTIC USE OF OCCUPATIONS

1. Occupations are a natural vehicle for facilitating development because they provide a naturally occurring nurturant. Since occupations are useful in facilitating normal development, they should be useful in assisting a person with abnormal developmental patterns.
2. Occupations are agents for learning skills through the processes of exploration, repetition, practice and problem solving. Since occupations facilitate initial learning they should be useful in facilitating relearning.
3. Interaction with occupations through play and work teaches a person

to organize and integrate skills into effective combinations for personal adaptation. Since occupations are useful in facilitating normal organization and integration they should be useful in assisting a person with maladaptive or nonadaptive behavior to become more adaptive.

4. Occupations range in complexity from simple to difficult and can involve only one or several performance components. Thus a person may be assisted in learning simple occupations which require few performance components or difficult occupations requiring many components, depending on the analysis of individual needs and abilities.

5. The performance of occupations is an important means by which people demonstrate to society their ability to function and adapt to the environment. A person with unmet needs may be able to satisfy those needs through the performance of occupational activities or tasks. Furthermore, a person who is considered a failure in meeting the demands of society and of the environment can become more successful by improving the level of performance in those occupational activities and tasks with are demanded by society or other environments.

6. Occupations help people orient to reality. A person who is not oriented to reality (confused, disoriented, hallucinating) can be helped to become more reality-oriented through the use of occupational activities and tasks.

ASSUMPTIONS ABOUT OCCUPATIONAL THERAPY

1. Change in occupation is effected by physical, biopsychological and sociocultural environment.

2. Change in an individual's occupations is effected by change in the total environment, individual skill acquisition, maintenance and loss and change in adaptive potential.

3. The rate and degree of change in an individual's occupations can be influenced by the intervention of occupational therapy.

4. Occupational therapy can be instrumental in facilitating positive change and preventing or diminishing the negative change in occupations.

5. The purpose of the intervention by occupational therapy is to promote the development or maintenance of the skills involved in performing occupations and prevent or reduce the dysfunction or incapacities which may result from illness or accident.

6. Occupational therapy as a discipline strives to promote the maximum occupational performance to which the individual is capable through skill development and acquisition consistent with the individual's needs.

7. Occupations used by the occupational therapist must be relevant and useful to the individual in relating to the environment.

8. Occupational therapists can analyze with the client those occupations which will be most useful to the individual.

9. Occupational therapists can analyze the skills needed to perform specific occupations.
10. Occupational therapists can assess problems in skill development and acquisition by evaluating the functional components of motor, sensory, cognitive, intrapersonal and interpersonal performance.
11. Occupational therapists can predict problems in occupational performance based on the analysis of problems in skill development and acquisition.
12. Occupational therapists can enable an individual to learn or relearn skills needed to perform the occupations which are needed by the individual.
13. Occupational therapists can assist the individual to integrate the skills needed to perform occupations.
14. Occupational therapists can enable an individual to adapt to the environment through the use of selected occupations.
15. Occupational therapists can assist the sociocultural environment to adapt to an individual through the use of selected occupations.
16. Occupational therapists can produce change in occupational performance, skill development and acquisition faster than a person could obtain the results using individual resources alone.
17. Occupational therapists can facilitate the development or redevelopment (establish or reestablish) of a sense of goal directedness and purposefulness of occupational performance.
18. Therapy (in occupational therapy) is the use of directed, purposeful occupations to influence positively a person's sense of well-being and thus the state of a person's health.
19. Directed purposeful occupations encourage the person to assume responsibility for meeting individual needs.
20. Directed, purposeful occupation is useful in orienting a person toward meeting responsibilities through increasing occupational performance levels and improving adaptive behavior.
21. Active doing (involvement) encourages the maintenance, development and redevelopment of occupations: specifically, self maintenance, productivity and leisure time skills.
22. Selected occupations can:
    a. Increase the level of specified development skills.
    b. Prevent loss of skills.
    c. Reintroduce or restore weakened or lost skills.
    d. Permit altered methods of performing skills.
    e. Maintain skills at an established level of performance.

Intervention Strategies

I. Media or agents
   A. Inanimate media
      1. Creative arts

A. *Materials*	B. *Process of*	C. *Product*
Pencil	Drawing	Drawing
Crayons	Painting	Painting
Paint	Designing	Design
Charcoal	Sketching	Sketch
Ink	Writing	Book, poem
Self/voice	Acting	Play
Instrument	Playing an instrument	Composition
Self/body	Dancing	Dance

      2. Manual skills/crafts

A. *Materials**	B. *Process of*	C. *Product*
Wood	Constructing	Woodworking project
Clay/plaster	Modeling	Ceramics project
Leather hides	Carving	Leatherwork project
Cloth	Cutting	Sewing project
Fiber (yarn, thread, cord)	Spinning Tying	Needlework project macrame project
Plastic	Etching	Plastics project
Metal	Bending, shaping	Metal work project
Sand/glass	Fusing	Enameling project
Reed	Weaving	Basketry project
Paper	Printing	Printing project

      3. Games and sports
         A. Games
            1. Table board games—chess
            2. Card games—bridge, poker, Old Maid
            3. Puzzles
            4. Knowledge and word games
            5. Target/skill games
            6. Tag/relay games
         B. Sports
            1. "Ball"
            2. "Net"
            3. Outings

* Materials and process may be combined in combinations other than these listed.

      4. Rods/fishing
      5. Guns/hunting
      6. Combative
      7. Track and field
      8. Water
      9. Winter/summer
4. Educational/learning
   A. Alphabets/letters
   B. Numbers/numerals
   C. Words/sentence recognition/reading
   D. Typing
   E. Manuscript printing
   F. Cursive writing
   G. Measurement
   H. Following commands
   I. Safety
5. Toys
   A. Construction blocks, erector sets
   B. Manipulation—take apart
   C. Nesting, stacking—boxes, rings
   D. Noise and music
   E. Action, self-propelled—wind-up toys, cars
   F. Role simulation—dolls, doll houses, stoves, dress up, woodworking
   G. Touch and feel—teddy bear, stuffed animals

B. Animate media
  1. Self
    A. Active friendliness—seek person out, make suggestion
    B. Autocratic—control person, make all decisions
  2. Dyad
    A. Companion—make some decisions, defer others
    B. Coequal partner—make decisions jointly
  3. Group
    A. Parallel
    B. Project
    C. Egocentric cooperative
    D. Cooperative
    E. Mature
  4. Animals
    A. House pets
    B. Farm animals
    C. Aquariums
  5. Plants
    A. Seeds
    B. Bulbs
    C. House plants
    D. Flowering plants
    E. Food plants

F. Bushes

G. Trees

II. Modality/agent groups

1. ADLs

A. Feeding

B. Dressing

C. Grooming hair, beard

D. Bathing/showering

E. Counting money

F. Shopping

G. Using public transportation

H. Driving a car/truck

I. Using the telephone

J. Locating resources—map reading, seeking directions

K. Budgeting

L. Banking

2. Productive activities

A. Work habits

1. Follow directions

2. Quality control

3. Perform procedures

4. Production output satisfactory

5. Interaction with supervisor

6. Interaction with peers

B. Job-seeking skills

1. Reading want ads

2. Going to employment office

3. Filling out application

4. Interviewing

5. Preparing a resume

3. Recreational/avocational activities

A. Determine interests

B. Determine current performance

C. Determine current level of skills and activities

D. Determine feasibility in terms of availability, relative costs

E. Select activities to pursue or discard

F. Determine need to learn new skills or redevelop old ones

G. Assist in acquiring equipment and supplies

H. Provide/organize time to perform the activities

4. Homemaking activities

A. Meal planning—help plan simple meals with basic nutrition included

B. Meal preparation—practice fixing meals

C. Cleaning/washing—organize cleaning/washing routine and practice steps

D. Budgeting—develop a basic budget

E. Minor repairing—replace light bulb or fuse, mend broken items

    F. Ironing—organization and practice
    G. Arranging/decorating—arrange furniture, hang curtains
    H. Storing/organizing—organize storage system
  5. Functional activities
    A. Reach, grasp and release
    B. Sitting and standing
    C. Moving by walking or wheelchair
    D. Stepping and climbing
    E. Maintaining static and dynamic balance
    F. Opening and closing doors, drawers, windows
III. Teaching methods
  1. Demonstration and performance
    A. Simultaneous imitation
    B. Delayed imitation
    C. One step demonstration—one step performance
    D. Multiple steps demonstrated then performed
  2. Exploration and discovery
    A. Unstructured situation "natural" environment
    B. Structured or planned situation
  3. Explanation and discussion
    A. Planning an activity
    B. Reviewing an activity
  4. Problem solving
    A. Gather data
    B. Assess data
    C. Select alternates
    D. Select a choice
    E. Implement choice
    F. Evaluate results
    G. Continue or revise
  5. Audiovisual aids
    A. Films (8 or 16 mm)
    B. Slide
    C. Video tapes
    D. Audio tapes
    E. Photographs
    F. Posters
    G. Bulletin boards
  6. Role playing and simulation
    A. Interpersonal situation
    B. Occupational performance
  7. Practice and repetition
    A. Distributed practice
    B. "Bunched" practice
  8. Behavioral management
    A. Self-selected reward
    B. Therapist-selected reward

      C. Type of reward
         1. Primary (food, water)
         2. Secondary (associated with primary)
         3. Generalized (money, tokens)

IV. Therapeutic approaches
    1. Normal developmental sequence analysis includes:
      A. Sensorimotor development
      B. Cognitive development
      C. Intrapersonal development
      D. Interpersonal development
    2. Normal activity sequence analysis includes:
      A. Performance at different ages
      B. Performance in different environments
      C. Performance determined by individual preference and habit
      D. Performance determined by sociocultural values and traditions
    3. Task analysis includes:
      A. Determining steps or processes
      B. Determining motion patterns
      C. Determining joint movements and specific muscles used
      D. Listing equipment used and in what order
    4. Graded activity analysis includes:
      A. Simple to complex
      B. Few steps to many steps
      C. Few tools/equipment to many tools/equipment
      D. Quick to finish to long time to finish
    5. Adapted activity analysis includes:
      A. Possibility of modifying existing equipment
      B. Possibility of changing to other equipment
      C. Possibility of omitting some steps in the task
      D. Possibility of condensing some steps in the sequence
      E. Possibility of changing the environment setting or arrangement
      F. Possibility of changing to a different environment
      G. Possibility of using a different position of the body
    6. Consulting
      A. Making suggestions about self maintenance occupations
      B. Making suggestions about productive occupations
      C. Making suggestions about leisure occupations
    7. Normal environment analysis includes:
      A. Home or immediate living environment
      B. Neighborhood
      C. Community
      D. City
      E. State
    8. Adapted environment analysis of methods to change:
      A. Home or immediate living environment
      B. Neighborhood

      C. Community

      D. City

      E. State

  9. One to one situation analysis includes:

      A. Type of roles client will assume

      B. Type of roles therapist will assume

      C. Environment in which the roles will be carried out

  10. Activity group analysis includes:

      A. Type of roles expected of members

      B. Type of group organization

      C. Type of environmental setting

  11. Time scheduling analysis includes:

      A. Minutes, partial hours, hours, days or weeks to be scheduled

      B. Type of occupations to be scheduled

      C. Review of past schedule

      D. Development of current schedules

      E. Plan for future schedules

  12. Progressive resistive exercise

      A. Add weight

      B. Increase number of practice sessions

      C. Work against gravity-incline plant

V. Specialized techniques

  1. One-handed techniques

      A. Alter task steps so that they can be done with one hand

      B. Use an object as a weight to stabilize

      C. Attach or impale part of the object to stabilize

      D. Alter the tools involved so that activity can be done with one hand

      E. Use the foot, knee, hip, mouth, shoulder or head to stabilize

  2. Work simplification and energy conservation together by location of performance

      A. Group activities

      B. Decrease time spent

      C. Decrease effort-energy expended

      D. Decrease number of steps in process

      E. Organize equipment—centralize or sequence

      F. Change motion patterns

      G. Change grip or holding patterns

  3. Prosthetic/orthotic training

      A. Teach good hygiene for stump care

      B. Teach signs of tissue breakdown

      C. Teach putting on harness and adjusting terminal device

      D. Teach operation of terminal device in relation to daily activities

      E. Provide opportunity for selected practice

  4. Joint protection

      A. Use largest weight-bearing joint available for lifting, stooping, bending and pulling, shoving

    B. Maintain a low center of gravity

    C. Maintain joint alignment

    D. Carry objects as close to the center of the body and at the center of gravity as possible

    E. Alternate sides of body, front or back when carrying

    F. Use carts, dollies, or other wheeled devices to substitute for carrying

    G. Organize objects within easy reach

    H. Use palm of hand for stabilizing rather than fingers

5. Adapted techniques

    A. Reorder the sequence of tasks

    B. Eliminate or add steps to the task

    C. Substitute a piece(s) of equipment or devices

    D. Alter the routine of habits

6. Adapted equipment

    A. Feeding

        1. Built-up or enlarged handles

        2. Extended handles

        3. Nonskid surfaces

        4. Lighten weight

        5. Decrease diameter

        6. One-handed tools or devices

    B. Dressing—simplified

        1. Enlarge button holes

        2. Velcro fasteners

        3. Larger zippers and pull tabs

        4. Larger size garment

        5. Practice boards, garments or dolls

    C. Communication aids

        1. Language boards

        2. Electric typewriters

        3. Symbolic languages

        4. Head sticks

        5. Switch on telephone

        6. Volume enhancer

    D. Adapted transportation

        1. Lifts for wheelchair

        2. Hand controls for brake and accelerator

        3. Smaller steering wheel or joy stick

        4. Remote electric door openers, locks and windows

        5. Removed or removable seats for wheelchairs

    E. Writing aids

        1. Grasp enhancers—larger diameter service or holder, triangle-shaped

        2. Grasp substitutes—splints

    F. Table adaptations

        1. Height, low or high—accommodate setting on floor in regular chair or wheelchair

    2. Size, small or large—work surface
    3. Shape—wrap around (cut out), square, rectangular
    4. Weight—heavy or light
    5. Composition—plastic, metal, wood
  G. Adapted chairs
    1. Foot boards and stops
    2. Lower or higher seat
    3. Curved or flat seat
    4. Square or triangle (corner)
    5. Side arms, present or absent
    6. Back, low, high or extendable
    7. Neck-head positioner
    8. Abduction bar
    9. Wings
   10. Seat short or long
   11. Seat, horizontal or slanted
   12. Seat, hard or soft
   13. Scoliosis pads
   14. Lower back, bar—increase lumbar curve
  H. Trays
    1. Lap or table
    2. Flat or incline (slant)
    3. No edge or edge
    4. Material—plastic, wood
7. Adapted therapy equipment
  A. Bilaterial tools—sander, saw
  B. Treadle or bicycle jig saw
  C. Practice boards—clothing fasteners, door fasteners
  D. Games—change size of pieces
  E. Slings—overhead, bilateral, weighted
  F. Vibrators—slow, fast
8. Activity configuration
  A. Listing activities
  B. Grouping activities by type of amount of time
  C. Determining interest level
  D. Determining ability level
  E. Selecting activities to learn
  F. Setting goals
9. Work/physical tolerance
  A. Change physical position such as sit or stand
  B. Change activity pattern—eliminate excessive reaching
  C. Stand or sit on "softer" surface
  D. Increase number of breaks
  E. Decrease amount of time, working
10. Learning techniques
  A. Forward chaining, steps $1 \rightarrow 2 \rightarrow 3$
  B. Backward chaining, last step first
  C. Easy to difficult

    D. Simple to complex

    E. Discrimination, matching, sorting, naming—perception before conception

    F. Self confirmation—gestalt appears if correctly done and all pieces fit together

11. Sensory integration techniques
    A. Vestibular stimulation
    B. Proprioception input
    C. Integration of two sides of body
    D. Development of praxis
    E. Vestibular bilateral integration
    F. Touch normalization
    G. Tactile discrimination

12. Sensorimotor
    A. Facilitation—activity which is rapid, arrhythmic
    B. Inhibition—activity which is slow, rhythmic

13. Splinting
    A. Types
        1. Static—prevent motion or change muscle tone in selected joints
        2. Dynamic—facilitate and guide motion in selected joints
    B. Functions
        1. Protection of joint from further injury—finger
        2. Prevention of joint deformity—ulnar deviation splint
        3. Substitution of one action for another—tenodesis splint
        4. Facilitation of correct motion—outrigger

14. Architectual barriers
    A. Doors too narrow
    2. Stairs—dangerous, too steep or undifferentiated riser
    3. Stairs, unnegotiable—no elevator or ramp for wheelchair
    4. Counters too high or too low
    5. Seats too high or too low
    6. Slippery floors or surface
    7. Deep pile carpet
    8. Throw rugs
    9. Faucets hard to grip and turn
    10. Grab bars and railings not available

Bibliography*

1. Allport G: *On Becoming*. New Haven, Conn, Yale University Press, 1955. (Occupational Therapy Process)
2. Bender L: *Psychopathology of Children with Organic Brain Disorders*. Springfield Ill, Charles C Thomas, 1956. (Perceptual Motor Model)
3. Bertalanffy LV: *General Systems Theory: Foundations, Developments, Application*. New York, George Braziller, 1968. (Model of Human Occupation)
4. Bobath K, Bobath B: Cerebral palsy. In Pearson PH, Williams CE: *Physical Therapy Services in the Developmental Disabilities*. Springfield Ill, Charles C Thomas, 1972. (Human Development through Occupation, Spatiotemporal Adaptation Model, Reflex Development)
5. Bruner J: Nature and uses of immaturity. In Bruner J, Jolly A, Sylva K: *Play: Its Role in Development and Evolution*. New York, Basic Books, 1976. (Model of Human Occupation and Doing and Purposeful Action)
6. Bruner J: *Toward a Theory of Instruction*. Cambridge, Mass, Harvard University Press, 1966. (Activity Therapy)
7. Buehler C: *Psychology for Contemporary Living*. New York, Hawthorn Books, 1968. (Model of Human Occupation)
8. Cruickshank W, Bice HV, Wallen NE: *Perception and Cerebral Palsy*. Syracuse, NY, Syracuse University Press, 1957. (Perceptual Motor Model)
9. Cumming J, Cumming E: *Ego and Milieu*. New York, Atherton Press, 1966. (Activity Therapy)
10. Dewey J: *Experience and Nature*. New York, Dover Books, 1958 (first published 1925). (Doing and Purposeful Action)
11. Dewey J: *The School and the Child*. London, Blackie and Son (year unknown). (Invalid Occupations]
12. Dobzhansky T: Introduction. In Mead M, Dobzhansky T, Toback E. *Science and the Concept of Race*. New York, Columbia University Press, 1969. (Neurobehavioral Model)
13. Dubos R: *Man Adapting*. New Haven, Conn, Yale University Press, 1965. (Adaptive Responses)
14. Erickson E: *Childhood and Society*. New York, WW Norton, 1950. (Occupational Behavior, Doing and Purposeful Action: Developmental Model)
15. Farber SD, Huss AJ: *Sensorimotor Evaluation and Treatment Procedures for Allied Health Personnel, 2nd ed*. Indianapolis, Indiana University Foundation, 1974. (Human Development through Occupation)
16. Fay T: The neurophysical aspects of cerebral palsy. *Arch Phys Med* 29:327–334, 1948. (Sensorimotor Model)
17. Flavell J: *The Developmental Psychology of Jean Piaget*. New York, Van Nostrand, 1963. (Spatiotemporal Adaptation)
18. Freud (see Hall C)
19. Frostig M, Lefever DW, Whittlesey JRB: *Marianne Frostig Developmental Test of Visual Perception, 3rd ed*. Palo Alto, Calif, Consulting Psychologists Press, 1961. (Perceptual Motor Model)
20. Gesell A: *The First Five Years of Life*. New York, Harper & Brothers, 1940. (Spatiotemporal Adaptation, Developmental Model, Neurobehavioral Model, Sensory Integration.)
21. Ginsburg H, Opper S: *Piaget's Theory of Intellectual Development: An Introduction*. Englewood Cliffs, NJ, Prentice Hall, 1968. (Neurobehavioral Model)
22. Ginzberg E, et al: Toward a theory of occupational choice. In Peters HJ, Hansen JC: *Vocational Guidance and Career Development*. New York, Macmillan, 1971. (Model of Human Occupation)
23. Glasser W: *Reality Therapy*. New York, Harper & Row, 1965. (Occupational Therapy Process)
24. Gordon IJ: *Human Development from Birth Through Adolescence*. New York, Harper & Row, 1969. (Spatiotemporal Adaptation)

---

* References are coded at the end by the name of the model in which the information is used as part of the frame of reference.

25. Hall C: *A Primer of Freudian Psychology.* New York, New American Library, 1974. (Developmental Model)
26. Harlow H: The nature of love. *Am Psychol* 13:673–685, 1958. (Sensory Integration)
27. Havighurst RJ: *Developmental Tasks and Education.* New York, David McKay, 1974. (Developmental Model)
28. Hebb DO: *The Organization of Behavior.* New York, John Wiley, 1949. (Perceptual Motor Model)
29. Held R, Hein A: Movement-producted stimulation in the development of visually guided behavior. *J Comp Physiol Psychol* 56:872–876, 1963. (Sensory Integration)
30. Herzburg F: *Work and the Nature of Man.* Cleveland, World Publishing Co, 1968. (Model of Human Occupation)
31. Hilgard E, Bower G: *Theories of Learning.* New York, Appleton-Century-Crofts, 1966. (Activity Therapy)
32. Homans G: *The Human Group.* New York, Harcourt, Brace and World, 1950. (Activity Therapy)
33. Hyde R: *Milieu Rehabilitation.* Providence, RI, Butler Health Center, 1967. (Activity Therapy)
34. Janet P: *La Medecine Psychologique.* Paris, 1924. (Philosophy of Occupation Therapy)
35. Jones M: *Social Psychiatry in Practice.* London, Penguin Books, 1968. (Activity Therapy)
36. Kabat H: New concepts and techniques of neuromuscular reeducation for paralysis. *Perm Found Med Bull* 8:121–143, 1950. (Sensorimotor Model)
37. Kabat H: Rhythmic Stabilization. *Perm Found Med Bull* 8:8–19, 1950. (Sensorimotor Model)
38. Kephart NC: *The Slow Learner in the Classroom.* Columbus, Ohio, Charles Merrill, 1960. (Perceptual Motor Model)
39. Keyser CJ: The nature of man. *Science* 54:207–213, 1921. (Philosophy of Occupation Therapy)
40. Korzybski A: *Manhood of Humanity: The Science and Art of Human Engineering.* New York, Dutton, 1921. (Philosophy of Occupation Therapy)
41. Lifton W: *Working with Groups.* New York, Wiley & Sons, 1961. (Activity Therapy)
42. Lorenz K: *Behind the Mirror: A Search for a Natural History of Human Knowledge.* New York, Harcourt, Brace, Jovanovich, 1977. (Adaptive Responses)
43. Maslow AH, Murphy G (Eds): *Maturation and Personality.* New York, Harper & Row, 1954. (Adaptive Response)
44. May R: *Existential Psychology.* New York, Random House, 1963. (Occupational Therapy Process)
45. McClelland D: *The Achieving Society.* Princeton, NJ, D. Van Nostrand Co., 1961. (Occupational Behavior)
46. Mills T: *The Sociology of Small Groups.* Englewood Cliffs, NJ, Prentice-Hall, 1963. (Activity Therapy)
47. Moore JC: Behavior, bias and the limbic system. *Am J Occup Ther* 30:11–19, 1976. (Human Development through Occupation)
48. Moore JC: *Concepts from the Neurobehavioral Sciences.* Dubuque, Iowa, Kendall Hunt, 1973. (Human Development through Occupation)
49. Moore JC: *Neuroanatomy Simplified: Some Basic Concepts for Understanding Rehabilitation.* Dubuque, Iowa, Kendall/Hunt, 1969. (Human Development through Occupation)
50. Mountcastle VB (see Rose JE)
51. Neff WS: *Work and Human Behavior.* New York, Atherton Press, 1968. (Model of Human Occupation)
52. Ostwald W: *Die Uberwindung des wissen schaftlichern materialismus and Naturphilosophie* (German only). (Philosophy of Occupation Therapy)
53. Pearce J, Newton S: *Conditions of Human Growth.* New York, Citadel Press, 1963. (Developmental Model)
54. Phelps WK: Description and differentiation of types of cerebral palsy. *Nerv Child* 8:107–127, 1949. (Sensorimotor Model)

55. Piaget J: *Play, Dreams and Imitation in Childhood.* New York, WW Norton, 1952. (Doing and Purposeful Action) (Also see Favell J, Wursten H, Ginsburg H)
56. Rose JE, Mountcastle VB: Touch and kinesthesis. In Field J, Mogoun HW: *Handbook of Physiology: Section Neurophysiology.* Washington, DC, American Physiological Society, pp 382–429. 1959, (Perceptual Motor Model)
57. Ruesch J: *Disturbed Communication.* New York, WW Norton, 1962. (Communication Process)
58. Ruesch J: *Therapeutic Communication.* New York, Robert Brunner & Co., 1962. (Communication Process)
59. Schilder P: *Contributions to developmental neurophychiatry.* New York, International Universities Press, 1964. (Sensory Integration)
60. Schilder P: *The Image and Appearance of the Human Body.* New York, International Universities Press, 1950. (Perceptual Motor Model)
61. Searles HF: *The Non Human Environment.* New York, International Universities Press, 1960. (Doing and Purposeful Action)
62. Sechehaye M: *Symbolic Realization.* New York, International Universities Press, 1951. (Recapitulation of Outogenesis)
63. Selye H: *The Stress of Life.* New York, McGraw Hill, 1956. (Adaptive Responses)
64. Skinner BF (see Hilgard E, Bower G)
65. Slavson SR: *Introduction to Group Therapy.* New York, International Universities Press, 1954. (Communication Process)
66. Smith MB: Competence and adaptation. *Am J Occup Ther* 28:11–15, 1974. (Model of Human Occupation)
67. Smith MB: Competence and socialization. In Clausen JA: *Socialization and Society.* Boston, Little Brown and Co., 1968. (Model of Human Occupation)
68. Spitz R: *The First Year of Life.* New York, International Universities Press, 1965. (Integrated Theory)
69. Strauss AA, Lehtinen LE: *Psychopathology and Education of the Brain Injured Child, Vol. 1.* New York, Grune & Stratton, 1947. (Perceptual Motor Model)
70. Sullivan HS: *Concepts of Modern Psychiatry.* New York, WW Norton, 1953. (Communication Process)
71. Sullivan HS: *The Interpersonal Theory of Psychiatry.* New York, WW Norton, 1953. (Communication Process)
72. Super DE: *The Psychology of Careers.* New York, Harper & Row, 1957. (Model of Human Occupation)
73. Tinbergen N: *The Study of Instinct.* Oxford, England, Oxford University Press, 1951. (Adaptive Responses)
74. Watson J (see Hilgard E, Bower G)
75. White RW: Motivation reconsidered: The concept of competence. *Psychol Rev* 66:297–333, 1959. (Occupational Behavior, Doing and Purposeful Action, Occupational Therapy Process)
76. White RW: The urge toward competence. *Am J Occup Ther* 25:271–274, 1971. (Doing and Purposeful Action)
77. Wursten H: On the relevancy of Piaget's theory to occupational therapy. *Am J Occup Ther* 28:213–217, 1971. (Developmental Model)
78. Zubek JP: Electroencephalographic changes during and after 14 days of perceptual deprivation. *Science* 139:480–492, 1963. (Adaptive Responses)

Author Index

533

Subject Index